Absolute Breast Imaging Review

Lucy Chow • Bo Li

Editors

Absolute Breast Imaging Review

Multimodality Cases for the Core Exam

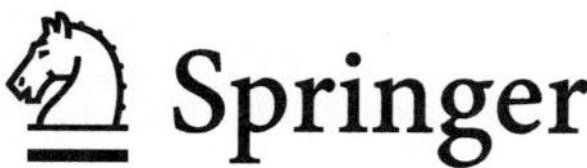

Springer

Editors
Lucy Chow
Department of Radiology
David Geffen School of Medicine at UCLA
Los Angeles, CA, USA

Bo Li
Department of Radiology
David Geffen School of Medicine at UCLA
Los Angeles, CA, USA

ISBN 978-3-031-08273-3   ISBN 978-3-031-08274-0   (eBook)
https://doi.org/10.1007/978-3-031-08274-0

This Springer imprint is published by the registered company Springer Nature Switzerland AG
The registered company address is: Gewerbestrasse 11, 6330 Cham, Switzerland

To my Michael, Teddy, and Marcel. You are my sun, my moon, and all my stars.

– Bo Li

To my devoted husband Anthony and beloved daughters Isabella and Chloe. To my parents John and Annie for their unwavering support. With them, anything is possible.

– Lucy Chow

The editors would also like to dedicate this book to their mentors, Dr. Lawrence Bassett and Dr. Nanette Debruhl.

Preface

As faculty members at an academic institution, we wanted to generate an educational resource for breast imaging fellows and radiology residents on the subject of breast imaging. Our goal was to create an informative and invaluable high yield breast imaging case review book to help with boards preparation and clinical practice.

We have collected numerous high-quality, multi-modality, breast imaging cases which directly align with the American Board of Radiology's critical concepts for the Breast Imaging Domain. The case presentations include mammography, ultrasound, and breast MRI technologies. Screening and diagnostic concepts as well as interventional and therapeutic procedures will be included. Within each chapter, cases will be presented as multiple-choice question format with detailed answer explanations. The contents of the book will help the reader test their knowledge and skills related to the clinical practice of breast imaging. Additional topics will also be addressed, such as indications for screening, regulations, physics, and quality and safety. We hope trainees at all levels of medical training find this text an integral part of board exam preparation and lifelong radiology learning.

Los Angeles, CA, USA
Los Angeles, CA, USA
Lucy Chow
Bo Li

Contents

Contributors

Hayet Amalou, MD Department of Radiology, David Geffen School of Medicine at UCLA, Los Angeles, CA, USA

Denise Andrews-Tang, MD Department of Radiology, David Geffen School of Medicine at UCLA, Los Angeles, CA, USA

Department of Radiology, Olive View-UCLA Medical Center, Sylmar, CA, USA

Parsa Asachi, PhD Department of Radiology, David Geffen School of Medicine at UCLA, Los Angeles, CA, USA

Kayla Blunt, PhD Department of Radiology, Morsani College of Medicine, University of South Florida Health, Tampa, FL, USA

Natalie Cain, MD Department of Radiology, David Geffen School of Medicine at UCLA, Los Angeles, CA, USA

Nina Capiro, MD Department of Radiology, David Geffen School of Medicine at UCLA, Los Angeles, CA, USA

James Chalfant, MD Department of Radiology, David Geffen School of Medicine at UCLA, Los Angeles, CA, USA

Tiffany L. Chan, MD Department of Radiology, David Geffen School of Medicine at UCLA, Los Angeles, CA, USA

Jennifer Choi, MD Department of Radiology, LAC+USC (GH), Los Angeles, CA, USA

Lucy Chow, MD Department of Radiology, David Geffen School of Medicine at UCLA, Los Angeles, CA, USA

Stephanie Histed Chung, MD Department of Diagnostic Radiology, Cooper University Hospital, Camden, NJ, USA

Jane Dascalos, MD Department of Radiology, David Geffen School of Medicine at UCLA, Los Angeles, CA, USA

Laura Doepke, MD Breast Imaging, Department of Radiology, Moffitt Cancer Center, Tampa, FL, USA

Iram Dubin, MD Department of Radiology, Olive View-UCLA Medical Center, Sylmar, CA, USA

Department of Radiology, David Geffen School of Medicine at UCLA, Los Angeles, CA, USA

Regan Ferraro, MD Rolling Oaks Radiology, Thousand Oaks, CA, USA

Cheryce Poon Fischer, MD Department of Radiology, David Geffen School of Medicine at UCLA, Los Angeles, CA, USA

Esha Gupta, MD Department of Radiology, David Geffen School of Medicine at UCLA, Los Angeles, CA, USA

Department of Radiology, Olive View-UCLA Medical Center, Sylmar, CA, USA

Melissa M. Joines, MD Department of Radiology, David Geffen School of Medicine at UCLA, Los Angeles, CA, USA

Stephanie Lee-Felker, MD Department of Radiology, West Los Angeles Veterans Affairs Medical Center, Los Angeles, CA, USA

Bo Li, MD Department of Radiology, David Geffen School of Medicine at UCLA, Los Angeles, CA, USA

Claire Lis, MD Department of Radiology, David Geffen School of Medicine at UCLA, Los Angeles, CA, USA

Yongkai Liu, PhD Departments of Radiology, and Physics & Biology in Medicine, Magnetic Resonance Research Labs, David Geffen School of Medicine, University of California, Los Angeles, Los Angeles, CA, USA

Hannah Milch, MD Department of Radiology, David Geffen School of Medicine at UCLA, Los Angeles, CA, USA

Shabnam Mortazavi, MD Department of Radiology, David Geffen School of Medicine at UCLA, Los Angeles, CA, USA

Steven R. Plimpton, MD Department of Radiology, David Geffen School of Medicine at UCLA, Los Angeles, CA, USA

Guita Rahbar, MD Department of Radiology, David Geffen School of Medicine at UCLA, Los Angeles, CA, USA

Department of Radiology, Olive View-UCLA Medical Center, Sylmar, CA, USA

Antionette Roth, MD Department of Radiology, Olive View-UCLA Medical Center, Sylmar, CA, USA

Mikhail Roubakha, MD Department of Radiology, David Geffen School of Medicine at UCLA, Los Angeles, CA, USA

Puja Shahrouki, MD Department of Radiology, David Geffen School of Medicine at UCLA, Los Angeles, CA, USA

Kyung Sung, PhD Radiology, Bioengineering, and Physics & Biology in Medicine, Magnetic Resonance Research Labs, David Geffen School of Medicine, University of California, Los Angeles, Los Angeles, CA, USA

Mariam Thomas, MD Department of Radiology, David Geffen School of Medicine at UCLA, Los Angeles, CA, USA

Department of Radiology, Olive View-UCLA Medical Center, Sylmar, CA, USA

Irene Tsai, MD Breast Imaging, UCI Department of Radiological Sciences, Orange, CA, USA

Craig Wilsen, MD Department of Radiology, David Geffen School of Medicine at UCLA, Los Angeles, CA, USA

Nazanin Yaghmai, MD Department of Radiology, David Geffen School of Medicine at UCLA, Los Angeles, CA, USA

Tiffany Yu, MD Department of Radiology, David Geffen School of Medicine at UCLA, Los Angeles, CA, USA

Bill Zhou, MD Department of Radiology, David Geffen School of Medicine at UCLA, Los Angeles, CA, USA

Regulations and Standards of Care

Laura Doepke, Esha Gupta, Hayet Amalou,
and James Chalfant

L. Doepke (✉)
Breast Imaging, Department of Radiology, Moffitt Cancer Center,
Tampa, FL, USA
e-mail: Laura.Doepke@moffitt.org

E. Gupta
Department of Radiology, David Geffen School of Medicine at UCLA, CA, USA

Department of Radiology, Olive View-UCLA Medical Center, Sylmar, CA, USA
e-mail: egupta@dhs.lacounty.gov

H. Amalou · J. Chalfant
Department of Radiology, David Geffen School of Medicine at UCLA,
Los Angeles, CA, USA
e-mail: hamalou@mednet.ucla.edu; jchalfant@mednet.ucla.edu

L. Chow, B. Li (eds.), *Absolute Breast Imaging Review*,
https://doi.org/10.1007/978-3-031-08274-0_1

1. What are the standard views for screening mammography?
   (a) Mediolateral view.
   (b) Mediolateral oblique view.
   (c) Craniocaudal view.
   (d) Both a and c.
   (e) Both b and c.

2. What is the most important component to be included in the view provided below?

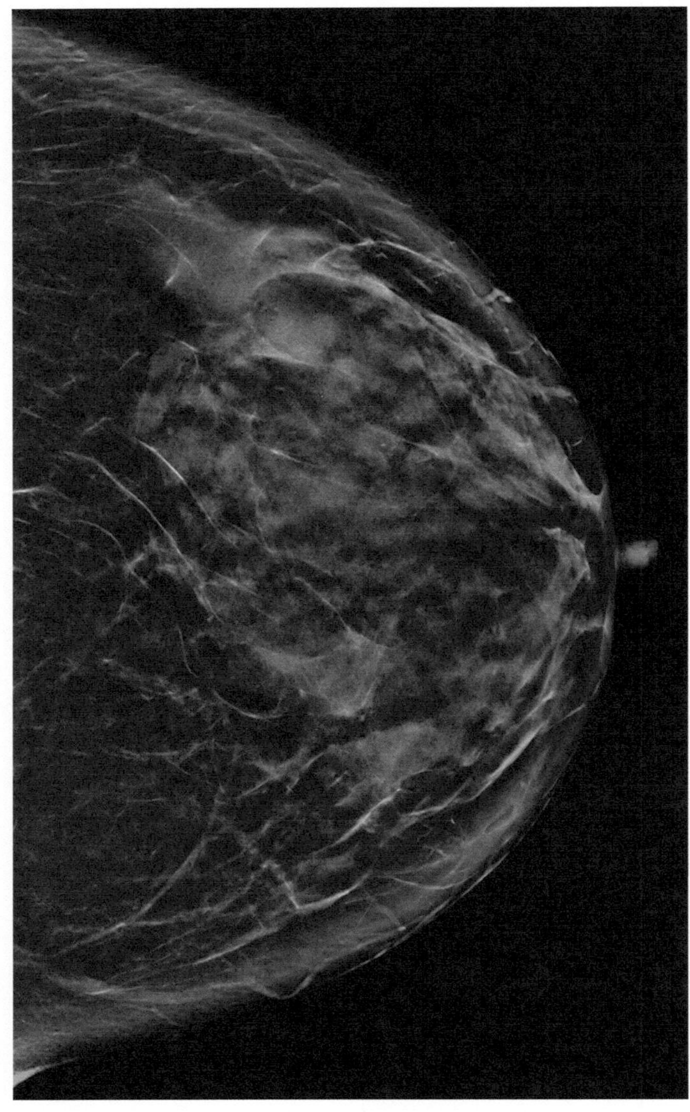

(a) Posterolateral tissue.
(b) Anterior third, nipple.
(c) Posteromedial tissue.
(d) Central tissue.

3. Figure a shows a close-up image of motion artifact on a mammogram which is corrected on Figure b. Which part of the breast is this artifact most evident on mammogram?

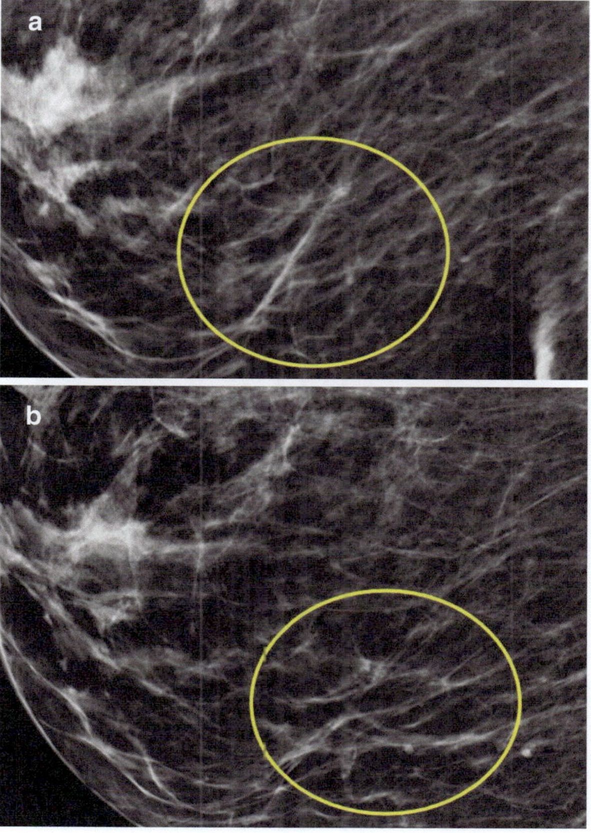

(a) Lateral breast on the craniocaudal view.
(b) Medial breast on the craniocaudal view.
(c) Superior breast on the mediolateral oblique view.
(d) Inferior breast on the mediolateral oblique view.

4. How many images are obtained on a standard screening mammogram on a patient with breast implants?
(a) 4.
(b) 6.
(c) 8.
(d) 10.

5. The view shown in the image below is used to:

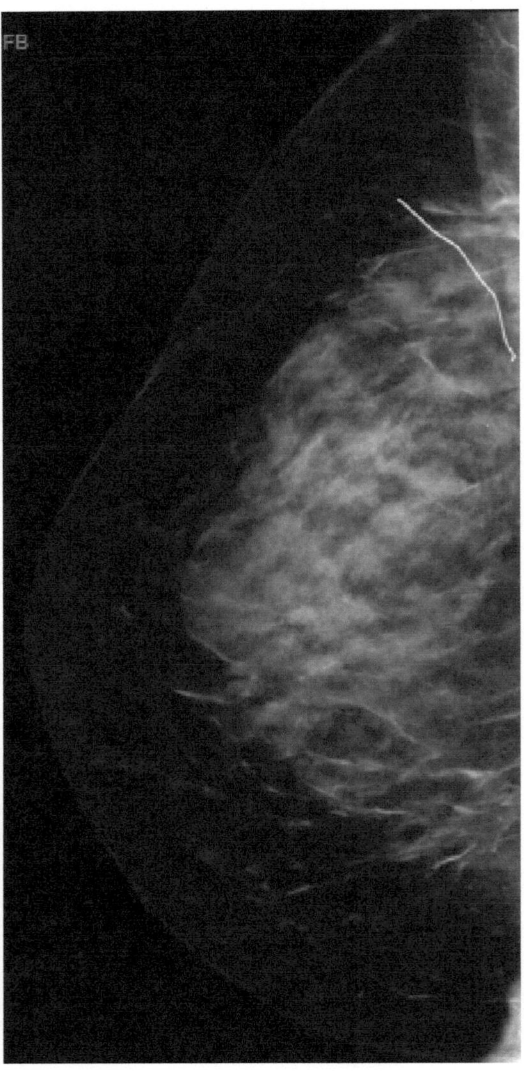

   (a) Evaluate the inferior posterior breast tissue with the detector closest to the feet.

   (b) Evaluate the superior posterior breast tissue with the detector closest to the feet.

   (c) Evaluate the inferior posterior breast tissue with the detector closest to the head.

   (d) Evaluate the superior posterior breast tissue with the detector closest to the head.

6a. What is the name of this view?

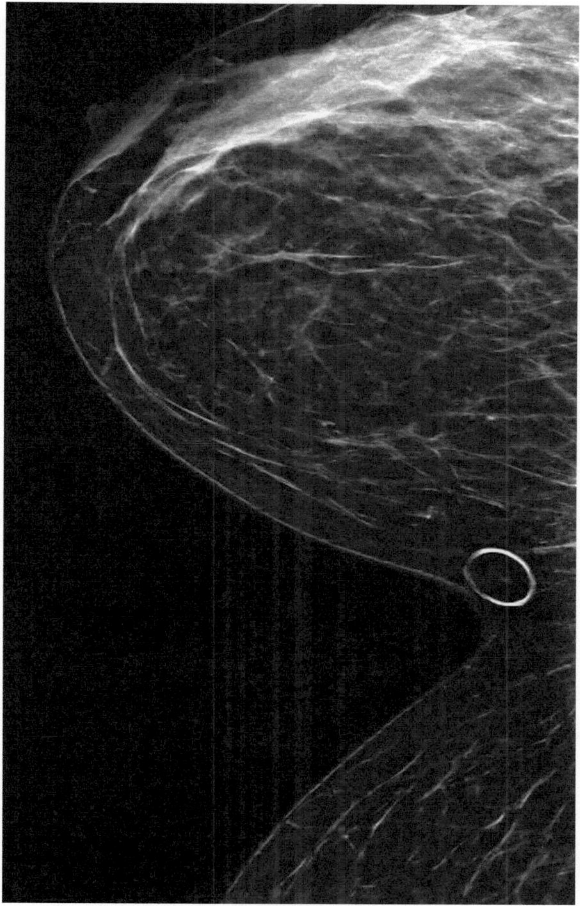

    (a) Mediolateral oblique view.
    (b) Exaggerated craniocaudal lateral view.
    (c) Craniocaudal view.
    (d) Cleavage view.

6b. The view shown in the above image is used to:
    (a) Evaluate the anterior and medial breast tissue with the beam directed superior to inferior.
    (b) Evaluate the posterior and medial breast tissue with the beam directed superior to inferior.
    (c) Evaluate the anterior and medial breast tissue with the beam directed inferior to superior.
    (d) Evaluate the posterior and medial breast tissue with the beam directed inferior to superior.

7. The image below was obtained during a diagnostic work up. Subsequent to this image being taken, a BB marker was placed on the group of calcifications (yellow circle) and a tangential image was obtained. Tangential views are used to evaluate:

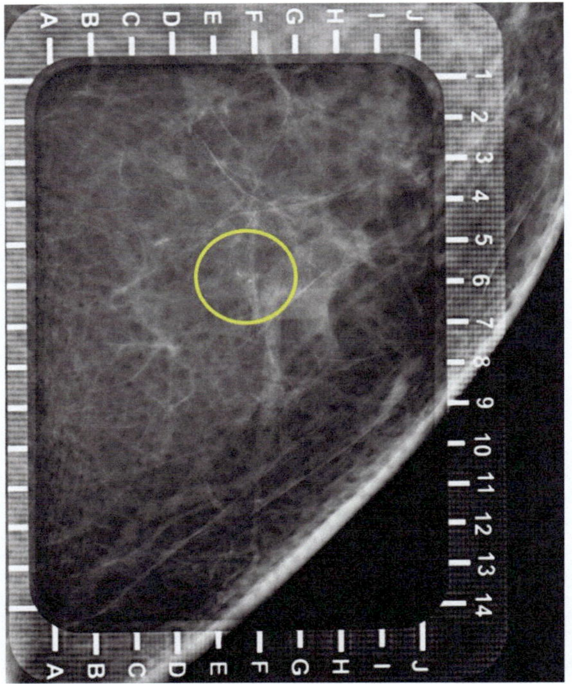

(a) Milk of calcium.
(b) Morphology of calcifications.
(c) If calcifications are dermal in location.
(d) Architectural distortion.

8. The image below demonstrates an artifact that can be seen with breast MRI. Which of the following can be a cause of the artifact identified?

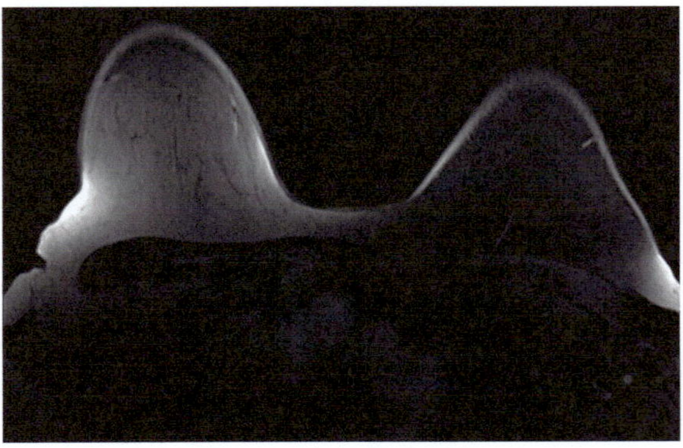

(a) Using a scanner with the phase-encoding direction in the anterior-posterior (AP) direction.
(b) Coil inhomogeneities.
(c) Missed uptake of gadolinium (extravasation, power injector malfunction).
(d) An RF coil tuned to the water peak.

9. Which of the following cannot be used to improve fat saturation on breast MRI? More than one answer choice may be correct.
(a) Shimming.
(b) Ensure center frequency is set to the water peak.
(c) Apply saturation pulse at a frequency of 3.5 ppm.
(d) Improve patient positioning.
(e) Increase the field of view.

10. The image below is from a contrast-enhanced MRI obtained on a patient with newly diagnosed right breast cancer. Which of the following describes how gadolinium-based contrast agents function?

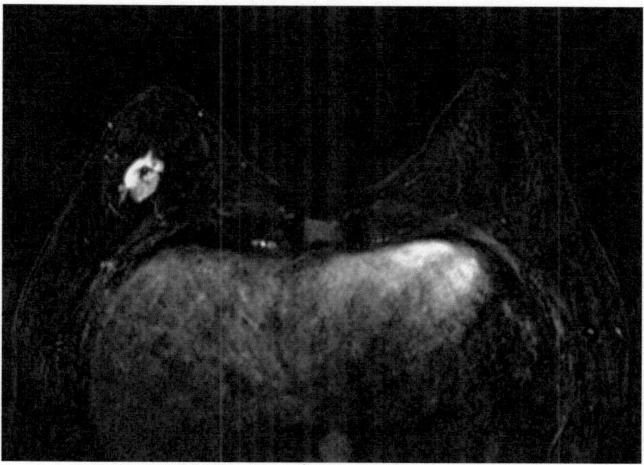

(a) Gadolinium diffuses into tumor cells at a slower rate than normal tissue.
(b) Gadolinium distorts the local magnetic field.
(c) Gadolinium causes protons to relax slower in the T1 and T2 weighting.
(d) Prolonged T1 values appear brighter on a T1-weighted scan.

11. The sequence in the below image:

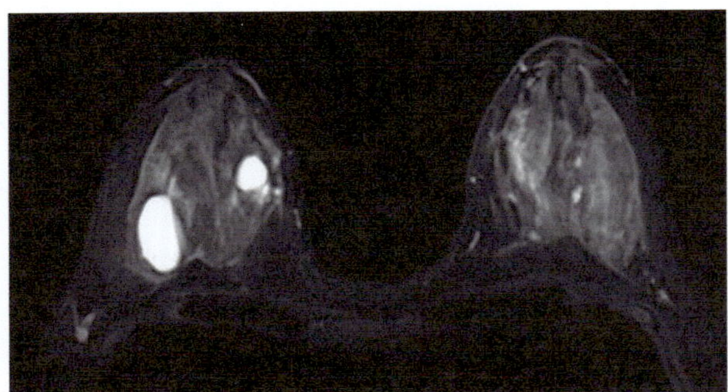

   (a) Uses contrast to evaluate the enhancement of a newly diagnosed breast cancer.
   (b) Will have short T2 values for fluid.
   (c) Uses a long TE and long TR.
   (d) Used to create a subtraction image during image processing.

12. The below image shows several ultrasound transducers. Breast ultrasound transducers:

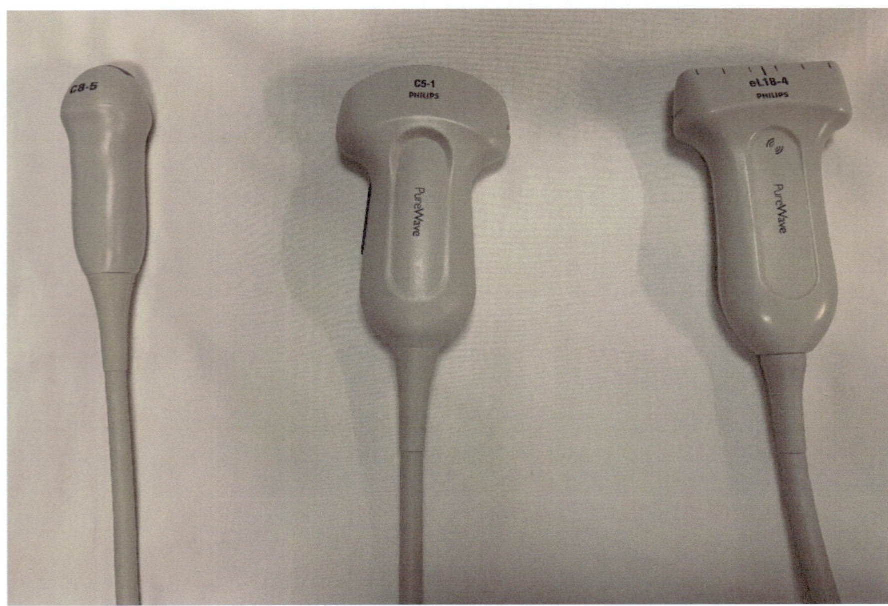

(a) Should be a curved array transducer.
(b) Center frequency should be at least 8 MHz according to the ACR practice guidelines.
(c) Can use a standoff device to evaluate deep lesions.
(d) Spatial resolution of the transducer is determined by axial and lateral resolution.

13. Spatial compound imaging uses:
    (a) Images obtained at a single angle to form a single image.
    (b) Only those sound beams that are propagated perpendicular to the transducer long axis.
    (c) Uses electronic beam steering to obtain multiple images to average out artifactual echoes.
    (d) Has no effect on ability to evaluate margins.

14. Most of the artifacts in breast ultrasound that diminish contrast resolution are caused by backscatter and:
    (a) Use of coded harmonics.
    (b) Side lobes.
    (c) Receiving higher frequency signals.
    (d) Digital encoding of the signal.

15. The below image shows an artifact seen with ultrasound images. This artifact (arrow):

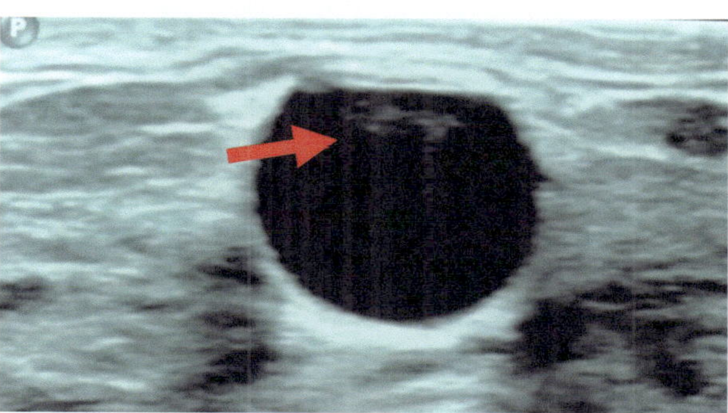

    (a) Is caused by reflections between two highly reflective interfaces in parallel.
    (b) Is caused by acoustic interference.
    (c) Can be increased with tissue harmonic imaging.
    (d) Can be reduced by increasing gain.

16. The image below demonstrates an artifact seen with digital breast tomosynthesis (DBT). This artifact:

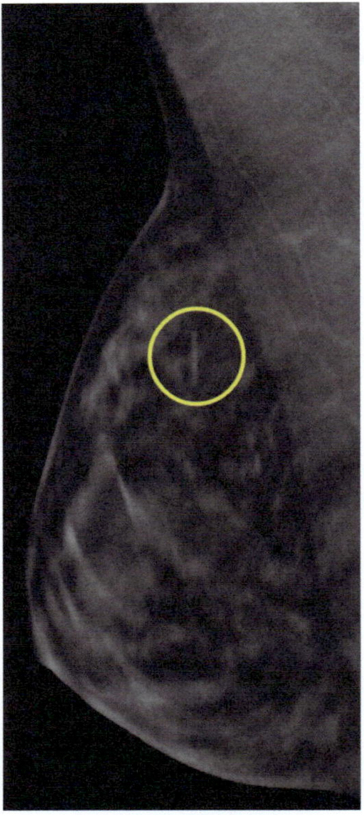

(a) Is caused by a large sweep angle.
(b) Is seen perpendicular to the direction of the X-ray tube sweep.
(c) Is caused by the large number of projections obtained during DBT.
(d) Is most evident when the DBT slice is in plane with objects high in density.

17. The image below demonstrates an artifact seen with tomosynthesis. This artifact:

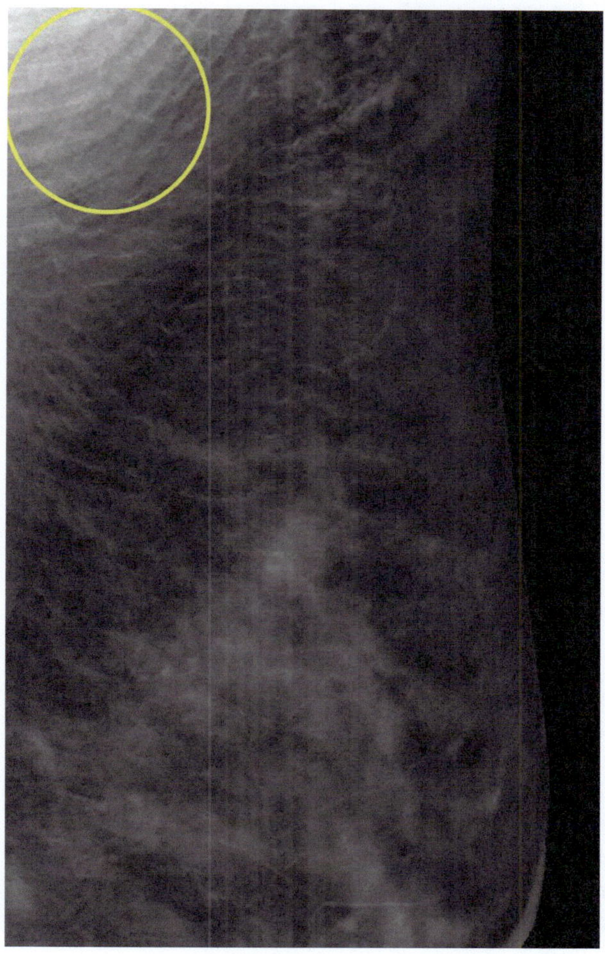

(a) Is caused by a limited detector size and small sweep angle.
(b) Appears as multiple lines on the synthesized image.
(c) Is related to "burn out" seen in dense or large breasts.
(d) Improves with metal reduction post-processing software.

18. Compared to standard views, the type of image shown below provides:

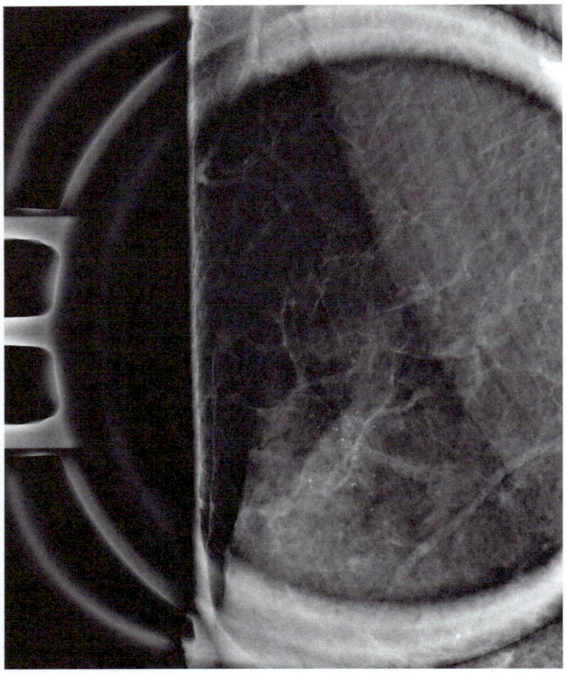

   (a) Fewer X-ray photons and a decrease in radiation.
   (b) Improved spatial resolution.
   (c) Increased noise.
   (d) Quality images by maximizing the penumbra.

19. Magnification views (such as the one seen in question 18) use a:
   (a) 0.1-mm focal spot.
   (b) 0.5-mm focal spot.
   (c) 1.0-mm focal spot.
   (d) 5.0-mm focal spot.

20. A 52-year-old female presents for a breast MRI. Axial T1-weighted image is shown below. Select the true statement.

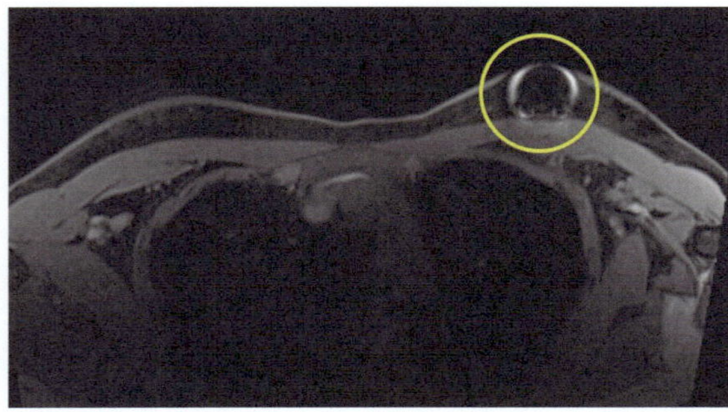

    (a) In axial breast MRI, phase-encoding direction is anterior to posterior.
    (b) The phase-encoding direction is anterior to posterior for sagittal breast MRI.
    (c) Type 2 chemical shift artifact is seen on breast MRI spin-echo sequences.
    (d) Metallic artifacts can be improved by decreasing field strength.

21. What is the purpose of a mammography medical outcomes audit?
    (a) To detect cases of inappropriate Medicare billing and reimbursement.
    (b) To ensure the reliability, clarity, and accuracy of the interpretation of mammograms.
    (c) To track national trends in breast cancer incidence and prevalence.
    (d) To guide annual reimbursement rate adjustments made by the Centers for Medicare and Medicaid Services.

22. What is a requirement for any mammography medical outcomes audit program?
    (a) Utilizes a peer review system to minimize false positive and false negative examinations.
    (b) Have a system to collect and review outcome data for all mammography examinations.
    (c) Establishes a system for corrective measures in the event an interpreting physician is performing outside of the MQSA benchmarks.
    (d) Collects basic statistical outcome data including sensitivity and specificity.

23. When should medical outcomes audit data be reviewed?
    (a) At least once every 12 months.
    (b) At least once every 24 months.
    (c) After each interpreting physician has interpreted 960 mammographic examinations.
    (d) Within 1 month of an MQSA inspection.

24. How should the medical outcomes audit data be analyzed?
    (a) Collectively for all interpreting physicians at the facility.
    (b) Individually for all interpreting physicians that meet MQSA continuing experience requirements.
    (c) Individually and collectively for all interpreting physicians at the facility.
    (d) Collectively for all board-certified interpreting physicians.

25. A screening mammogram is interpreted as BI-RADS Category 1 on 8/1/2020. Several months later, the patient feels a palpable lump and undergoes diagnostic evaluation. Subsequent percutaneous biopsy on 2/15/2021 demonstrates invasive ductal carcinoma. For a medical outcomes audit, which statistical term best describes the 8/1/2020 screening mammogram?
    (a) True positive.
    (b) True negative.
    (c) False positive.
    (d) False negative.

26. A screening mammogram is interpreted as BI-RADS Category 2 on 10/1/2020. The patient subsequently develops unilateral spontaneous bloody nipple discharge and undergoes diagnostic evaluation. Percutaneous biopsy on 10/15/2021 demonstrates ductal carcinoma in situ. For a medical outcomes audit, which statistical term best describes the 10/1/2020 screening mammogram?
    (a) True positive.
    (b) True negative.
    (c) False positive.
    (d) False negative.

27. A screening mammogram is interpreted as BI-RADS Category 0 on 9/1/2020. The subsequent diagnostic evaluation is interpreted as BI-RADS Category 4, and percutaneous biopsy on 9/15/2020 demonstrates invasive ductal carcinoma. For a medical outcomes audit, which statistical term best describes the 9/1/2020 screening mammogram?
    (a) True positive.
    (b) True negative.
    (c) False positive.
    (d) False negative.

28. A screening mammogram is interpreted as BI-RADS Category 0 on 3/1/2020. The subsequent diagnostic evaluation is interpreted as BI-RADS Category 4, and percutaneous biopsy on 3/15/2020 demonstrates sclerosing adenosis. The patient does not undergo any additional biopsies or surgeries in the next year. For a medical outcomes audit, which statistical term best describes the 3/1/2020 screening mammogram?
    (a) True positive.
    (b) True negative.
    (c) False positive.
    (d) False negative.

29. Which of the following tissue diagnoses is considered a true positive for audit purposes?
    (a) Atypical ductal hyperplasia.
    (b) Ductal carcinoma in situ.
    (c) Lobular carcinoma in situ.
    (d) Papilloma.

30. What is the definition of PPV1 (positive predictive value 1)?
    (a) Percentage of all positive screening examinations that receive a BI-RADS Category 4 or 5 upon diagnostic evaluation.
    (b) Percentage of all screening examinations that result in a tissue diagnosis of cancer within 1 year.
    (c) Percentage of all examinations that result in biopsy.
    (d) Percentage of all positive screening examinations that result in a tissue diagnosis of cancer within 1 year.

31. Which of the following best describes PPV2 (positive predictive value 2)?
    (a) (True negative)/(true negative + false negative).
    (b) (True positive)/(true positive + false positive).
    (c) (True positive)/(true positive + false negative).
    (d) (True negative)/(true negative + false positive).

32. Which of the following best describes PPV3 (positive predictive value 3)?
    (a) (True positive + false positive)/(true negative + false negative).
    (b) (False positive)/(number of biopsies).
    (c) (True positive)/(number of biopsies).
    (d) (True positive + false positive)/(number of BI-RADS 4 or 5 interpretations).

33. What is the definition of sensitivity?
    (a) Probability of interpreting an examination as positive when cancer exists.
    (b) Probability of interpreting an examination as positive when cancer does not exist.
    (c) Probability of interpreting an examination as negative when cancer does not exist.
    (d) Probability of interpreting an examination as negative when cancer exists.

34. What is the definition of specificity?
    (a) (True positive)/(false positive + false negative).
    (b) (True positive)/(true positive + false negative).
    (c) (True negative)/(true positive − false negative).
    (d) (True negative)/(true negative + false positive).

35. A breast imaging facility performs 3,000 screening mammograms within a one-year period. Radiologist 1 recalls 175 patients resulting in 9 positive biopsies. Radiologist 2 recalls 125 patients resulting in 5 positive biopsies. What is the facility's cancer detection rate?
    (a) 4.7 per 1,000.
    (b) 5.1%.
    (c) 10 per 1,000.
    (d) 4.7%.

36. A 44-year-old female presents for her annual screening mammogram. Compared to her screening mammogram from 1 year prior, there is a new spiculated mass in the right breast. A subsequent biopsy demonstrates invasive ductal carcinoma. Which term applies to this scenario?
    (a) Incident cancer.
    (b) Prevalent cancer.
    (c) Interim cancer.
    (d) Occult cancer.

37. Based on the most recent version of the BI-RADS Atlas (5th edition), what is an acceptable screening mammography cancer detection rate (per 1,000 examinations)?
    (a) ≥ 2.5.
    (b) ≥ 14.3.
    (c) ≥ 34.1.
    (d) ≥ 50.9.

38. Based on the most recent version of the BI-RADS Atlas (5th edition), what is an acceptable abnormal interpretation (recall) rate?
    (a) 1–3%.
    (b) 5–12%.
    (c) 17-22%.
    (d) 20–25%.

39. Based on the most recent version of the BI-RADS Atlas (5th edition), what is an acceptable PPV1 (positive predictive value 1)?
    (a) 1–2%.
    (b) 3–8%.
    (c) 15–20%.
    (d) 20–40%.

40. Based on the most recent version of the BI-RADS Atlas (5th edition), what is an acceptable PPV2 (positive predictive value 2)?
    (a) 1–5%.
    (b) 12–15%.
    (c) 20–40%.
    (d) 40–60%.

41. What does MQSA stand for?
    (a) Mammography Quality Standards Act.
    (b) Mammography Quantity Service Award.
    (c) Mammography Quality Survey Accreditation.
    (d) Mammography Quality Standards Action.

42. Which organization oversees the regulation of mammography quality standards in the USA?
    (a) American College of Radiology.
    (b) Food and Drug Administration.
    (c) National Institutes of Health.
    (d) Regulated by each state independently.

43. What does the EQUIP (Enhancing Quality Using the Inspection Program) require?
    (a) Periodic clinical image quality review.
    (b) Repeat analysis QC.
    (c) Daily review of mammography.
    (d) Written procedure for corrective action.

44. How often should a physicist visit the site to check equipment?
    (a) Daily.
    (b) Weekly.
    (c) Quarterly.
    (d) Annually.

45. What does MQSA requires of each mammography facility?
    (a) Have a mechanism to file serious consumer complaints.
    (b) Give screening mammography results to patients within one week.
    (c) Have a physicist visit monthly to check equipment.
    (d) Communicate pathology results to patients.

46. The patient must receive a written summary of the mammogram results within how many days of performing the mammogram?
    (a) 1.
    (b) 7.
    (c) 14.
    (d) 30.

47. The MQSA requires a radiologist to have interpreted at least how many mammograms in the 24 months prior to the annual MQSA inspection to maintain certification?
    (a) 240.
    (b) 480.
    (c) 720.
    (d) 960.

48. To meet MQSA requirements, how many mammographic examinations should the interpreting radiologist have interpreted within any 6-month period during the last 2 years of residency?
    (a) 240.
    (b) 480.
    (c) 720.
    (d) 960.

49. How many category 1 CME credits are required by the MQSA within a 36-month period for continued certification of a radiologist?
    (a) 60.
    (b) 30.
    (c) 15.
    (d) 25.
    (e) 100.

50. According to the MQSA, how often should phantom imaging be obtained for quality control?
    (a) Daily.
    (b) Weekly.
    (c) Semiannually.
    (d) Annually.

51. If a "suspicious" or "highly suspicious" finding is reported, the facility is expected to contact the referring health care provider within how many days?
    (a) 1.
    (b) 2.
    (c) 5.
    (d) 10.
    (e) 30.

52. For the small ACR Mammography phantom, how many fibers, masses, and specks must be visualized in order to pass?
    (a) 3 fibers, 3 masses, 3 specks.
    (b) 4 fibers, 3 masses, 3 specks.
    (c) 4 fibers, 4 masses, 4 specks.
    (d) 5 fibers, 4 masses, 5 specks.

53. How often must repeat analysis be tested?
    (a) Daily.
    (b) Weekly.
    (c) Quarterly.
    (d) Annually.

54. Each facility must establish a system to track:
    (a) Positive mammographic findings.
    (b) Negative mammographic findings.
    (c) Short-term follow-up mammograms.
    (d) Benign mammographic findings.

55. Each facility must establish a protocol for:
    (a) Cleaning mammography equipment.
    (b) Performing mammographic examinations.
    (c) Scheduling appointments for new patients.
    (d) Mailing lay letters.

56. Who is held responsible for the QC and QA?
    (a) Lead Interpreting Physician.
    (b) Physicist.
    (c) Designated QC (Quality Control) Technologist.
    (d) Designated QA (Quality Assurance) Technologist.

57. If an interpreting physician has not previously been trained, how many hours of initial training are required prior to independently using any new mammographic modality?
    (a) 2.
    (b) 8.
    (c) 24.
    (d) 48.

58. A valid certificate issued by the MQSA must be:
    (a) Kept safely in a folder.
    (b) Given to each patient.
    (c) Displayed prominently.
    (d) Displayed at only one facility.

59. How often is a compression force measurement performed for quality control?
    (a) Daily.
    (b) Weekly.
    (c) Monthly.
    (d) Semiannually.

Answers

1. e. Both b and c.

   A standard screening mammogram includes a craniocaudal and mediolateral oblique view.

2. c. Posteromedial tissue.

   A well-positioned craniocaudal view must include the posteromedial tissue as this is the one component of the breast that may be excluded from the MLO view. If done correctly, the technologist can include the posteromedial breast tissue without medially exaggerated views, which exclude the deep lateral breast. The measurement of the posterior nipple line on the craniocaudal view (line from the nipple to the edge of the image) should be within 1 cm of the length found on the MLO view. Another indicator of a well-positioned craniocaudal view is visualization of the pectoralis muscle but this is only included in approximately 30% of adequate craniocaudal views [1, 2].

3. d. Inferior breast on the mediolateral oblique view.

The inferior (and subareolar) breast on the mediolateral oblique view is most susceptible to motion unsharpness and inadequate compression. The breast is supported by an immobilized surface both superiorly and inferiorly on the craniocaudal view. The inferior breast on the mediolateral oblique view is more prone to sagging and is not supported. Comparing the mediolateral oblique view to the craniocaudal view can help in assessing sharpness or motion artifact [3].

4. c. 8.

For a standard screening mammogram, 8 images are obtained on a patient with implants. This includes left and right craniocaudal and mediolateral oblique views with the implant included and the implant displaced. For those patients who opt for tomosynthesis at our institution, 3D is only applied to the displaced views. The implant included view is most useful to see the far posterior breast tissue. The implant displaced views are accomplished by moving the implant superiorly and posteriorly while the breast tissue is pulled anteriorly and then compressed within the paddle [4].

5. d. Evaluate the superior posterior breast tissue with the detector closest to the head.

A from below (FB) or caudocranial view is obtained to evaluate superior posterior findings. The detector is closest to the head in this view which decreases the source to object distance and the tissue of interest is not displaced by the compression paddle. This can be especially useful for patients who are difficult to position (i.e., kyphotic patients) or in identifying calcifications or other targets of interest on diagnostic workup or for needle localizations [5].

6a. d. Cleavage view.

6b. b. Evaluate the posterior and medial breast tissue with the beam directed superior to inferior.

The cleavage view is used to evaluate the posterior and medial breast with the beam directed superior to inferior. Both breasts are included in this view but the breast of interest should be closest to the top of the monitor when viewed by the radiologist [6].

7. c. If calcifications are dermal in location.

Tangential views are often used to evaluate whether calcifications are dermal in location. The clinical implication of this is important, since dermal calcifications are considered benign and do not warrant follow up or stereotactic biopsy. A tangential view is performed by initially deciding which view (CC or ML) has the group of calcifications closest to the skin. The technologist then images the breast, in that view, with a paddle used for needle localization (either fenestrated or open with crosshairs). Once the group of calcifications is identified with this image, a BB marker is placed over the group of calcifications and then a tangential view is obtained to the marker (see image below) [4].

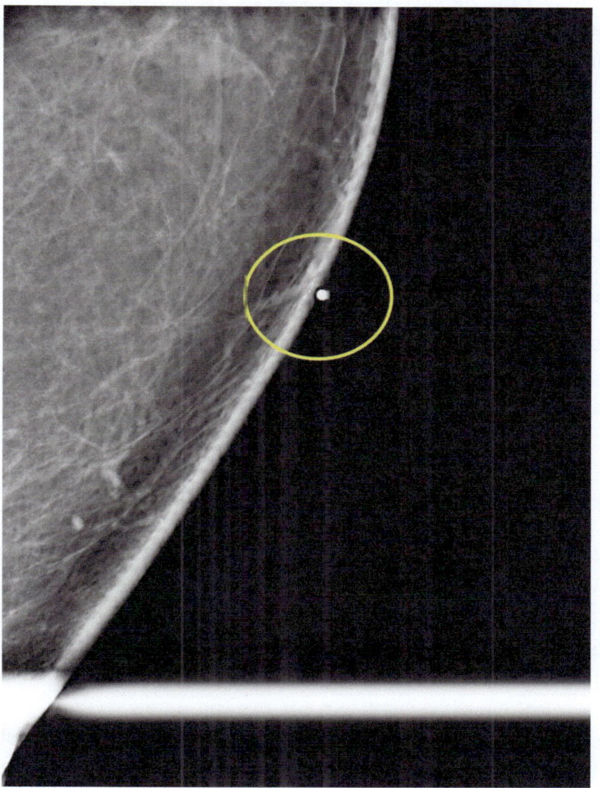

8. b. Coil inhomogeneities.

The image demonstrates inadequate fat suppression, which is an artifact seen with MRI. This can be caused by coil inhomogeneities or an RF coil tuned to the fat peak. Coil inhomogeneities are often seen when larger patients are too close to the coil surface. Attempts should be made to minimize this by repositioning the patient within the coil. The clinical implication of this is that areas of incomplete saturation can be misinterpreted as enhancement and lead to false-positive diagnoses. Lastly, this can occur with inhomogeneity of the magnetic field which should be corrected with magnet shimming.

There are a number of other artifacts that can occur with breast MRI including: motion or misregistration, missed uptake of gadolinium, chemical shift artifacts, and susceptibility artifacts related to diamagnetic/paramagnetic structures such as metallic clips. Motion artifacts in breast MRI are often related to cardiac motion which can result in ghosting, particularly if the phase-encoding direction is in the anterior-posterior direction. A phase-encoding direction that is transverse, or left to right, can reduce this artifact. A chemical shift artifact occurs when the fat signal is mismapped in the readout direction. This is usually related to lower bandwidth and can be remedied by increasing bandwidth. Surgical clips or other diamagnetic/paramagnetic structures can cause susceptibility artifact which is often seen as a signal void [7].

9. c. (Apply saturation pulse at a frequency of 3.5 ppm) and e (Increase the field of view).

   Breast MRI images use fat saturation to increase the detection of breast cancer. Inhomogeneous fat saturation can be caused by several factors. These include magnetic field inhomogeneity, fat saturation pulse not applied at the water peak, improper patient positioning within the breast coil, and too large a field of view.

   To ensure proper fat saturation, it is important to make sure the patient's breast is centered in the breast coil. Field inhomogeneity may also be improved by shimming the magnet. Also, verify that the center peak is set to water frequency [8].

10. b. Gadolinium distorts the local magnetic field.

   Gadolinium-based contrast agents distort the local magnetic field secondary to its paramagnetic effects. It primarily causes T1 shortening. Because of neoangiogenesis in breast cancers, the vessels have a higher perfusion rate and are more porous. As a result, gadolinium diffuses into tumor tissue at a faster rate [9].

11. c. Uses a long TE and long TR.

   The image is a T2-weighted image without contrast and with fat saturation. These images are useful in evaluating for the presence of fluid-filled structures such as cysts (seen in the image of the question stem), hematomas, or areas of edema in the breast. As they are non-contrast sequences, they are not used to evaluate enhancement curves or in the creation of subtraction images (where the T1 fat saturation pre-contrast images are subtracted from the T1 fat saturation post-contrast images).

Although there can be some variation in the number and types of sequences obtained with a full-length breast MRI, the following is an example of the protocol which is used at our institution:

Localizer (Scout), T1-weighted images without contrast and without fat saturation, T2-weighted images without contrast and with fat saturation, Dynamic T1-weighted images with fat saturation, without contrast and with contrast [10].

12. d. Spatial resolution of the transducer is determined by axial and lateral resolution.

Breast ultrasound transducers should be linear array, high resolution, and operating with at least 12 MHz center frequency (preferably higher) with electronic focusing or automatic adjustment of focusing. Standoff devices are used to evaluate superficial lesions, particularly dermal lesions. The axial (Z) and lateral (X and Y) resolution determine the overall spatial resolution and good resolution in all three planes are required for high-resolution breast ultrasound [11, 12].

13. c. Uses electronic beam steering to obtain multiple images to average out artifactual echoes.

Spatial compound imaging uses electronic beam steering to obtain multiple images to average out artifactual echoes. The images are acquired at different angles which helps to better characterize margins and internal echogenicity [13].

14. b. Side lobes.

Coded harmonics is used to diminish artifacts and improve contrast resolution in breast ultrasound. The majority of these artifacts are caused by backscatter and side lobes. Coded harmonics uses a signal that is digitally encoded. It has the ability to transmit the beam at a lower frequency and receive at a higher center frequency so that adequate penetration is present for deep lesions in the breast or on the chest wall. The result is a higher signal-to-noise ratio image with less artifacts [14].

15. a. Is caused by reflections between two highly reflective interfaces in parallel.

Reverberation is caused by reflections between two highly reflective interfaces in parallel. It is seen as several parallel lines which are brighter toward the skin and become less intense at deeper locations within the breast. It is most commonly encountered in breast ultrasound on imaging of cysts and can mimic debris which may lead to unnecessary short-term follow-ups or even interventions such as aspirations or biopsies. This artifact can be minimized by decreasing the gain, using tissue harmonic imaging, using more than one window or altering the area of interest.

Speckle causes tissue to appear more granular and is caused by acoustic interference. It essentially reduces resolution (both spatial and contrast) and can be minimized by using speckle reduction imaging which is found on most current ultrasound equipment and is usually a proprietary to the seller or brand of the equipment involved in post-processing. Tissue harmonic imaging and spatial compounding can also minimize speckle [15].

16. b. Is seen perpendicular to the direction of the X-ray tube sweep.

The image demonstrates a blurring ripple artifact which has a direct relationship with the limited number of projections obtained during tomosynthesis. Because the number of projections is limited, the ability to suppress anatomic noise is limited leading to blurring ripple artifacts which are seen perpendicular to the direction of the X-ray tube sweep. High-density objects can cause a blurring ripple artifact, however, this artifact is not seen when the DBT slice is in plane with the object of high density (i.e., metallic objects such as clips). The artifact is manifest when immediately out of plane with the object by appearing less defined and wider than the actual size of the object. The further away the section from the object can cause even more elongation of the object, also known as the "slinky" artifact. Blurring ripple artifact is also seen as a halo or streak around metallic densities on synthetic mammogram [16].

17. a. Is caused by a limited detector size and small sweep angle.

There are a few artifacts that are specific to tomosynthesis. These include: truncation or stair-step artifacts, blurring ripple artifacts, and artifacts related to resolution of superficial tissue and loss of skin.

Truncation artifacts (seen in this image) are related to limited detector size and small sweep angle and directly relate to objects on the edge of the detector contributing data which is not uniform. This data at the edge of the detector is not within the volume that is reconstructed however it still contributes data and leads to a truncation or stair-step artifact. The stair-step appearance is only seen on the individual tomosynthesis images and is summarized as a single line on the synthetic images. Another truncation artifact is when the attenuation of the X-ray beam is overestimated at the image margins leading to a "bright edge." The use of a larger detector or a tilt of the detector concentric to the sweep angle of the X-ray tube can limit truncation artifacts. Metal reduction post-processing software improves blurring ripple artifacts.

Artifacts related to poor resolution of superficial tissue and loss of skin are often seen in dense breast tissue or large breasts. The doses of radiation needed in these patients are often higher which leads to "burn out" of the dermis or subcutaneous tissue as higher energy levels reach the detector in these areas causing saturation and loss of resolution [16].

18. b. Improved spatial resolution.

19. a. 0.1 mm focal spot.

Magnification views are most often used to evaluate calcifications. They use a small (0.1 mm) focal spot and use magnification values between 1.4 and 2.0. They improve spatial resolution and decrease noise at the cost of increased radiation. Quality images are obtained by minimizing the penumbra or blurring at the edge of the image caused by a finite focal spot [4, 17].

20. d. Metallic artifacts can be improved by decreasing field strength.

The image demonstrates susceptibility artifact associated with metal within a chest wall port-a-cath.

Increasing receiver bandwidth can improve metal artifact/magnetic susceptibility artifact (or one can use a lower field strength magnet or spin-echo sequence). Phase encoding is typically done in the anterior to posterior direction for body MRI. With breast MRI, phase encoding is left to right in the axial plane and superior to inferior in the sagittal plane, in order to avoid pulsation artifact. Chemical shift artifact is common in breast MRI due to the presence of multiple fat–fluid interfaces anatomically in the breast, but type 2 chemical shift artifact only occurs on gradient-echo sequences [8, 18, 19].

21. b. To ensure the reliability, clarity, and accuracy of the interpretation of mammograms.

The purpose of the mammography medical outcomes audit is to ensure the reliability, clarity, and accuracy of mammogram interpretation [20].

22. b. Have a system to collect and review outcome data for all mammography examinations.

Facilities must have a system to collect and review outcome data for all mammography examinations [20].

23. a. At least once every 12 months.

A review of medical outcomes audit data should be performed at least once every 12 months [20].

24. c. Individually and collectively for all interpreting physicians at the facility.

Analysis should be made individually and collectively for all interpreting physicians at the facility [20].

25. d. False negative. False negative (FN): Tissue diagnosis of cancer within 1 year of a negative examination [21].

26. b. True negative. True negative (TN): No known tissue diagnosis of cancer within 1 year of a negative examination [21].

27. a. True positive. True positive (TP): Tissue diagnosis of cancer within 1 year after a positive examination.

BI-RADS Category 0 is considered a positive screening mammogram. Therefore, the initial screening mammogram, in this case, is considered a true positive, as it led to a subsequent diagnosis of cancer within 1 year [21].

28. c. False positive (FP): No known tissue diagnosis of cancer within 1 year.

BI-RADS Category 0 is considered a positive screening mammogram. Therefore, the initial screening mammogram, in this case, is considered a false positive, as there is no known tissue diagnosis of cancer within 1 year. The BI-RADS Category of the diagnostic evaluation does not change whether the screening examination is a true or false positive [21].

29. b. Ductal carcinoma in situ.

For the purposes of an audit, ductal carcinoma in situ and primary invasive breast carcinoma are considered true-positive diagnoses of cancer [21].

While MQSA regulations require certain basic elements of a medical outcomes audit program, the BI-RADS Atlas (5th edition) recommends the collection and analysis of several additional parameters as part of a clinically relevant audit. Some relevant definitions include: [21].

Positive screening mammography: BI-RADS Category 0 (screening examination for which additional diagnostic imaging is recommended prior to the next routine screening examination). Use of BI-RADS Category 3, 4, and 5 assessments for screening mammography is discouraged but would also be included.

Negative screening mammography: BI-RADS Category 1 or 2.

Positive diagnostic mammography: BI-RADS Category 4 or 5 (diagnostic examination for which tissue diagnosis is recommended).

Negative diagnostic mammography: BI-RADS Category 1, 2, or 3.

True positive (TP): Tissue diagnosis of cancer within 1 year after a positive examination. For the purposes of an audit, ductal carcinoma in situ and primary invasive breast carcinoma are considered true positive diagnoses of cancer.

True negative (TN): No known tissue diagnosis of cancer within 1 year of a negative examination.

False negative (FN): Tissue diagnosis of cancer within 1 year of a negative examination.

False positive (FP): No known tissue diagnosis of cancer within 1 year.*

*This is a simplified definition. There are three separate definitions of a false-positive examination depending on whether the examination was a screening or diagnostic study and whether a biopsy was subsequently performed.

TP+TN+FP+FN = total number of examinations

	Biopsy +	Biopsy −
Imaging +	TP	FP
Imaging −	FN	TN

30. d. Percentage of all positive screening examinations that result in a tissue diagnosis of cancer within 1 year.

PPV1 = Percentage of all positive screening examinations that result in a tissue diagnosis of cancer within 1 year = TP/(number of positive screening examinations) = TP/(TP+FP) [21]

31. b. (True positive)/(true positive + false positive).

PPV2 = Percentage of all diagnostic examinations recommended for tissue diagnosis or surgical consultation (BI-RADS Category 4 or 5) that result in a tissue diagnosis of cancer within 1 year = TP/(number of diagnostic examinations recommended for tissue diagnosis) = TP/(TP+FP) [21]

32. c. (True positive)/(number of biopsies).

PPV3 = Percentage of all known biopsies done as a result of positive diagnostic examinations (BI-RADS Category 4 or 5) that resulted in a tissue diagnosis of cancer within 1 year (also known as biopsy yield of malignancy or positive biopsy rate) = TP/(number of biopsies) = TP/(TP+FP) [21]

Positive predictive value (PPV):

There are three separate definitions of PPV. PPV1 is a metric designed to evaluate screening examinations, while PPV2 and PPV3 are metrics designed to evaluate diagnostic examinations (although some research studies have also applied these terms to screening examinations). Since these terms have different definitions, the TP and FP values used to calculate them are also different [21].

PPV1 = Percentage of all positive screening examinations that result in a tissue diagnosis of cancer within 1 year

PPV1 = TP/(number of positive screening examinations)

PPV1 = TP/(TP+FP)

PPV2 = Percentage of all diagnostic examinations recommended for tissue diagnosis or surgical consultation (BI-RADS Category 4 or 5) that result in a tissue diagnosis of cancer within 1 year

PPV2 = TP/(number of diagnostic examinations recommended for tissue diagnosis)

PPV2 = TP/(TP+FP)

PPV3 = Percentage of all known biopsies done as a result of positive diagnostic examinations (BI-RADS Category 4 or 5) that resulted in a tissue diagnosis of cancer within 1 year (also known as biopsy yield of malignancy or positive biopsy rate)

PPV3 = TP/(number of biopsies)

PPV3 = TP/(TP+FP)

Positive Predictive Value

	Biopsy +	Biopsy −	
Imaging +	TP	FP	$\dfrac{TP}{(TP+FP)}$
Imaging −	FN	TN	

33. a. Probability of interpreting an examination as positive when cancer exists.

Sensitivity = TP/(TP+FN) = Probability of interpreting an examination as positive when cancer exists [21]

34. d. (True negative)/(true negative + false positive).

Specificity = TN/(TN+FP) = Probability of interpreting an examination as negative when cancer does not exist [21]

Sensitivity

	Biopsy +	Biopsy −
Imaging +	TP	FP
Imaging −	FN	TN

$$\frac{TP}{(TP+FN)}$$

Specificity

	Biopsy +	Biopsy −
Imaging +	TP	FP
Imaging −	FN	TN

$$\frac{TN}{(TN+FP)}$$

35. a. 4.7 per 1,000.

The cancer detection rate is the number of cancers detected at imaging per 1,000 patients examined (14 positive biopsies / 3,000 screening mammograms = 4.7 per 1,000) [21].

36. a. Incident cancer.

Incident cancers are those found at a subsequent screening examination performed at or close to the recommended screening interval. *Prevalent cancers* are those found at first-time screening examination. The other answers are distractors [21].

37. a. ≥ 2.5.

The most recent version of the BI-RADS Atlas (5th edition) presents audit analysis benchmarks in two ways [21], and both sets of numbers are commonly referenced. One set of benchmarks is based on an article by Carney et al., which suggests acceptable ranges of performance [22]. Benchmarks based on 2006 data from the Breast Cancer Surveillance Consortium (BCSC) are also included in the BI-RADS Atlas and all fall within these acceptable ranges [23].

≥ 2.5 per 1,000 is considered an acceptable range. The BCSC mammography screening benchmark is 4.7 per 1,000 [21–23].

38. b. 5–12%.

5–12% is considered an acceptable range. The BCSC mammography screening benchmark is 10.6% [21–23].

39. b. 3–8%.

3–8% is considered an acceptable range. The BCSC mammography screening benchmark is 4.4% [21–23].

40. c. 20–40%.

20–40% is considered an acceptable range. The BCSC mammography screening benchmark is 25.4% [21–23].

41. a. Mammography Quality Standards Act.

The Mammography Quality Standards Act was passed on October 27, 1992, to establish national quality standards for mammography [24].

42. b. Food and Drug Administration.

The FDA developed and implements the MQSA regulations [24].

43. a. Periodic clinical image quality review.

The EQUIP initiative was introduced by the MQSA to emphasize clinical image quality. Periodic clinical image quality reviews are discussed at the time of the MQSA inspection and are to have been done since the last inspection. This review needs to be performed at least annually and written documentation is required. Repeat and reject rates are not required for EQUIP and are not directly linked to poor-quality images presented for interpretation to an interpreting radiologist. A daily review of mammography is not considered as a periodic review of sample images. A separate dedicated review of images is necessary for EQUIP. Facilities are not required to create a written procedure for the facility's system of corrective action. A facility may verbally explain its system to the inspector. Whether written or verbal, the system must include mechanisms for ongoing interpreting physician feedback and documenting and assessing corrective actions [25].

44. d. Annually.

The medical physicist must evaluate the facility's quality control program and complete the QC test summary within the 45 days provided to obtain clinical and phantom images as part of a new unit's Annual Survey Report submitted to the ACR with the full application and/or testing materials. After the initial certification, the physicist is annually required to perform the manufacturer-specified QC or the QC outlined in the 2018 ACR Digital Mammography QC Manual and provide a written report of the survey's findings to the responsible physician(s) and professional(s) responsible [26].

45. a. Have a mechanism to file serious consumer complaints.

MQSA requires that each facility should develop a system for collecting and resolving serious consumer complaints. If a complaint cannot be resolved at the facility, the consumer should contact the facility's accreditation body [27].

46. d. 30.

Within 30 days of the examination, the facility is required to communicate the results to the referring health care provider and to the patient in a lay letter. If a patient is self-referred, the report must be given to the patient [28].

47. d. 960.

To stay certified, the radiologist must continue to interpret or multi-read at least 960 mammographic exams over a 24-month period [28].

48. a. 240.

To immediately begin independent interpretation of mammograms following a residency program, medical residency graduates of 2014 or later must have interpreted 240 mammographic examinations under direct supervision within any 6-month period during the last 2 years of the medical residency [28].

49. c. 15.

For initial certification, at least 60 hours of documented Category 1 CME in mammography is required (40 hours if before 1999). The radiologist must have at least 15 Category 1 CME credits within a 36-month period for continued certification [28].

50. b. Weekly.

The phantom image must be performed each week on the units where mammograms are performed. The test does not need to be performed on the same day each week [28].

51. c. 5.

If the assessment is BI-RADS Category 4 or 5, the facility is required to communicate the results as soon as possible to the referring health care provider and to the patient in a lay summary. It is expected that this is accomplished within 5 business days. The facility is required to have an established communication system in place [29].

52. b. 4 Fibers, 3 masses, 3 specks.

Per ACR guidelines, in order to pass the small ACR Mammography Phantom, there must be no clinically significant artifacts and the 4 largest fibers, the 3 largest speck groups, and the 3 largest masses must be visualized. A speck can be mistaken for a calcification [30].

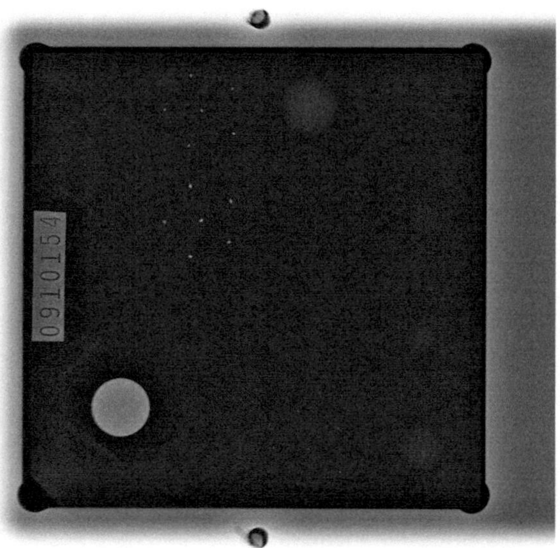

53. c. Quarterly.

Repeat analysis is performed quarterly to determine the cause of repeated mammograms. Analysis of this data helps to improve efficiency and reduce patient radiation. The overall repeat rate should be 2% or less. For the rate to be meaningful, at least 250 patients should be included. If the repeat rate is above 2%, the source of the problem should be identified, and corrective action should be taken within 30 days. These steps are part of quality control [30].

54. a. Positive mammographic findings.

MQSA lets the facility decide how to track "positive mammographic findings" which refers to "suspicious" (BI-RADS Category 4) and "highly suggestive of malignancy" (BI-RADS Category 5). This system may be manual or computerized. This must include tracking of mammograms, whether biopsies were performed and if the biopsies were benign or malignant. If biopsies were recommended and no results were obtained, the facility must document attempts to find this information [28].

55. a. Cleaning mammography equipment.

There must be a written facility-specific procedure for cleaning mammography equipment. This must address cleaning contaminated mammography equipment to prevent the transmission of blood-borne pathogens and infectious diseases. There must be documentation that the infection control procedures were performed when the mammography equipment was contaminated. Written protocols are not required for performing mammographic examinations, scheduling appointments, and printing lay letters [31].

56. a. Lead Interpreting Physician.

The lead interpreting physician (LIP), usually a radiologist, has the overall responsibility that all MQSA requirements of QA and QC for the facility are met. The LIP appoints a lead QC technologist and medical physicist to ensure an effective QC program. The LIP must review the mammography facility's QC at least quarterly [30].

57. b. 8.

All mammography personnel must have 8 hours of training in a new mammography modality. For residents and fellows, the training should be documented in the residency or fellowship letter. The training does not need to be provided by the manufacturer [32].

58. c. Displayed prominently.

An MQSA certificate should be displayed prominently to indicate that the facility is certified. All certificates must be valid and not expired to legally provide mammography [29].

59. d. Semiannually.

Every 6 months, compression force is tested to ensure that the mammography unit can provide adequate compression and does not allow too much pressure. A towel is placed on the breast support surface and a bathroom scale is placed under the compression paddle. The maximum compression force is measured. The measured force must be between 25 and 45 lbs. [30].

References

1. Zuley M, Braner B. Positioning in mammography. Chapter 6. In: Bassett LW, Mahoney MC, Apple SK, D'Orsi CJ, editors. Breast imaging. Philadelphia: Elsevier; 2010. p. 113–5.
2. Bassett LW, Doepke L. Clinical image evaluation. Chapter 7. In: Bassett LW, Mahoney MC, Apple SK, D'Orsi CJ, editors. Breast imaging. Philadelphia: Elsevier; 2010. p. 122–3.
3. Accreditation Case Review: Mammography and Stereotactic Biopsy. https://www.sbi-online.org/Portals/0/Breast%20Imaging%20Symposium%202016/Final%20Presentations/105A%20Parkinson%20-%20Accreditation%20Case%20Review%201%20-%20FINAL.pdf. (2016). Accessed December 6 2021.
4. Zuley M, Braner B. Positioning in mammography. Chapter 6. In: Bassett LW, Mahoney MC, Apple SK, D'Orsi CJ, editors. Breast imaging. Philadelphia: Elsevier; 2010. p. 119.
5. Zuley M, Braner B. Positioning in mammography. Chapter 6. In: Bassett LW, Mahoney MC, Apple SK, D'Orsi CJ, editors. Breast imaging. Philadelphia: Elsevier; 2010. p. 117.
6. Zuley M, Braner B. Positioning in mammography. Chapter 6. In: Bassett LW, Mahoney MC, Apple SK, D'Orsi CJ, editors. Breast imaging. Philadelphia: Elsevier; 2010. p. 118.
7. Oshiro T, Schultze-Haakh H, Little J. Magnetic resonance equipment and techniques. Chapter 11. In: Bassett LW, Mahoney MC, Apple SK, D'Orsi CJ, editors. Breast imaging. Philadelphia: Elsevier; 2010. p. 189–92.
8. Harvey JA, Hendrick RE, Coll JM, Nicholson BT, Burkholder BT, Cohen MA. Breast MR imaging artifacts: how to recognize and fix them. Radiographics. 2007;27(Suppl 1):S131–45. https://doi.org/10.1148/rg.27si075514.
9. Oshiro T, Schultze-Haakh H, Little J. Magnetic resonance equipment and techniques. Chapter 11. In: Bassett LW, Mahoney MC, Apple SK, D'Orsi CJ, editors. Breast imaging. Philadelphia: Elsevier; 2010. p. 185–6.
10. Oshiro T, Schultze-Haakh H, Little J. Magnetic resonance equipment and techniques. Chapter 11. In: Bassett LW, Mahoney MC, Apple SK, D'Orsi CJ, editors. Breast imaging. Philadelphia: Elsevier; 2010. p. 181–7.
11. Comstock C. Ultrasound equipment. Chapter 9. In: Bassett LW, Mahoney MC, Apple SK, D'Orsi CJ, editors. Breast imaging. Philadelphia: Elsevier; 2010. p. 146–52.
12. Equipment: Breast Ultrasound. https://accreditationsupport.acr.org/support/solutions/articles/11000045910-equipment-breast-ultrasound. (2019). Accessed December 6 2021.
13. Comstock C. Ultrasound equipment. Chapter 9. In: Bassett LW, Mahoney MC, Apple SK, D'Orsi CJ, editors. Breast imaging. Philadelphia: Elsevier; 2010. p. 148–9.
14. Rapp CL, Stavros AT. Coded harmonics in breast ultrasound: does it make a difference? J Diagn Med Sonogr. 2001;17(1):22–8. https://doi.org/10.1177/87564790122250093.
15. Baad M, Lu ZF, Reiser I, Paushter D. Clinical significance of US artifacts. Radiographics. 2017;37(5):1408–23. https://doi.org/10.1148/rg.2017160175.
16. Tirada N, Li G, Dreizin D, Robinson L, Khorjekar G, Dromi S, et al. Digital breast tomosynthesis: physics, artifacts, and quality control considerations. Radiographics. 2019;39(2):413–26. https://doi.org/10.1148/rg.2019180046.
17. Takahashi S, Sakuma S. Principles of magnification radiography. In: Magnification radiography. Berlin, Heidelberg: Springer; 1975. p. 2.
18. Yitta S, Joe BN, Wisner DJ, Price ER, Hylton NM. Recognizing artifacts and optimizing breast MRI at 1.5 and 3 T. AJR Am J Roentgenol. 2013;200(6):W673–82. https://doi.org/10.2214/AJR.12.10013.
19. AuntMinnie,com's Board Review: https://www.auntminnie.com/index.aspx?sec=olce&sub=br
20. United States Food and Drug Administration: Medical outcomes audit program. https://www.accessdata.fda.gov/cdrh_docs/presentations/pghs/Medical_Outcomes_Audit_Program.htm. (2021). Accessed December 6 2021.
21. D'Orsi CJ, Sickles EA, Mendelson EB, Morris EA, et al. ACR BI-RADS® Atlas, Breast Imaging Reporting and Data System. 5th rev. ed. Reston, VA: American College of Radiology; 2013.

22. Carney PA, Sickles EA, Monsees BS, Bassett LW, Brenner RJ, Feig SA, et al. Identifying minimally acceptable interpretive performance criteria for screening mammography. Radiology. 2010;255(2):354–61. https://doi.org/10.1148/radiol.10091636.
23. Rosenberg RD, Yankaskas BC, Abraham LA, Sickles EA, Lehman CD, Geller BM, et al. Performance benchmarks for screening mammography. Radiology. 2006;241(1):55–66. https://doi.org/10.1148/radiol.2411051504.
24. "Mammography Quality Standards Act Regulations." October 2002. https://www.fda.gov/radiation-emitting-products/regulations-mqsa/mammography-quality-standards-act-regulations
25. "Mammography Quality Standards Act (MQSA) Enhancing Quality Using the Inspection Program (EQUIP) Frequently Asked Questions – Facilities." June 2018. https://www.fda.gov/media/101293/download
26. "Guidance Document: Mammography Facility Surveys, Mammography Equipment Evaluations, and Medical Physicist Qualification Requirements under MQSA." September 2005. https://www.fda.gov/regulatory-information/search-fda-guidance-documents/mammography-facility-surveys-mammography-equipment-evaluations-and-medical-physicist-qualification#4
27. "Consumer Information (MQSA)." https://www.fda.gov/radiation-emitting-products/mammography-quality-standards-act-and-program/consumer-information-mqsa." Accessed March 25th 2021.
28. "Compliance Guidance: The Mammography Quality Standards Act Final Regulations: Preparing for MQSA Inspections; Final." November 2001. https://www.fda.gov/regulatory-information/search-fda-guidance-documents/compliance-guidance-mammography-quality-standards-act-final-regulations-preparing-mqsa-inspections
29. "Frequently Asked Questions about MQSA." https://www.fda.gov/radiation-emitting-products/consumer-information-mqsa/frequently-asked-questions-about-mqsa Accessed March 25th 2021.
30. Berns EAPD, Butler PF, et al. Digital mammography quality control manual. 2nd ed. Reston, VA: American College of Radiology; 2018. p. 39–48.
31. "MQSA Inspection Procedures Version 7.0." June 2015. Page 88. https://www.fda.gov/media/79764/download
32. "Frequently Asked Questions about DBT and MQSA Training Requirements." https://www.fda.gov/radiation-emitting-products/facility-certification-and-inspection-mqsa/frequently-asked-questions-about-dbt-and-mqsa-training-requirements. Accessed March 25th 2021.

BI-RADS Terminology

2

Claire Lis, Hannah Milch, Jane Dascalos,
and Denise Andrews-Tang

C. Lis (✉) · H. Milch · J. Dascalos
Department of Radiology, David Geffen School of Medicine at UCLA, Los Angeles, CA,
USA
e-mail: clis@mednet.ucla.edu; hmilch@mednet.ucla.edu; jdascalos@mednet.ucla.edu

D. Andrews-Tang
Department of Radiology, David Geffen School of Medicine at UCLA, Los Angeles, CA,
USA

Department of Radiology, Olive View-UCLA Medical Center, Sylmar, CA, USA
e-mail: dandrews@dhs.lacounty.gov

© The Author(s), under exclusive license to Springer Nature
Switzerland AG 2022
L. Chow, B. Li (eds.), *Absolute Breast Imaging Review*,
https://doi.org/10.1007/978-3-031-08274-0_2

1. Match the following images with the following calcification morphology: vascular, popcorn, rim, rod-like.

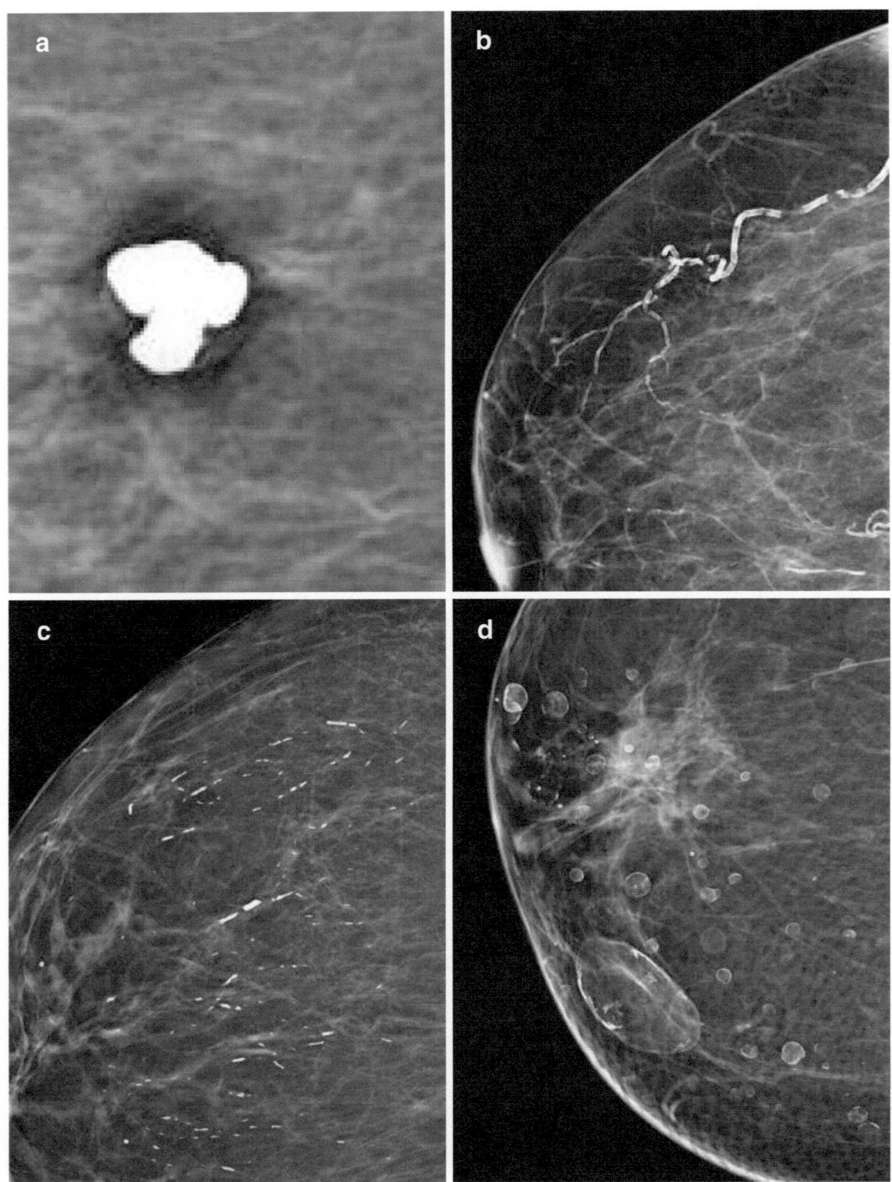

    (a) A—rim; B—rod-like; C—vascular; D—popcorn.
    (b) A—vascular; B—rim; C—rod-like; D—popcorn.
    (c) A—popcorn; B—rod-like; C—vascular; D—rim.
    (d) A—popcorn; B—vascular; C—rod-like; D—rim.

2. Match the following images with the following calcification morphology: suture, coarse heterogeneous, round, dystrophic, amorphous.

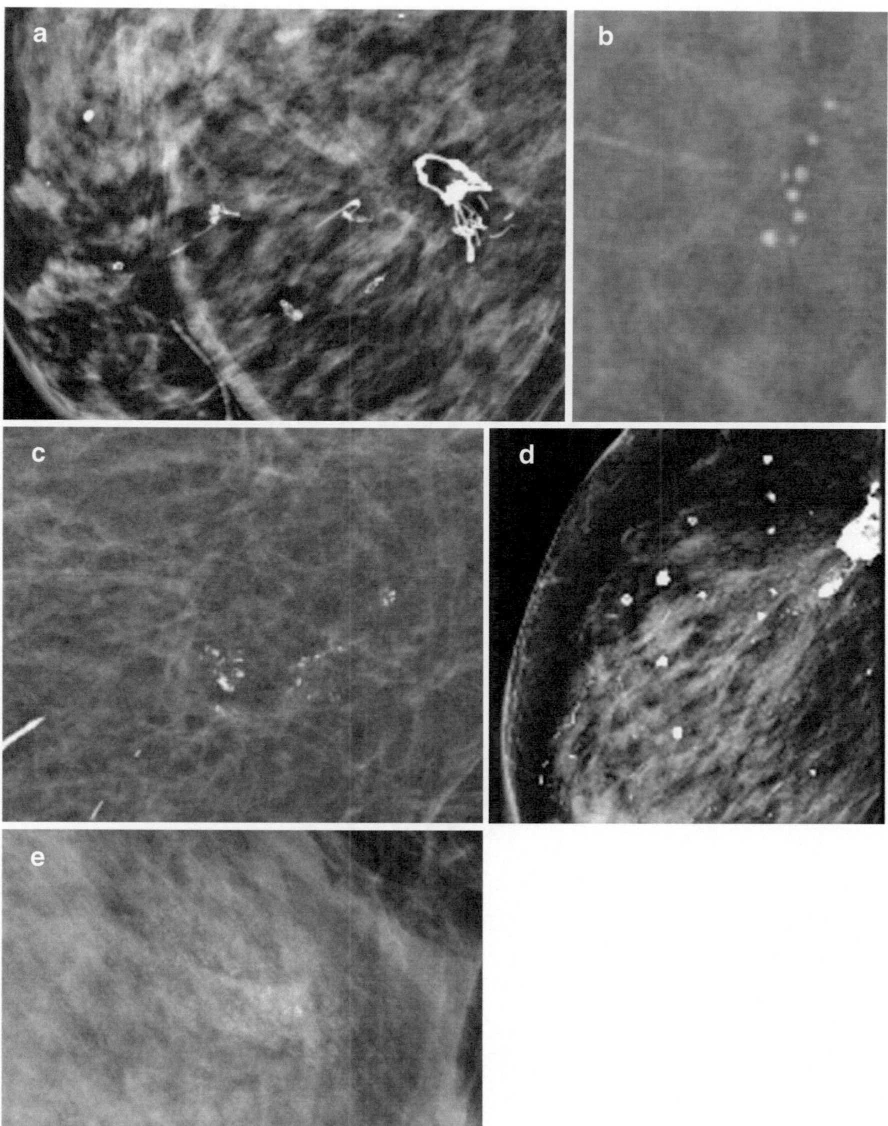

(a) A—amorphous; B—dystrophic; C—round; D—coarse heterogeneous; E—suture.

(b) A—round; B—amorphous; C—dystrophic; D—suture; E—coarse heterogeneous.

   (c) A—coarse heterogeneous; B—dystrophic; C—amorphous; D—suture; E—round.

   (d) A—suture; B—round; C—coarse heterogeneous; D—dystrophic; E—amorphous.

3. Match the following images with the following calcification distribution patterns: grouped, regional, segmental, diffuse, linear.

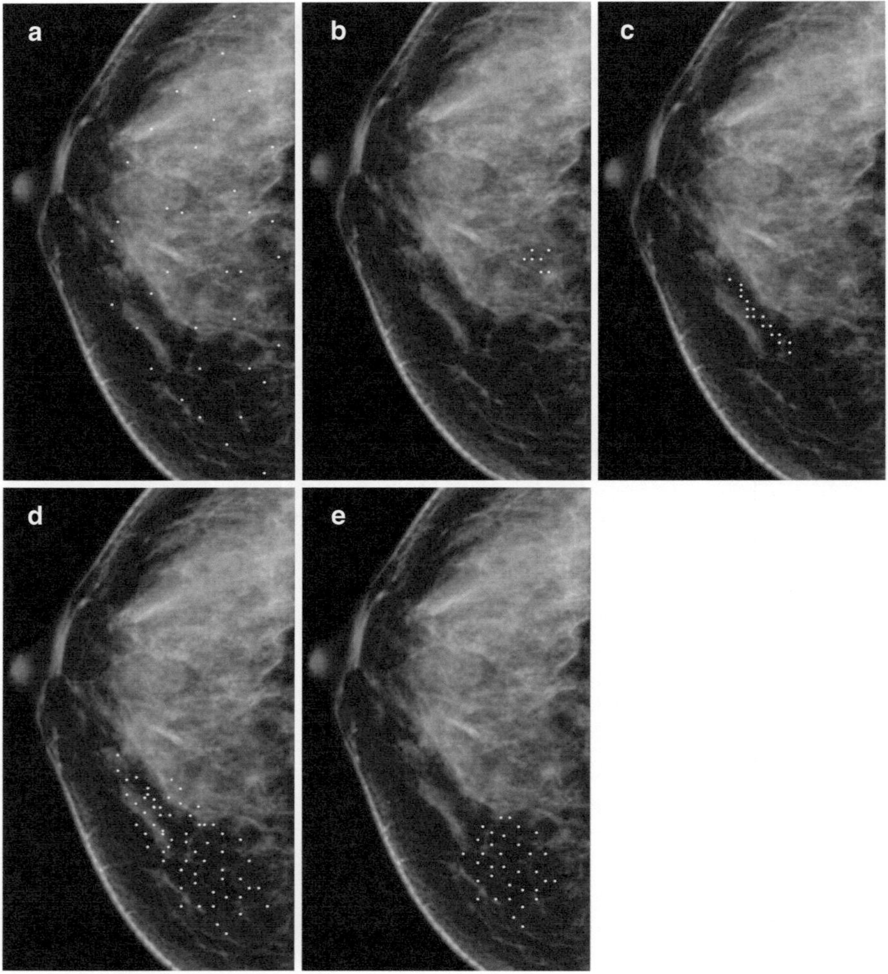

   (a) A—diffuse; B—linear; C—grouped; D—regional; E—segmental.

   (b) A—diffuse; B—grouped; C—linear; D—segmental; E—regional.

   (c) A—regional; B—segmental; C—linear; D—diffuse; E—grouped.

   (d) A—regional; B—grouped; C—segmental; D—linear; E—diffuse.

4. A patient presents for a diagnostic mammogram for a finding seen on a screening mammogram, shown below. It is present on CC and MLO view. How should this finding be described according to the BI-RADS lexicon?

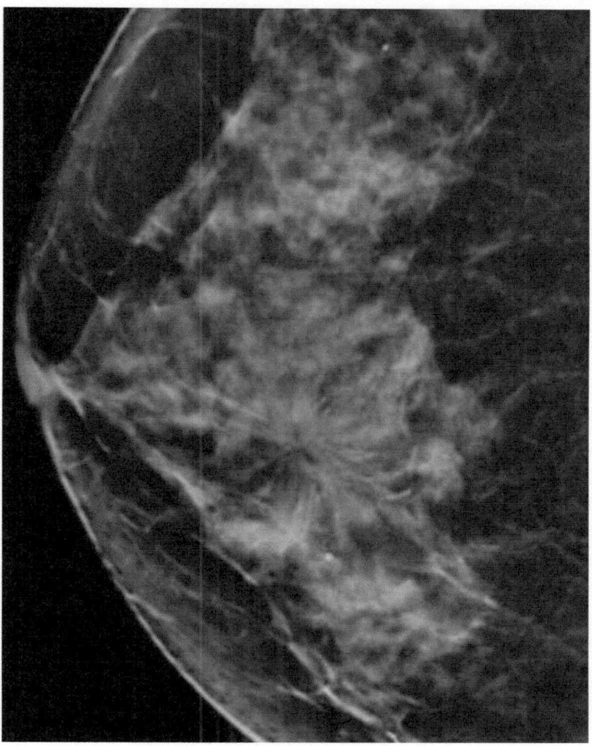

(a) Asymmetry.
(b) Architectural distortion.
(c) Focal density.
(d) Geographic abnormality.

5. A patient underwent diagnostic evaluation for a mass seen on screening mammography. On diagnostic evaluation, the mass was assigned a BI-RADS category 4B. What is the likelihood of malignancy corresponding to BI-RADS category 4B?
(a) >2% to ≤10%.
(b) >25% to <75%.
(c) >10% to ≤50%.
(d) >50% to <95%.

6. Identify the following mass shapes:

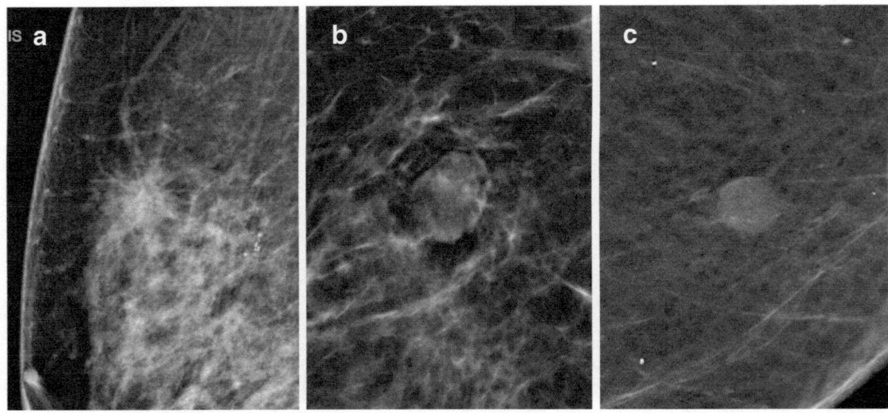

   (a) A—irregular; B—oval; C—round.
   (b) A—round; B—ovoid; C—oval.
   (c) A—irregular; B—ovoid; C—round.
   (d) A—irregular; B—round; C—ovoid.

7. Match the following images with the following margin types: circumscribed, obscured, microlobulated, and indistinct.

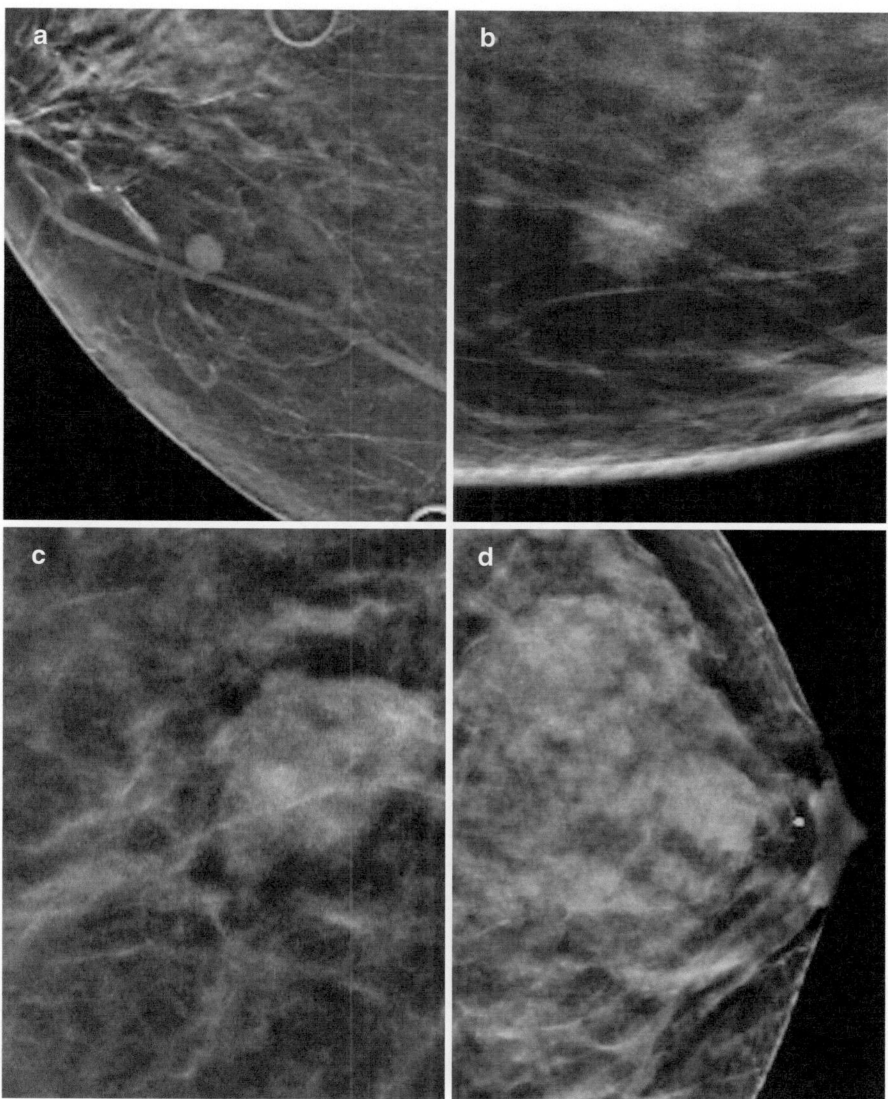

(a) A—circumscribed; B—obscured; C—indistinct; D—microlobulated.
(b) A—circumscribed; B—indistinct; C—microlobulated; D—obscured.
(c) A—circumscribed; B—indistinct; C—obscured; D—microlobulated.
(d) A—circumscribed; B—microlobulated; C—indistinct; D—obscured.

8. A patient underwent diagnostic evaluation for a palpable mass, shown below. What is the echogenicity of the mass?

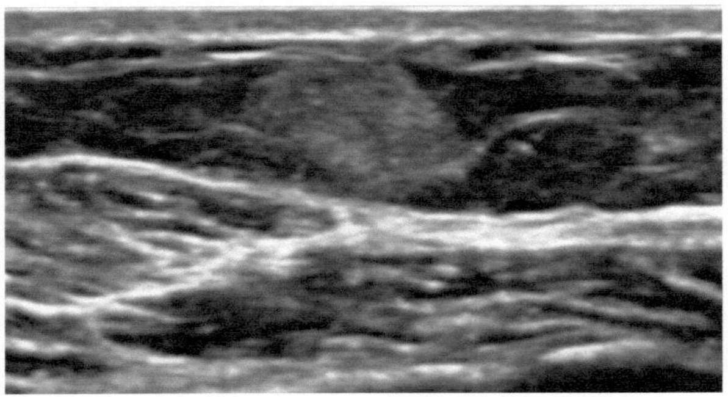

    (a) Hypoechoic.
    (b) Hyperechoic.
    (c) Isoechoic.
    (d) Mixed hypoechoic/hyperechoic.

9. What are the margins of the finding seen on the ultrasound image below?

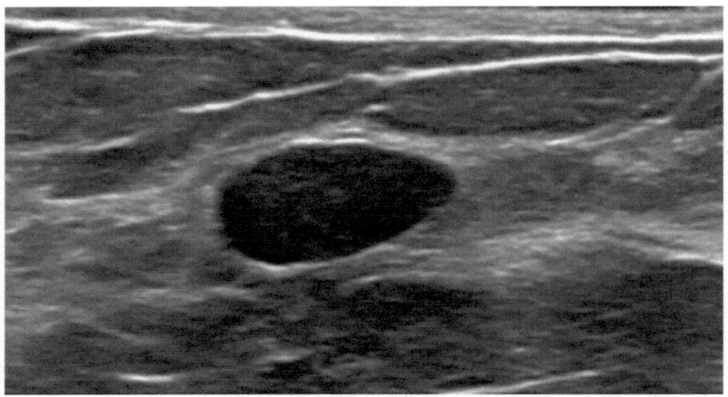

    (a) Circumscribed.
    (b) Indistinct.
    (c) Parallel.
    (d) Spiculated.

10. What are the margins of the mass seen on the ultrasound image below?

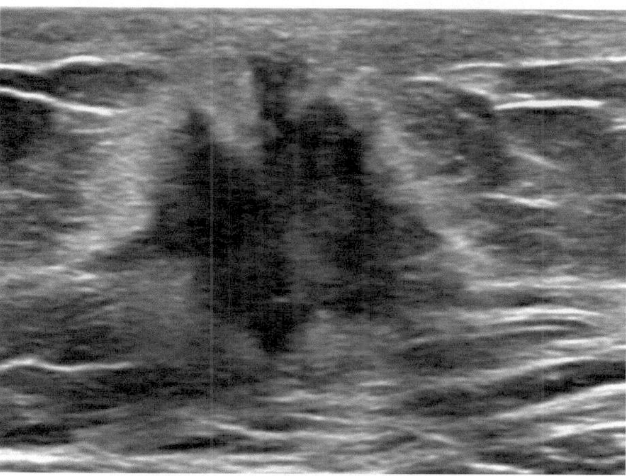

    (a) Circumscribed.
    (b) Indistinct.
    (c) Parallel.
    (d) Spiculated.

11a. A 40-year-old woman presents for diagnostic work-up of new calcifications seen on baseline screening mammogram. Which is the appropriate term to describe this calcification pattern?

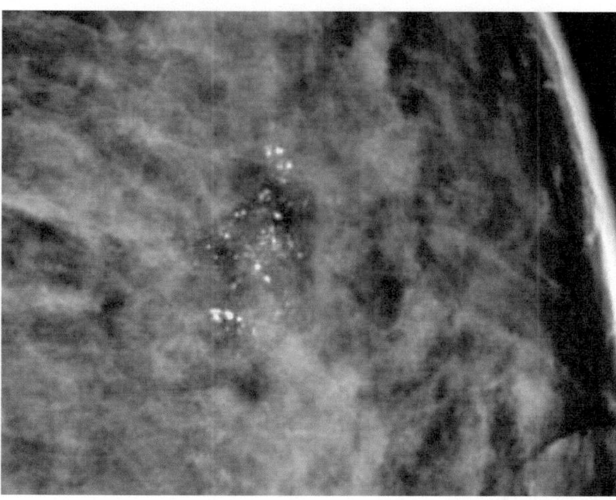

    (a) Fine pleomorphic.
    (b) Milk of calcium.
    (c) Rod like.
    (d) Dystrophic.

11b. What is the appropriate BI-RADS category for these calcifications?
    (a) BI-RADS Category 0.
    (b) BI-RADS Category 2.
    (c) BI-RADS Category 3.
    (d) BI-RADS Category 4.

11c. What is the most appropriate next step?
    (a) Return to annual screening mammogram.
    (b) Follow-up in 6 months.
    (c) Stereotactic biopsy.
    (d) Refer to surgery for excisional biopsy.

12a. A 55-year-old woman presents for her annual screening mammogram. What is the appropriate description for breast tissue density? [1]

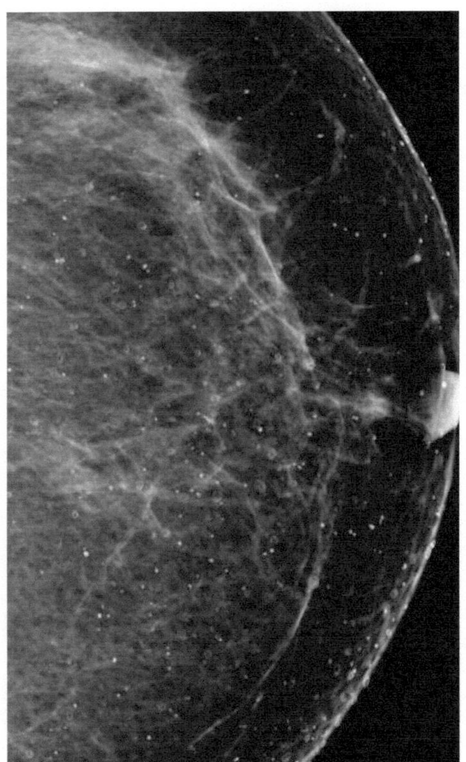

    (a) Almost entirely fatty.
    (b) Scattered areas of fibroglandular density.
    (c) Heterogeneously dense.
    (d) Extremely dense.

12b. What is the most appropriate BI-RADS category for the calcifications seen on
the screening mammogram?
(a) BI-RADS Category 0.
(b) BI-RADS Category 2.
(c) BI-RADS Category 3.
(d) BI-RADS Category 4.

13a. A 50-year-old woman presents for diagnostic evaluation of calcifications
detected on screening mammography. Which are the appropriate terms to
describe the calcification morphology and distribution on the diagnostic mammogram below?

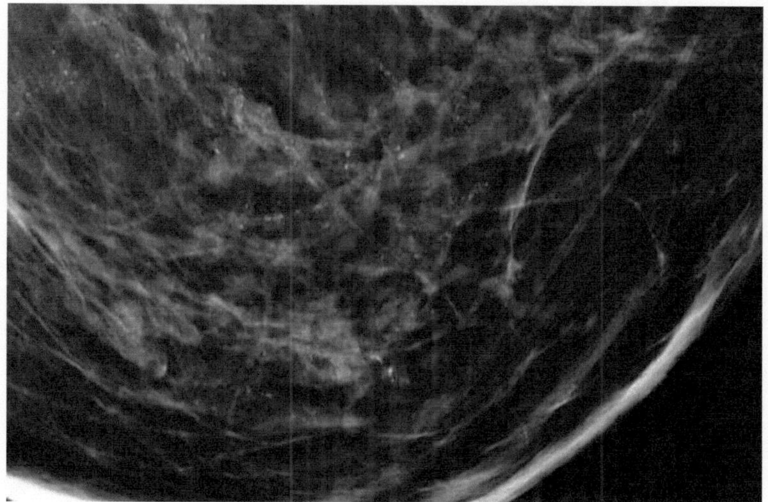

(a) Fine linear branching, segmental.
(b) Popcorn, grouped.
(c) Large rod-like, linear.
(d) Ground glass, diffuse.

13b. What is the appropriate BI-RADS category for the above finding?
(a) BI-RADS Category 2.
(b) BI-RADS Category 3.
(c) BI-RADS Category 4.
(d) BI-RADS Category 6.

14a. A 58-year-old woman presents for diagnostic evaluation of a palpable mass in the right breast.
The calcifications span over 3 cm. The distribution of these calcifications is best described as:

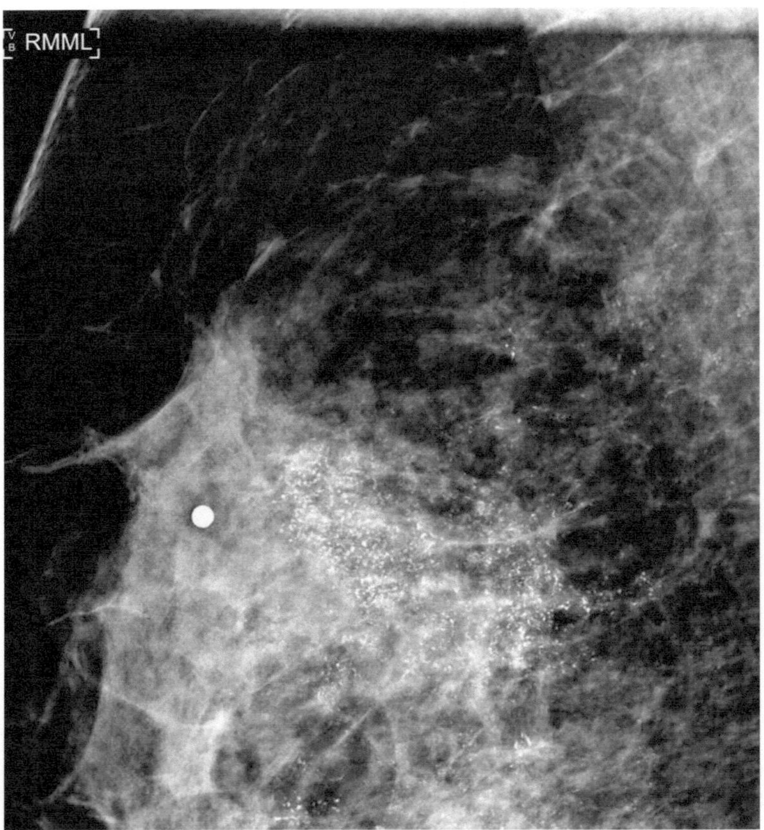

(a) Grouped.
(b) Clumped.
(c) Regional.
(d) Extensive.

14b. Breast ultrasound of the palpable mass was obtained, shown below. Which ultrasound descriptors best characterize this mass?

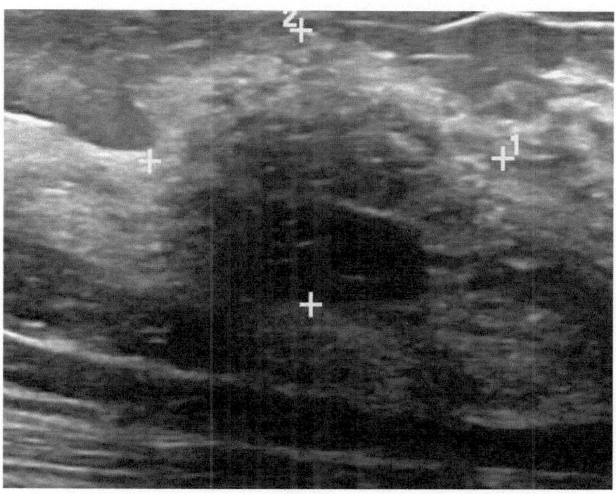

    (a) Circumscribed, posterior enhancement.
    (b) Microlobulated, posterior enhancement.
    (c) Indistinct, posterior shadowing.
    (d) Angular, posterior shadowing.

14c. MRI was obtained for further evaluation, shown below. Which of the following best describes the finding and enhancement characteristics?

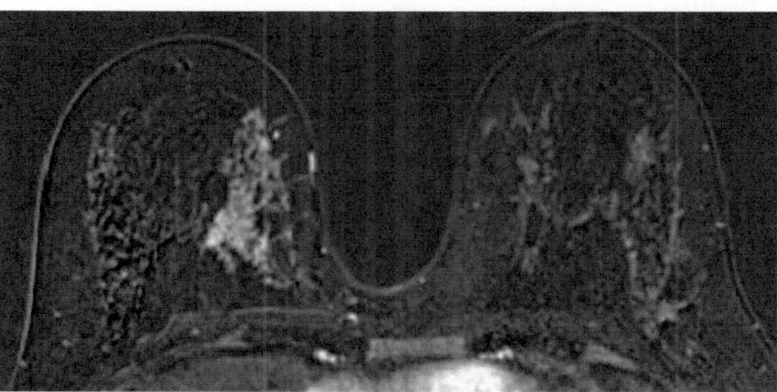

    (a) Irregular mass, homogenous enhancement.
    (b) Spiculated mass, rim enhancement.
    (c) Focal non-mass enhancement.
    (d) Segmental non-mass enhancement.

15a. A 42-year-old woman presents with a palpable mass in the left breast. Ultrasound evaluation of the mass was performed, shown below. Which ultrasound descriptors best characterize this mass?

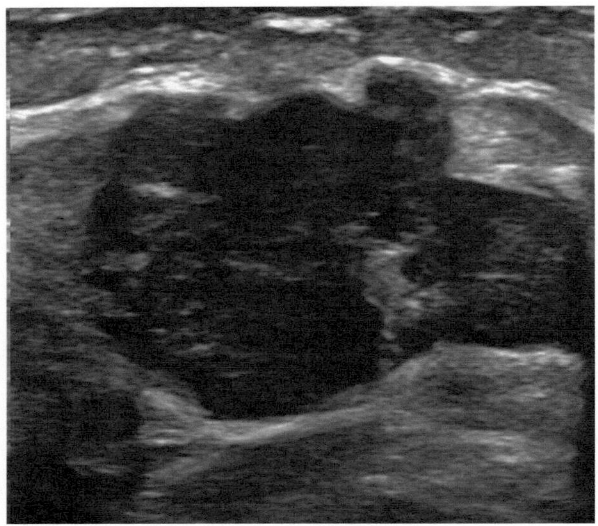

(a) Indistinct, complex cystic and solid, no posterior features.
(b) Spiculated, heterogenous, posterior shadowing.
(c) Circumscribed, anechoic, posterior enhancement.
(d) Microlobulated, hypoechoic, combined posterior enhancement, and shadowing.

15b. MRI was performed for further evaluation, shown below. Axillary ultrasound showed enlarged lymph nodes. What is the appropriate BI-RADS category?

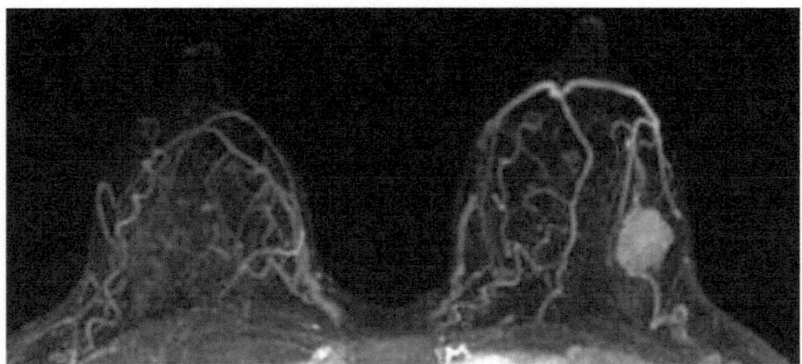

(a) BI-RADS Category 2.
(b) BI-RADS Category 3.
(c) BI-RADS Category 5.
(d) BI-RADS Category 6.

16. A 45-year-old woman presents for diagnostic tomosynthesis for a palpable abnormality, which revealed a breast mass as shown below. Which of the following features increases suspicion for malignancy in this patient?

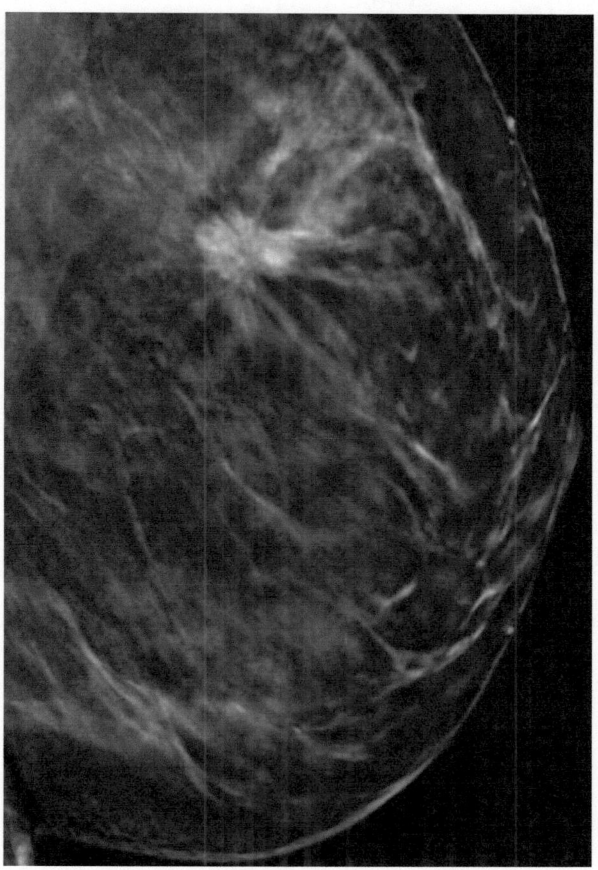

(a) Spiculations.
(b) Nipple retraction.
(c) Calcifications.
(d) Skin thickening.

17a. A 46-year-old woman presents for diagnostic evaluation for findings on her screening mammogram. Ultrasound evaluation was performed. Which ultrasound descriptors best characterize this mass?

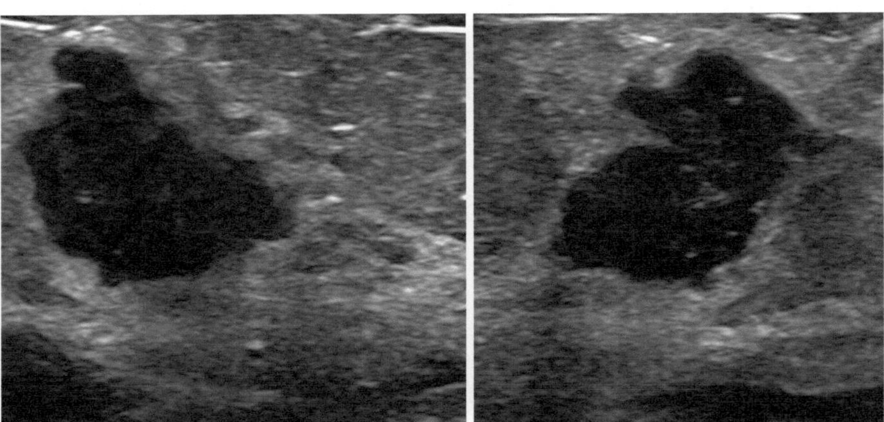

- (a) Parallel, circumscribed.
- (b) Not parallel, angular.
- (c) Parallel, spiculated.
- (d) Not parallel, indistinct.

17b. MRI was obtained for further evaluation, shown below. Which of the following best describes the finding and enhancement characteristics in the right breast?

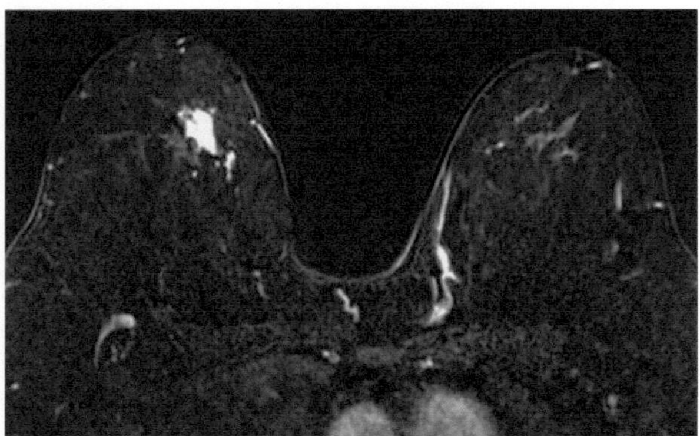

- (a) Round circumscribed mass with rim enhancement.
- (b) Focal non-mass enhancement.
- (c) Irregular mass with homogeneous enhancement.
- (d) Linear non-mass enhancement.

18a. A 27-year-old woman presents for diagnostic evaluation of a palpable abnormality in the right breast. Ultrasound was performed, shown below. Which of the following best characterizes this finding?

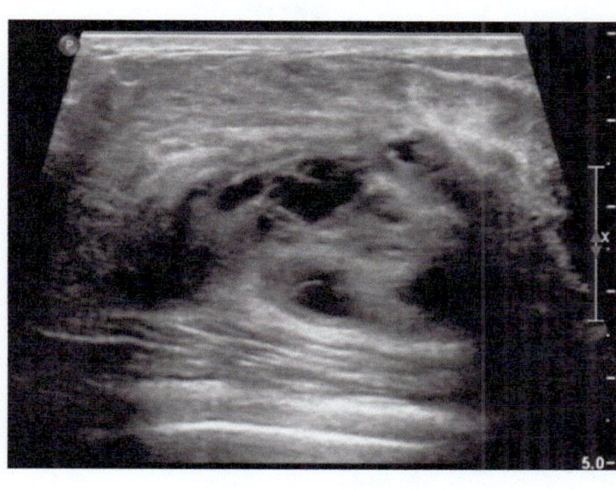 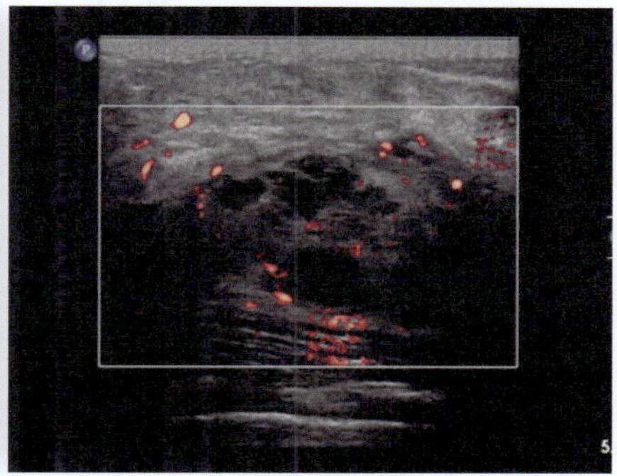

    (a) Clustered microcysts.
    (b) Arteriovenous malformation.
    (c) Microlobulated mass.
    (d) Complex cystic and solid mass.

18b. What is the appropriate BI-RADS category?
    (a) BI-RADS Category 1.
    (b) BI-RADS Category 2.
    (c) BI-RADS Category 3.
    (d) BI-RADS Category 4.

19. A 51-year-old female presents with a palpable abnormality in the superior aspect of the right breast, indicated by the arrow. Mammogram and ultrasound were performed, shown below. What is the appropriate BI-RADS category?

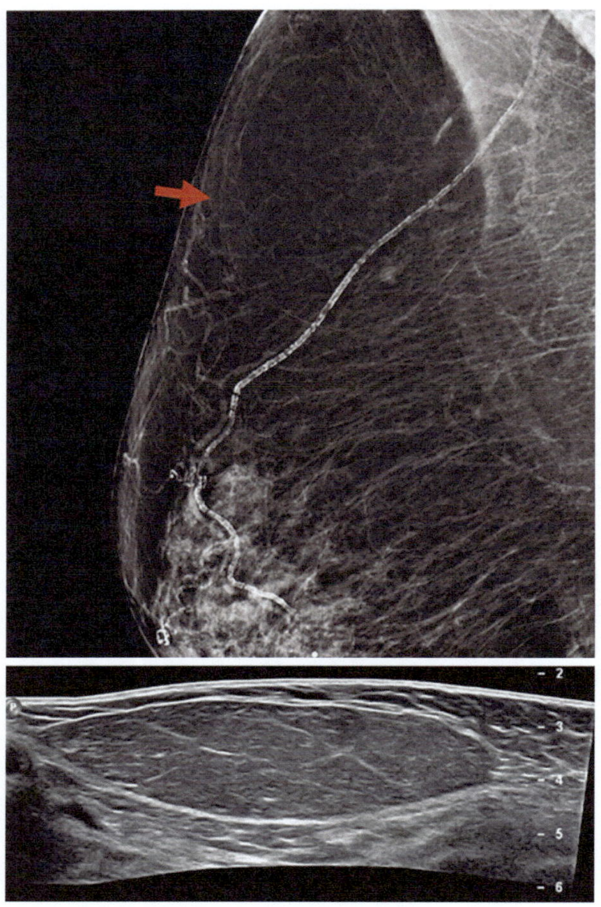

(a) BI-RADS Category 2.
(b) BI-RADS Category 3.
(c) BI-RADS Category 4a.
(d) BI-RADS Category 4c.

20. A 60-year-old woman presents for breast MRI for further evaluation of calcifications seen on mammography. Which of the following best describes the finding and enhancement characteristics in the left breast?

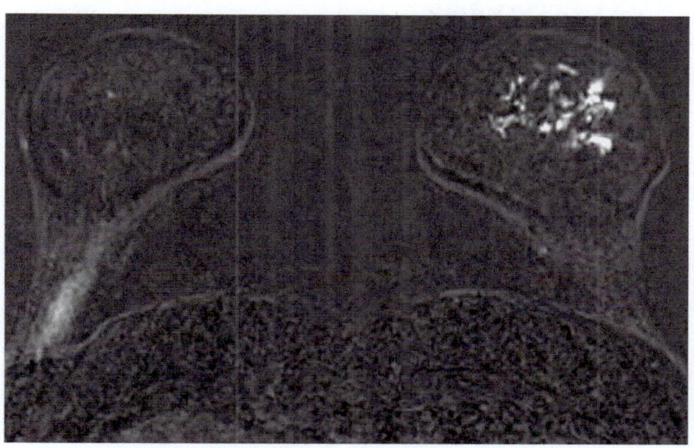

   (a) Irregular mass with dark internal septations.
   (b) Regional clumped non-mass enhancement.
   (c) Round mass with heterogenous enhancement.
   (d) Focal non-mass enhancement.

21. A 36-year-old woman presents with a palpable mass in the breast. Ultrasound evaluation was performed, shown below. What is the appropriate BI-RADS category for this finding?

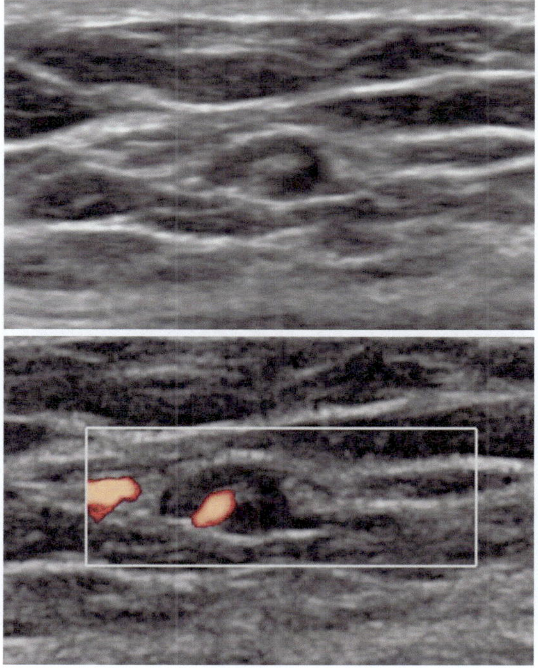

(a) BI-RADS Category 2.
(b) BI-RADS Category 3.
(c) BI-RADS Category 4.
(d) BI-RADS Category 5.

22a. A patient presents for diagnostic evaluation for calcifications seen on a screening mammogram. Diagnostic mammogram (CC and ML views) and ultrasound correlate are shown below. Which of the following best describes the calcifications seen on mammogram?

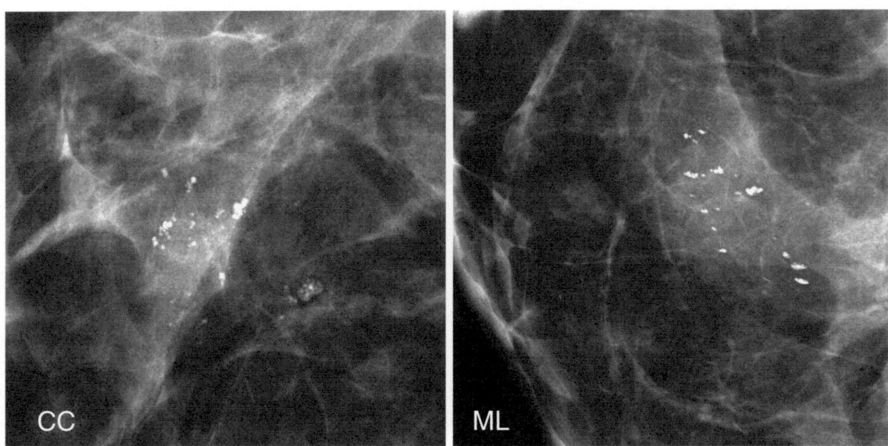

(a) Fine linear branching.
(b) Milk of calcium.
(c) Rod like.
(d) Dystrophic.

22b. Which of the following best describes the findings on ultrasound?

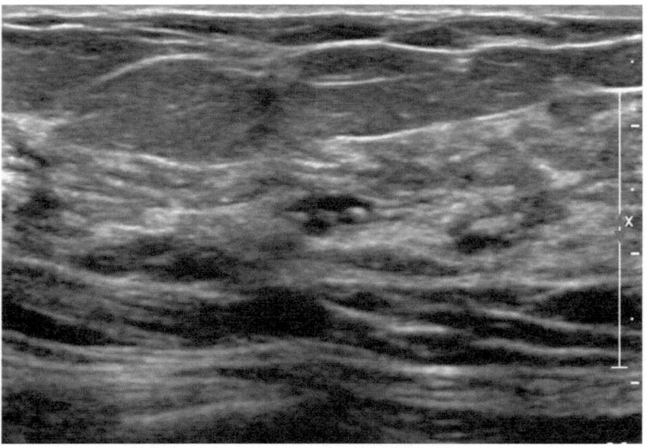

    (a) Clustered microcysts.
    (b) Anechoic simple cyst.
    (c) Indistinct hypoechoic mass.
    (d) Spiculated heterogenous mass.

22c. What is the most appropriate BI-RADS category for this finding?
    (a) BI-RADS Category 0.
    (b) BI-RADS Category 3.
    (c) BI-RADS Category 5.
    (d) BI-RADS Category 6.

23. A patient underwent CT chest following a motor vehicle collision, and a mass
was found in the right breast, shown on coronal projections below. The patient
has a large amount of bruising in the area of the mass seen on ultrasound. A
follow-up ultrasound was obtained, shown below. What is the appropriate
BI-RADS category for this finding?

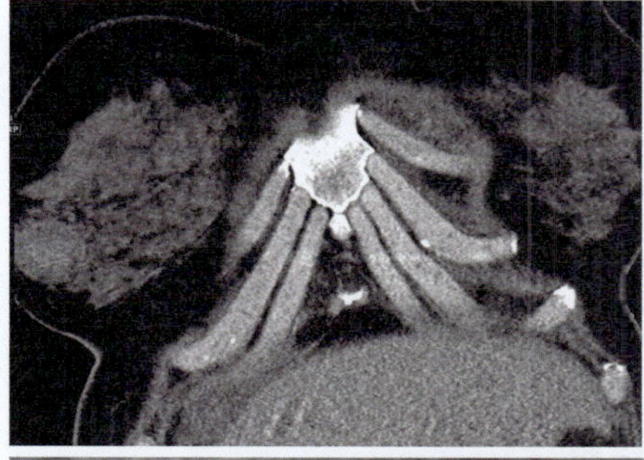

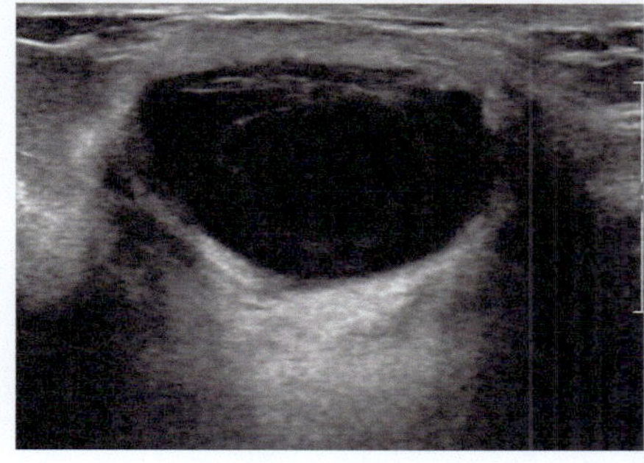
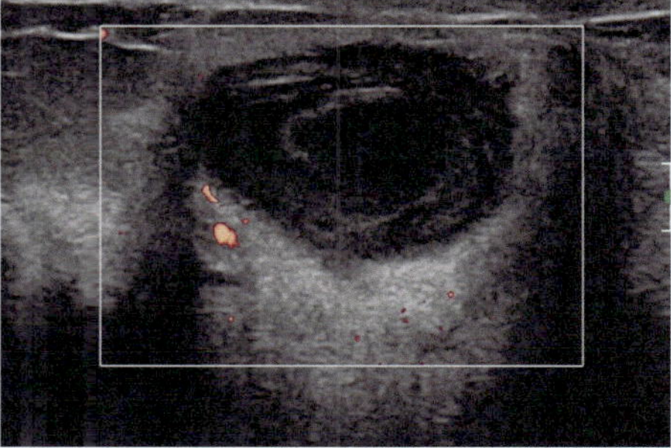

    (a) BI-RADS Category 0.
    (b) BI-RADS Category 2.
    (c) BI-RADS Category 3.
    (d) BI-RADS Category 4.

24. A patient presents for breast MRI for further evaluation of a biopsy-proven malignancy in the left breast, shown below. What is the appropriate BI-RADS category for the MRI of the known malignancy shown?

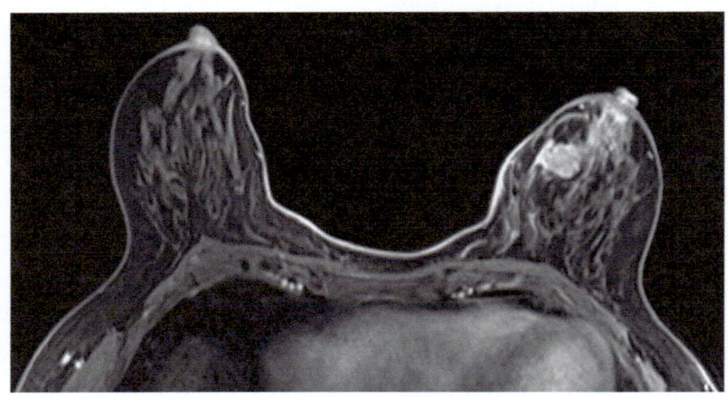

   (a) BI-RADS Category 3.
   (b) BI-RADS Category 4.
   (c) BI-RADS Category 5.
   (d) BI-RADS Category 6.

25a. A 73-year-old woman presents with a palpable abnormality in the left breast, ultrasound is shown below. Which of the following ultrasound features is demonstrated?

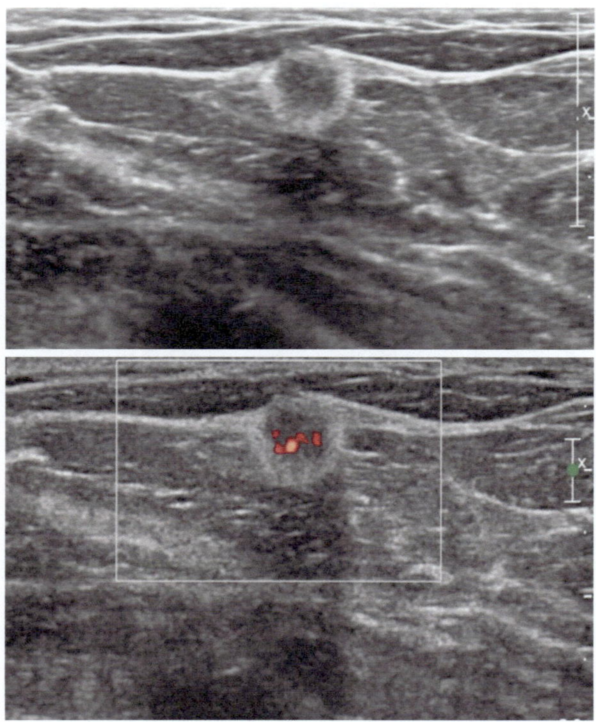

    (a) Oval shape.
    (b) Posterior acoustic enhancement.
    (c) Indistinct margins.
    (d) Spiculated margins.

25b. What is the appropriate BI-RADS category for this finding?
    (a) BI-RADS Category 2.
    (b) BI-RADS Category 3.
    (c) BI-RADS Category 4.
    (d) BI-RADS Category 6.

26. What is one of the advantages of utilizing screening tomosynthesis over screening mammography?
    (a) Screening tomosynthesis can help differentiate cysts from masses.
    (b) Screening tomosynthesis has a higher sensitivity in detecting calcifications.
    (c) Screening tomosynthesis can help differentiate true asymmetries from superimposition of normal breast tissue.
    (d) Screening tomosynthesis can replace the need for further diagnostic work-up of calcifications due to improved visualization.

27a. A 55-year-old woman was recalled for further evaluation of calcifications seen on a screening mammogram (indicated by the arrow on tomosynthesis slice 1/50). Based on the diagnostic mammogram images provided, what is the most appropriate BI-RADS category for the calcifications?

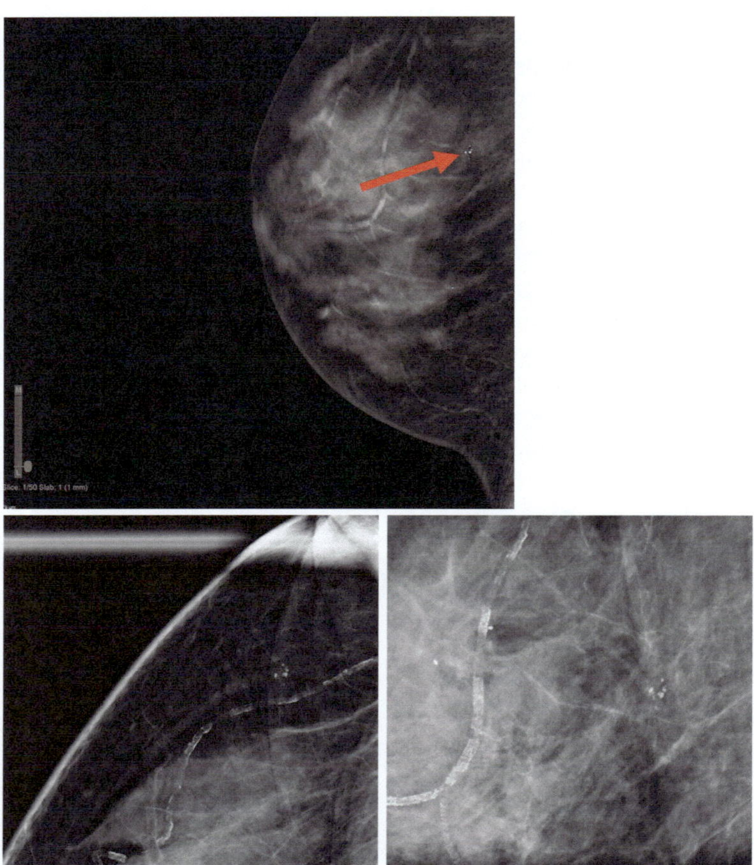

    (a) BI-RADS Category 0.
    (b) BI-RADS Category 2.
    (c) BI-RADS Category 3.
    (d) BI-RADS Category 4.

27b. What is the most appropriate next step?
    (a) Follow-up in 6 months.
    (b) Stereotactic biopsy.
    (c) Refer to surgery for excisional biopsy.
    (d) Return to routine screening mammogram.

28. Which of the following scenarios should **NOT** receive BI-RADS assessment category 3?
    (a) Solitary group of punctate calcifications on mammography.
    (b) Indeterminate finding.
    (c) A finding with greater than 0% but ≤2% likelihood of malignancy.
    (d) Oval circumscribed mass with parallel orientation.
    (e) A complicated cyst.

29. What is the recommended length of follow-up for a finding receiving BI-RADS assessment category 3?
    (a) Until the finding decreases in size.
    (b) 1–2 years of stability.
    (c) 2–3 years of stability or until any time that the radiologist deems it benign.
    (d) 2–4 years of stability or until the finding increases in size.

30. A screening mammogram is negative for malignancy, however, there is a suggestion of implant rupture and MRI is recommended. What is the appropriate BI-RADS assessment category for the screening mammogram?
    (a) BI-RADS Category 0.
    (b) BI-RADS Category 2.
    (c) BI-RADS Category 3.
    (d) BI-RADS Category 4.

31. You are interpreting a breast MRI for a patient with a known malignancy in the right breast, confirmed by recent ultrasound-guided biopsy. In addition to the known malignancy, the breast MRI demonstrates a suspicious mass in the left breast. What is the final overall BI-RADS assessment category?
    (a) BI-RADS Category 0.
    (b) BI-RADS Category 2.
    (c) BI-RADS Category 3.
    (d) BI-RADS Category 4.
    (e) BI-RADS Category 6.

32. A patient with known malignancy undergoes MRI following neoadjuvant chemotherapy. The mass seen on the MRI before chemotherapy has now resolved and the MRI does not demonstrate any suspicious mass or area of abnormal enhancement. What is the most appropriate BI-RADS assessment category?
    (a) BI-RADS Category 0.
    (b) BI-RADS Category 1.
    (c) BI-RADS Category 2.
    (d) BI-RADS Category 3.
    (e) BI-RADS Category 4.
    (f) BI-RADS Category 6.

33. Which of the following terms is used to describe a discrete area of fibroglandular density that is visible on only one mammographic projection?
    (a) Asymmetry.
    (b) Focal asymmetry.
    (c) Mass.
    (d) Architectural distortion.

34. Two years ago, a 43-year-old woman underwent diagnostic work-up of an asymmetry seen on prior screening examination, and the finding was determined to be superimposition of normal fibroglandular tissue. She presents again today for screening mammogram. The asymmetry is seen again, and is now larger and more conspicuous than on prior examination. What is the most appropriate BI-RADS category for today's screening examination?
    (a) BI-RADS Category 0.
    (b) BI-RADS Category 2.
    (c) BI-RADS Category 3.
    (d) BI-RADS Category 4.

35. A woman presents for her screening mammogram in 2017 which was assigned BI-RADS 1, shown below. She presented 3 years later for screening mammogram, shown below. Which of the following best describes the finding?

2017

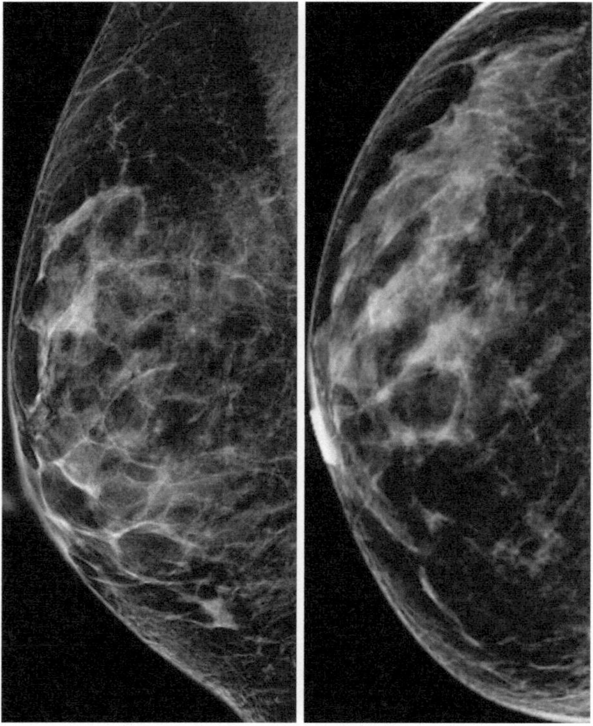

2020

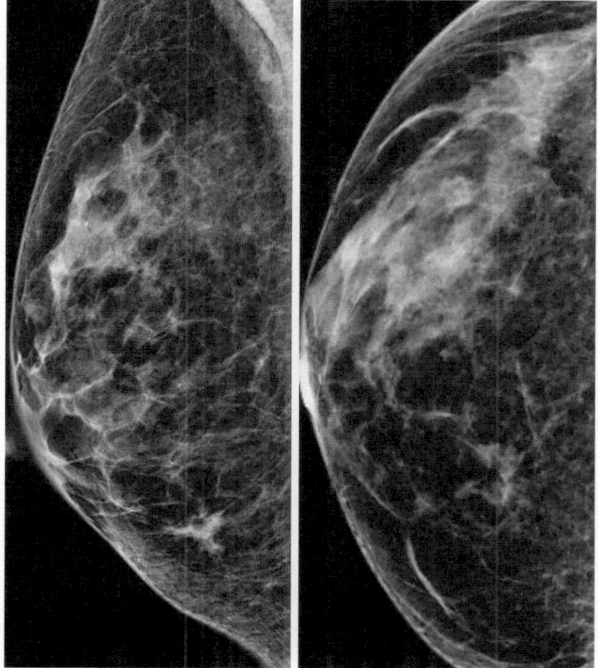

(a) Asymmetry.
(b) Global asymmetry.
(c) Developing asymmetry.
(d) Focal asymmetry.

Answers

1. d. A—popcorn; B—vascular; C—rod-like; D—rim.

   Popcorn calcifications are large, dense, and well-defined produced by involuting fibroadenomas. Vascular calcifications are linear calcifications that form parallel tracks, which are formed within the wall of the blood vessel. Large rod-like calcifications are benign calcifications that are formed within ectatic ducts, and are associated with plasma cell mastitis. They are thick and linear, and may be branching. As opposed to fine linear branching calcifications, they are usually >1 mm in diameter. Rim, or eggshell, calcifications are thin benign calcifications that conform to the shape of an oval or sphere, and contain central lucency. They are usually less than 1 mm in thickness, and are associated with fat necrosis, oil cysts, or simple cysts [2, 3].

2. d. A—suture; B—round; C—coarse heterogeneous; D—dystrophic; E—amorphous.

   Suture calcifications are benign, smooth, linear, or curvilinear (often forming loops), which can be seen after breast surgery and radiation if suture material does not fully resorb, forming a nidus for calcification. Coarse heterogeneous calcifications are irregular, conspicuous microcalcifications that are usually 0.5–1 mm. Coarse heterogeneous calcifications can be benign or malignant. Round calcifications are typically benign calcifications formed in the acini of the terminal ductal lobular units, and include punctate calcifications but can also be >0.5 mm. Dystrophic calcifications are benign calcifications with an irregular, coarse, or "lava-shaped" appearance and typically >1 mm. They can be seen following trauma or radiation. Amorphous calcifications are small, powdery, indistinct or cloud-like calcifications, which do not conform to a distinct shape [2].

3. b. A—diffuse; B—grouped; C—linear; D—segmental; E—regional.

   Grouped distribution is defined as a cluster of at least 5 calcifications within 1 cm from each other, in an area at most 2 cm in greatest linear dimension. Segmental distribution is defined as corresponding to ducts and branches of a segment or lobe. Regional distribution is greater than 2 cm, can occupy greater than one quadrant, and do not correspond with the expected distribution of a ductal unit. Diffuse distribution is defined as scattered randomly throughout the breast. Linear distribution is suggestive of deposition along ducts, and similar to segmental distribution, however, less extensive [2].

4. b. Architectural distortion.

An asymmetry is a discrete area of fibroglandular density that is visible on only one mammographic projection. Architectural distortion is an area of parenchymal distortion (spiculations radiating from a point, focal retraction, or straightening at the edge of the parenchyma), which is not associated with a mass. Architectural distortions are suspicious findings in the absence of trauma or prior surgery. Focal density and geographic abnormality are not terms included in the BI-RADS atlas [2].

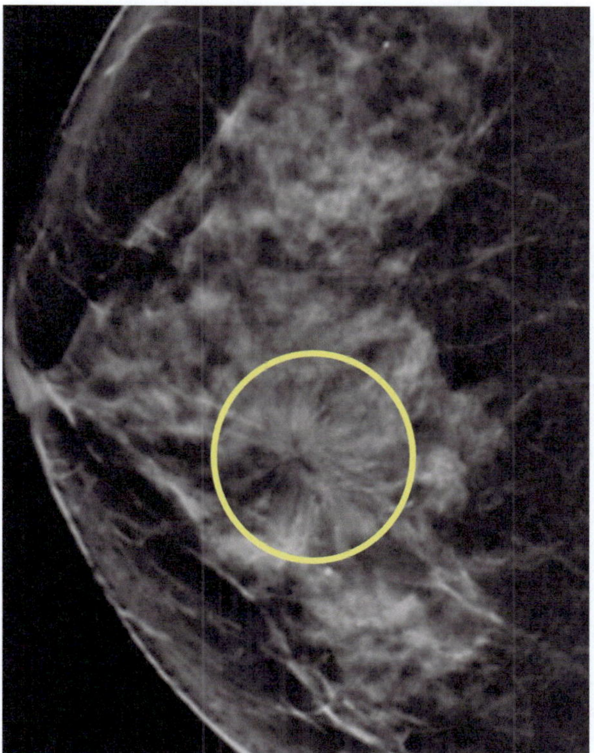

5. c. >10% to ≤50%.

A BI-RADS Category 4B corresponds with a moderate level of suspicion for malignancy and has a >10% to ≤50% likelihood of malignancy. BI-RADS Category 4A corresponds with a low level of suspicion for malignancy and has a >2% to ≤10% likelihood of malignancy. BI-RADS Category 4C corresponds with a high level of suspicion for malignancy and has a >50% to <95% likelihood of malignancy [2].

6. a. A—irregular; B—oval; C—round.

The shape of mass A is irregular, which is a suspicious finding. The shape of mass B is oval. The shape of mass C is round. Ovoid is not a term used in the BI-RADS atlas [2, 4].

7. b. A—circumscribed; B—indistinct; C—microlobulated; D—obscured.

The margins of mass A are circumscribed, defined as more than 75% of the circumference being well defined. The margins of mass B are indistinct, defined as none of the circumference being well defined, which is usually a suspicious finding. The margins of mass C are microlobulated, defined as small undulations along the borders, which is usually a suspicious finding. The margins of mass D are obscured, defined as more than 25% of the circumference hidden by adjacent fibroglandular tissue [2].

8. b. Hyperechoic.

The mass shown is uniformly brighter than the subcutaneous fat, therefore it is hyperechoic [2, 4].

9. a. Circumscribed.

The finding has circumscribed margins, rather than indistinct or spiculated margins. Parallel is a term used to describe orientation, not margins. The finding is anechoic and circumscribed, consistent with a benign simple cyst [2, 4].

10. d. Spiculated.

The mass has a stellate appearance, consistent with a spiculated mass [2, 4].

11a. a. Fine pleomorphic.

Fine pleomorphic calcifications vary in shape and size, and are more conspicuous than amorphous calcifications, with the appearance of "shards of glass" or "crushed stone." Pleomorphic calcifications are suspicious for malignancy, but can also be seen with high risk lesions such as atypical ductal hyperplasia or benign etiologies such as fibrocystic change [2].

11b. d. BI-RADS Category 4.

BI-RADS 4 is the category for findings that are "suspicious for malignancy" (2–94% probability of malignancy). The calcifications are fine-pleomorphic and grouped, and therefore suspicious for malignancy. Biopsy is indicated for the findings [2].

11c. c. Stereotactic Biopsy.

Return to annual screening mammogram and follow-up in 6 months would not be appropriate in this case because the calcifications are suspicious for malignancy. Stereotactic biopsy would be the appropriate next step for further work-up. Excisional biopsy is not indicated for initial tissue sampling, as the calcifications are well visualized on mammogram and can be targeted with stereotactic biopsy [2].

12a. b. Scattered areas of fibroglandular density.

The mammogram demonstrates scattered areas of fibroglandular density. See below for examples of almost entirely fatty, heterogeneously dense, and extremely dense. Heterogeneously dense breasts may obscure small masses, and extremely dense breasts lower the sensitivity of mammography [3].

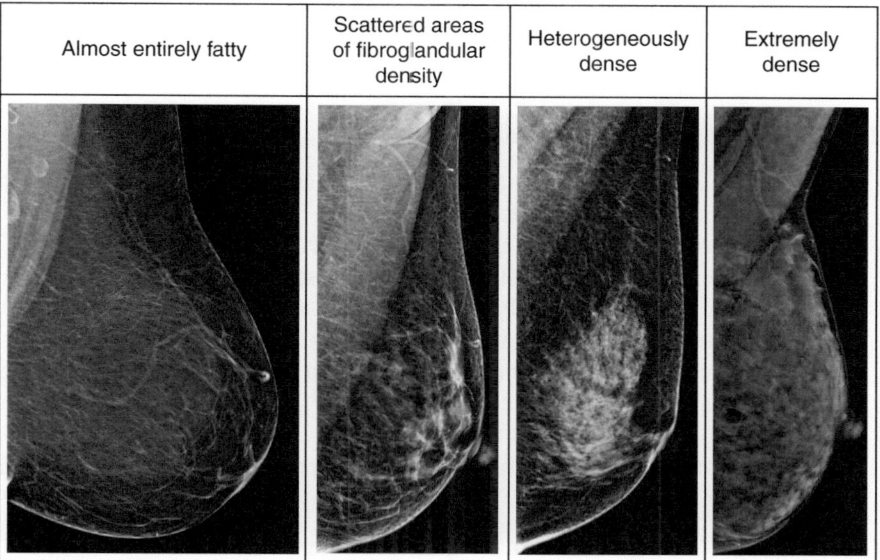

12b. b. BI-RADS Category 2.

The calcifications are diffuse, and are seen along the skin surface, consistent with benign dermal calcifications. Additional diagnostic imaging is not needed in this case, and so BI-RADS 2 is the appropriate category [2].

13a. a. Fine linear branching, segmental.

Fine linear branching calcifications are thin (<0.5 mm), linear or curvilinear irregular calcifications associated with filling, or "casting" of a duct. Fine linear branching calcifications are suggestive of malignancy. Segmental distribution is defined as corresponding to ducts and branches of a segment or lobe. The calcifications are fine linear branching and segmental, and are suspicious for malignancy [2]. Ground glass is not a BI-RADS term.

13b. c. BI-RADS Category 4.

The calcifications are fine linear branching in a segmental distribution. Both the morphology and the distribution are suspicious for malignancy. Biopsy is indicated (BI-RADS 4) [2].

14a. c. Regional.

These fine pleomorphic calcifications are best described as regional from the following choices. Regional distribution describes a large area of calcifications greater than 2 cm. Extensive is not part of the BI-RADS lexicon for calcification distribution. Clumped is an internal enhancement pattern used to describe non-mass enhancement in breast MRI [2].

14b. c. Indistinct, posterior shadowing.

The margins of the mass are indistinct, and not clearly demarcated from the surrounding tissue. In addition, the mass is heterogeneous in echogenicity, with punctate calcifications, and posterior acoustic shadowing, all of which are suspicious features [2, 4].

14c. d. Segmental non-mass enhancement.

The MRI demonstrates non-mass enhancement and does not meet criteria for a mass, as there are ill-defined and non-convex borders. Non-mass enhancement is also defined as having areas of intervening fat. The distribution of non-mass enhancement is best characterized as segmental, as it has a triangular or conical appearance with the apex directed toward the nipple, suggestive of ductal involvement. Focal distribution of non-mass enhancement is characterized to an area < 25% of a breast quadrant, and the image is more consistent with segmental distribution [2].

15a. d. Microlobulated, hypoechoic, combined posterior enhancement, and shadowing.

Although the shape of this mass is irregular, the margins of the mass would be considered microlobulated rather than spiculated. The mass is predominately hypoechoic, and there is combined posterior shadowing and enhancement. These features increase suspicion for malignancy. A circumscribed, anechoic mass with posterior enhancement would be consistent with a simple cyst. The margins of the mass can be outlined, and are therefore not indistinct [2, 4].

15b. c. BI-RADS Category 5.

MRI demonstrates an enhancing irregular mass in the left breast, which makes this mass highly suspicious for malignancy [2].

16. a. Spiculations.

The mass demonstrates spiculated margins, or lines radiating from the mass. Spiculations implies a suspicious finding. Although nipple retraction can be associated with malignancy, there is no definite nipple retraction seen here. There are no definite calcifications seen here. The skin in this patient is normal in appearance [2].

17a. b. Not parallel, angular.

The mass is taller than wide, and is not parallel. The mass has sharp angular margins. These findings are suspicious for malignancy. Parallel masses are wider than tall. Spiculated margins are characterized as having sharp lines that radiate from the mass. Indistinct margins are characterized by having a poorly defined margin which is not clearly demarcated from the surrounding tissue [2, 4].

17b. c. Irregular mass with homogeneous enhancement.

The mass in the right breast has irregular margins, and uniform homogeneous internal enhancement. The mass in the right breast is not round and circumscribed. The finding in the right breast would not be considered non-mass enhancement, as it is a space occupying lesion with convex borders [2].

18a. d. Complex cystic and solid mass.

The mass has both solid and cystic components, as well as internal vascularity. The margins of this mass are relatively smooth and circumscribed, rather than microlobulated. Clustered microcysts are more cystic than solid, with thin avascular septations. An arteriovenous malformation may have the appearance of a cystic and solid mass on grayscale ultrasound imaging, however, the cystic appearing components would have vascular flow, which is not seen here [2–4].

18b. d. BI-RADS Category 4.

Complex cystic and solid masses are suspicious for malignancy [2].

19. a. BI-RADS Category 2.

BI-RADS 2 is the category for benign findings. The finding is a circumscribed, isoechoic mass on ultrasound, which corresponds to a fat containing circumscribed mass on mammogram. The finding is most consistent with a lipoma, which is a benign finding [2].

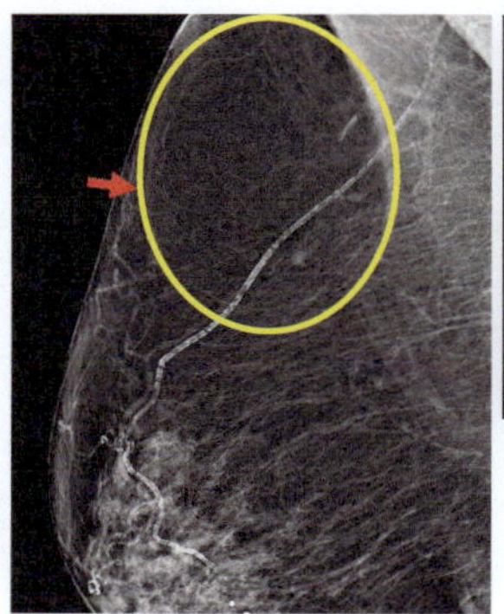
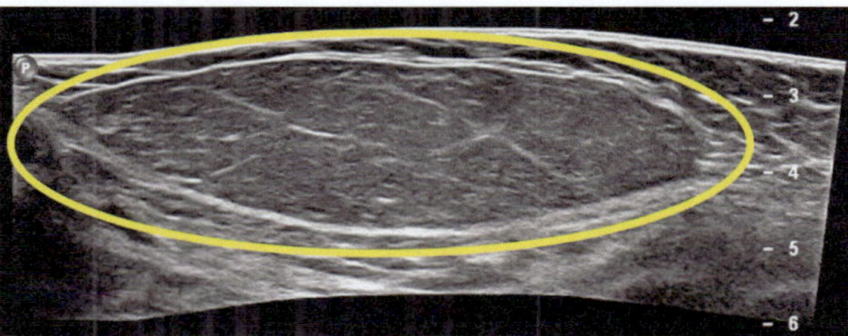

20. b. Regional clumped non-mass enhancement.

The finding does not meet criteria for a mass; it is not a space occupying lesion, there are no clear margins, and there are areas of intervening fat. Therefore, it is consistent with non-mass enhancement. Dark internal septations are typically benign and can be seen with fibroadenomas, but the appearance here is more consistent with areas of intervening fat. This finding is most consistent with non-mass enhancement, with a regional distribution. Regional distribution does not conform to a ductal or segmental pattern, but is larger than a focal distribution which is defined as <25% of a quadrant. Clumped non-mass enhancement describes enhancement of varying shapes with some confluent areas, as seen here. Clumped non-mass enhancement is a suspicious finding [2].

21. a. BI-RADS Category 2.

BI-RADS 2 is the category for benign findings. The ultrasound demonstrates a normal appearing lymph node, with a normal reniform appearance, normal echogenic fatty hilum with normal hilar vascular flow, and normal cortical thickness < 3 mm. Therefore, this is a benign finding [2].

22a. b. Milk of calcium.

Milk of calcium calcifications are benign calcification deposits within cysts. They often appear round, amorphous, or "smudged" on CC views, and crescent or "tea-cup" shaped on ML views, as they conform to the shape of cysts with positional changes. The calcifications are crescent shaped on ML view, and are associated with clustered microcysts, therefore consistent with milk of calcium [2].

22b. a. Clustered microcysts.

Clustered microcysts are clustered anechoic cystic masses, individually <2–3 mm, with thin intervening septations and no discrete solid component. The mass in the image is an example of clustered microcysts, and is also noted to contain punctate echogenic foci which represent calcifications, also seen on mammography [2].

22c. b. BI-RADS Category 3.

Clustered microcysts are typically associated with benign findings including fibrocystic change and apocrine metaplasia. They are often assessed as benign (Category 2), or probably benign (Category 3) if new or if there is diagnostic uncertainty [2]. If new, especially in a postmenopausal woman, the margins and associated calcifications should be carefully assessed [5].

23. b. BI-RADS Category 2.

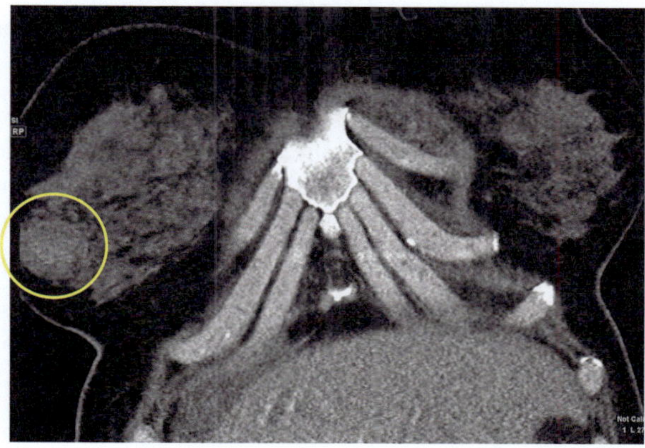

On CT, a mildly hyperattenuating mass is seen. This corresponds to a circum-scribed mass with lace-like internal echogenicity on the ultrasound. The cyst is avascular, and internal echoes are in a pattern characteristic of a hematoma. Given the history of trauma and bruising, this mass represents a hematoma. Further imaging is not required for diagnostic evaluation. Hematomas are benign and usually self-resolving, and so BI-RADS 2 is the appropriate category [2].

24. d. BI-RADS Category 6.

BI-RADS 6 is the category for biopsy-proven malignancy, described in the question stem [2].

25a. c. Indistinct margins.

The mass is round. This mass demonstrates posterior acoustic shadowing, rather than enhancement. Posterior acoustic enhancement can be seen classi-cally with simple cysts. The margins of the mass are indistinct, and demon-strates an echogenic rim or echogenic halo (a white band surrounding the mass). These findings raise suspicion for malignancy. Although these margins are indistinct, there are not clear spiculations arising from the mass [2, 4].

25b. c. BI-RADS Category 4.

BI-RADS 4 is the category for findings that are "suspicious for malignancy." This mass has suspicious features including, round shape, not parallel orienta-tion, indistinct margins with an echogenic rim, posterior shadowing, and internal vascularity. Therefore, it is categorized as a BI-RADS 4 lesion [2].

26. c. An asymmetry may represent a true abnormality obscured by isodense fibroglandular tissue, or it may represent superimposition of normal breast tissue. Tomosynthesis slices can help to differentiate overlapping normal breast tissue [6].

a. Although breast tomosynthesis can help delineate mass margins due to removal of superimposed breast tissue, tomosynthesis cannot definitively distinguish masses from cysts. Even masses with circumscribed margins should not be assumed to be benign (unless multiple and bilateral), and still require further evaluation with ultrasound [6].

b. Early studies evaluating the performance of breast tomosynthesis have demonstrated no statistically significant difference in detection of calcifications [6].

d. Calcifications may appear enhanced on tomosynthesis synthetic images, which are designed to preserve high-attenuating voxels. Synthesized images may also contain artifacts which may be mistaken for calcifications. Conversely, calcifications may appear less defined due to the arc pathway of the X-ray tube causing slight blurring of microcalcifications [6].

27a. b. BI-RADS Category 2.

These calcifications appear slightly heterogeneous on the CC and ML magnification views however they are visualized on the first tomosynthesis slice as demonstrated on the tomosynthesis scroll bar therefore they are dermal calcifications. Dermal calcifications are benign and no further evaluation if required. Additional diagnostic imaging is not needed in this case, and so BI-RADS 2 is the appropriate category [2].

27b. d. Return to routine screening mammogram.

Dermal calcifications are benign, so return to screening mammogram is the appropriate course. Follow-up in 6 months and biopsy are not indicated for benign calcifications [2].

28. b. Indeterminate finding.

The BI-RADS atlas specifically states that BI-RADS Category 3 should not be used for indeterminate findings, such as findings where the radiologist cannot decide between BI-RADS Category 2 and BI-RADS Category 4. BI-RADS Category 3 is reserved for specific situations where the likelihood of malignancy is 0–2%, such as a solitary group of punctate calcifications on mammography or an oval circumscribed mass with parallel orientation seen on ultrasound. BI-RADS Category 2 or 3 is appropriate for a complicated cyst seen ultrasound [2].

29. c. 2–3 years of stability or until any time that the radiologist deems it benign.

The BI-RADS atlas recommends 2–3 years of imaging follow-up for a probably benign finding that has received BI-RADS Category 3. The follow-up interval is usually every 6 months for the first year, and then can continue every 6 months or be extended to annual follow-up. If, at any time, the interpreting radiologist determines the finding has 0% likelihood of malignancy, the assessment can be changed to BI-RADS Category 2 [2].

30. b. BI-RADS Category 2.

The BI-RADS assessment category is intended to describe the likelihood of malignancy. If there is concern for implant rupture but there is no mammographic evidence of malignancy, the correct assessment is BI-RADS Category 2, because implant rupture is a benign finding. The interpreting radiologist can then add a sentence recommending MRI to further evaluate the implant [2].

31. d. BI-RADS Category 4.

The final BI-RADS assessment category should be determined based on the most actionable item according to the following hierarchy, from lowest to highest: 1, 2, 3, 6, 0, 4, 5. The newly seen suspicious mass in the left breast (BI-RADS Category 4) is the most actionable finding and requires biopsy, and therefore the final overall BI-RADS assessment Category is 4. The known malignancy in the right breast (BI-RADS assessment Category 6) has already been confirmed and is known by the referring physician [2].

32. f. BI-RADS Category 6.

Even though there is no imaging abnormality on the MRI, the final assessment category should be BI-RADS 6. This situation is an exception to the central BI-RADS principle which states that the final assessment category should be assigned based on the imaging findings. Current practice dictates that even patients with a complete imaging response to therapy proceed with surgery. Therefore, it could cause confusion to the treatment team to provide a final assessment of negative or benign [2].

33. a. Asymmetry.

An asymmetry is a discrete area of fibroglandular density that is visible on only one mammographic projection [2].

34. a. BI-RADS Category 0.

BI-RADS Category 0 is the category for imaging that is incomplete or requires additional diagnostic imaging. Although an asymmetry most often reflect summation of normal fibroglandular tissue, when an asymmetry appears larger or more conspicuous than on previous examinations, the likelihood of malignancy is significantly increased. Such finding have been termed "developing asymmetry." Developing asymmetry on screening examination should be worked up further with diagnostic imaging, and so BI-RADS Category 0 is the most appropriate choice [2].

35. c. Developing asymmetry.

An asymmetry is a term to describe a discrete unilateral fibroglandular density which is seen in one or more projections, and that does not meet criteria for a mass. Asymmetries are further subdivided into the following categories: asymmetry, focal asymmetry, global asymmetry, and developing asymmetry. An asymmetry is seen in only one mammographic projection. A focal asymmetry is seen in two mammographic projections. A global asymmetry is visible in two mammographic projections and involves more than one quadrant. A developing asymmetry is a focal asymmetry that is enlarging or more conspicuous than on prior examinations. The case is an example of a developing asymmetry in the lower inner quadrant of the right breast [2, 3].

References

1. Eghtedari M, Chong A, Rakow-Penner R, Ojeda-Fournier H. Current status and future of BI-RADS in multimodality imaging, from the *AJR* special series on radiology reporting and data systems. AJR Am J Roentgenol. 2021 Apr;216(4):860–73. https://doi.org/10.2214/AJR.20.24894.
2. D'Orsi CJ, Sickles EA, Mendelson EB, Morris EA, et al. ACR BI-RADS® Atlas, Breast Imaging Reporting and Data System. 5th rev. ed. Reston, VA: American College of Radiology; 2013.
3. Rao AA, Feneis J, Lalonde C, Ojeda-Fournier H. A pictorial review of changes in the BI-RADS fifth edition. Radiographics. 2016;36(3):623–39. https://doi.org/10.1148/rg.2016150178.
4. Lee J. Practical and illustrated summary of updated BI-RADS for ultrasonography. Ultrasonography. 2017;36(1):71–81. https://doi.org/10.14366/usg.16034.
5. Goldbach AR, Tuite CM, Ross E. Clustered microcysts at breast US: outcomes and updates for appropriate management recommendations. Radiology. 2020;295(1):44–51. https://pubs.rsna.org/doi/full/10.1148/radiol.2020191505.
6. Lee CH, Destounis SV, Friedewald SM, Newell MS. Digital breast tomosynthesis (DBT) guidance (a supplement to ACR BI-RADS® mammography). Reston, VA: American College of Radiology; 2013.

Screening Mammogram

3

Nazanin Yaghmai, Tiffany Yu, Regan Ferraro,
and Guita Rahbar

N. Yaghmai (✉) · T. Yu
Department of Radiology, David Geffen School of Medicine at UCLA,
Los Angeles, CA, USA
e-mail: nyaghmai@mednet.ucla.edu; ttyu@mednet.ucla.edu

R. Ferraro
Rolling Oaks Radiology, Thousand Oaks, CA, USA

G. Rahbar
Department of Radiology, David Geffen School of Medicine at UCLA,
Los Angeles, CA, USA

Department of Radiology, Olive View-UCLA Medical Center, Sylmar, CA, USA
e-mail: grahbar@mednet.ucla.edu

© The Author(s), under exclusive license to Springer Nature
Switzerland AG 2022
L. Chow, B. Li (eds.), *Absolute Breast Imaging Review*,
https://doi.org/10.1007/978-3-031-08274-0_3

1. The American College of Radiology (ACR) recommends annual breast cancer screening for an average-risk woman beginning at what age?
   (a) 30.
   (b) 40.
   (c) 50.
   (d) 60.

2. What is the lifetime risk of developing breast cancer for an average-risk woman?
   (a) <5%.
   (b) <15%.
   (c) <25%.
   (d) <35%.

3. Screening mammography is appropriate for which of the following individuals?
   (a) A 50-year-old asymptomatic female with a history of one first-degree relative with breast cancer diagnosed in her 50s.
   (b) A 40-year-old asymptomatic female with a "probably benign" finding identified at a diagnostic exam 6 months prior.
   (c) A 60-year-old male with bilateral palpable retroareolar masses.
   (d) A 35-year-old breastfeeding female with strong family history of breast cancer and left-sided breast pain, swelling, and redness.
   (e) A 55-year-old asymptomatic female with smoking history and incidentally noted right breast mass on low-dose lung cancer screening chest CT.

4. Which of the following factors places a woman in the high-risk category for breast cancer screening?
   (a) History of fibroadenoma.
   (b) First-degree relative with history of breast cancer diagnosed in her 70s.
   (c) History of cigarette smoking.
   (d) A 31-year-old untested daughter whose mother has a BRCA gene mutation.

5. A 38-year-old female is diagnosed with biopsy-proven lobular carcinoma in situ. At what age should she begin breast cancer mammography screening?
   (a) 38 years of age.
   (b) 40 years of age.
   (c) 45 years of age.
   (d) 50 years of age.

6a. A 25-year-old female with a confirmed BRCA1 mutation and no personal history of breast cancer presents to her primary care doctor with questions regarding breast cancer screening. This patient meets criteria for which of the following breast cancer screening risk categories?
   (a) Low-risk.
   (b) Average-risk.
   (c) Intermediate-risk.
   (d) High-risk.

6b. Based on her risk category, at what age should she start breast cancer screening with mammography?
   (a) At the time of BRCA1 mutation detection.
   (b) At age 30 years.
   (c) At age 40 years.
   (d) At age 50 years.

6c. What breast screening modality(ies) is (are) indicated for this patient?
   (a) Mammography only.
   (b) Mammography with molecular breast imaging.
   (c) Mammography with breast MRI or ultrasound.
   (d) Mammography with dedicated FDG-PET breast.

7. A 40-year-old female with an average risk for breast cancer and extremely dense breasts presents for baseline screening. In addition to mammography, she inquires about a whole breast screening ultrasound. Which of the following is an indication for screening ultrasound?
   (a) Palpable mass in woman aged under 30 years.
   (b) High-risk and unable to tolerate MRI.
   (c) Breast cancer screening during pregnancy.
   (d) Fatty breasts.

8. Which of the following statements is true regarding breast cancer screening and dense breast tissue?
   (a) Dense breast tissue lowers the sensitivity of mammography and increases breast cancer risk compared to patients with fatty breast tissue.
   (b) Dense breast notification laws suggest women with dense breast tissue are informed of risks related to dense breast tissue.
   (c) Screening breast ultrasound performed with mammography decreases the false-positive rate of breast cancer.
   (d) Screening breast MRI is indicated.

9. A 33-year-old female with no known increased risk factors for breast cancer presents with a palpable mass which is ultimately diagnosed as invasive ductal carcinoma. She undergoes lumpectomy followed by radiation therapy. Which of the following statements is true?
   (a) Based on her individual risk factors, she should be screened with annual mammography and FDG-PET.
   (b) Based on her age, she should start screening with breast MRI and transition to mammography at age 40 years.
   (c) Based on her history, she should start breast cancer screening 6–12 months post-radiation.
   (d) Screening is not recommended since she is aged under 40 years.

10. In which of the following scenarios is screening mammography indicated during pregnancy?
    (a) A 35-year-old pregnant female with high-risk of breast cancer.
    (b) A 40-year-old pregnant female with bloody nipple discharge.
    (c) A 32-year-old pregnant female with palpable breast mass.
    (d) A 28-year-old lactating female with average-risk for breast cancer.

11. What is the earliest age at which it is recommended that patients with a BRCA gene mutation begin annual breast cancer screening with contrast-enhanced breast MRI?
    (a) 20 years old.
    (b) 25 years old.
    (c) 30 years old.
    (d) 35 years old.

12. Which of the following is NOT considered a risk factor for breast cancer?
    (a) Age.
    (b) Early menstrual periods before the age of 12 years.
    (c) Fatty breasts.
    (d) First pregnancy after the age of 30 years.

13. The imaging finding indicated by the circle:

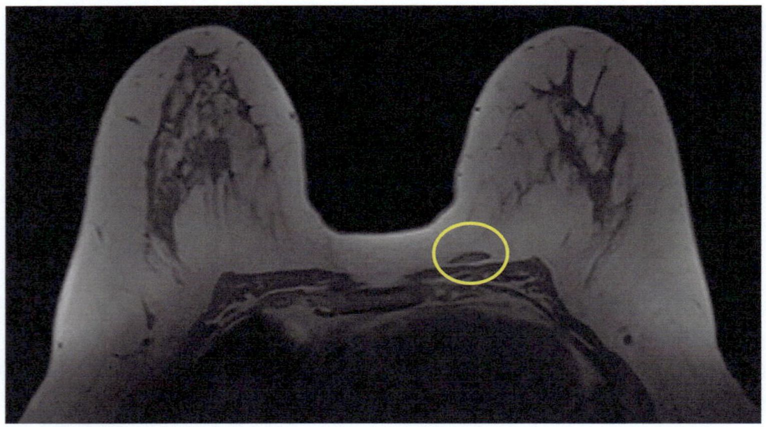

    (a) Could be suspicious in a patient with cancer.
    (b) Represents a normal anatomical variant.
    (c) Is most often bilateral.
    (d) Is easily seen on MLO views.

14. Which of the following is true regarding an increase in breast density detected on screening mammogram

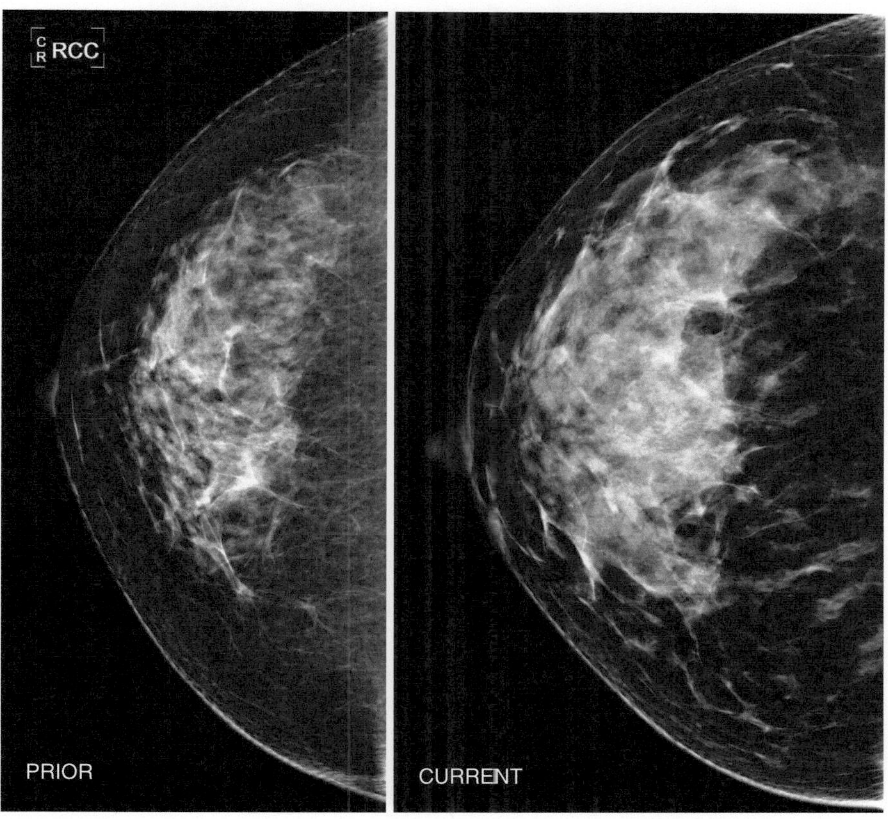

(a) Tamoxifen causes an increase in breast density.
(b) This finding could be explained by a typical age-related change in breast density.
(c) This finding is typical after a period of weight gain.
(d) If unilateral, additional diagnostic workup is indicated.

15. Which of the following is true regarding accessory breast tissue:

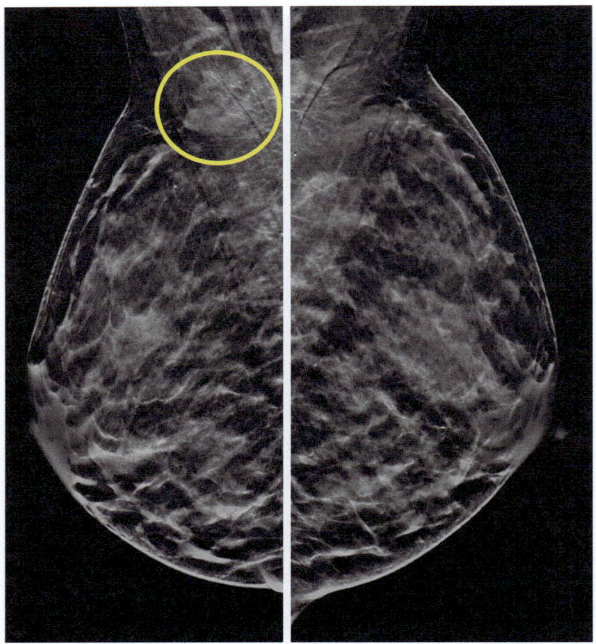

(a) It results from abnormal migration during embryologic development.
(b) It most commonly occurs in the axilla, but may be present anywhere along the "milk line".
(c) Incidence is approximately 70%.
(d) It is not responsive to hormonal stimulation as typical breast tissue and any symptom associated with accessory breast tissue should be considered suspicious.

16. An 18-year-old patient presents with a hard, palpable breast lump. Targeted ultrasound was performed directly over her area of concern. What is the next step?

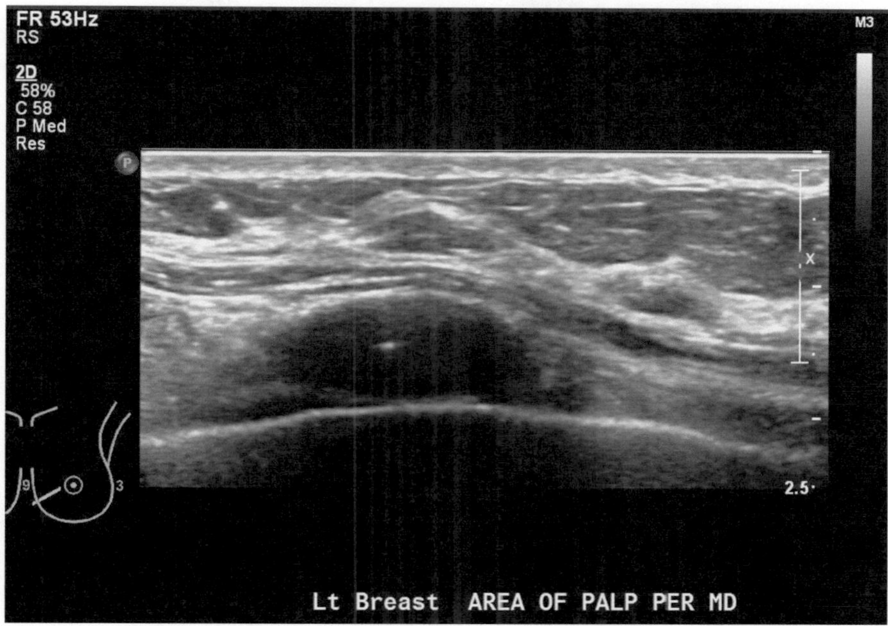

(a) Reassure the patient that the mass she is feeling is a normal anatomical structure.
(b) Recommend cross-sectional imaging to better characterize the mass.
(c) Perform a biopsy.
(d) Refer the patient to a breast surgeon.

17. When is the optimal timing to perform a breast screening MRI in relationship to a patient's menstrual cycle?
(a) Week 1 (days 1–7).
(b) Week 2 (days 7–14).
(c) Week 3 (days 14–21).
(d) Week 4 (days 21–28).

18. Which of the following is FALSE regarding the structures indicated by the arrows?

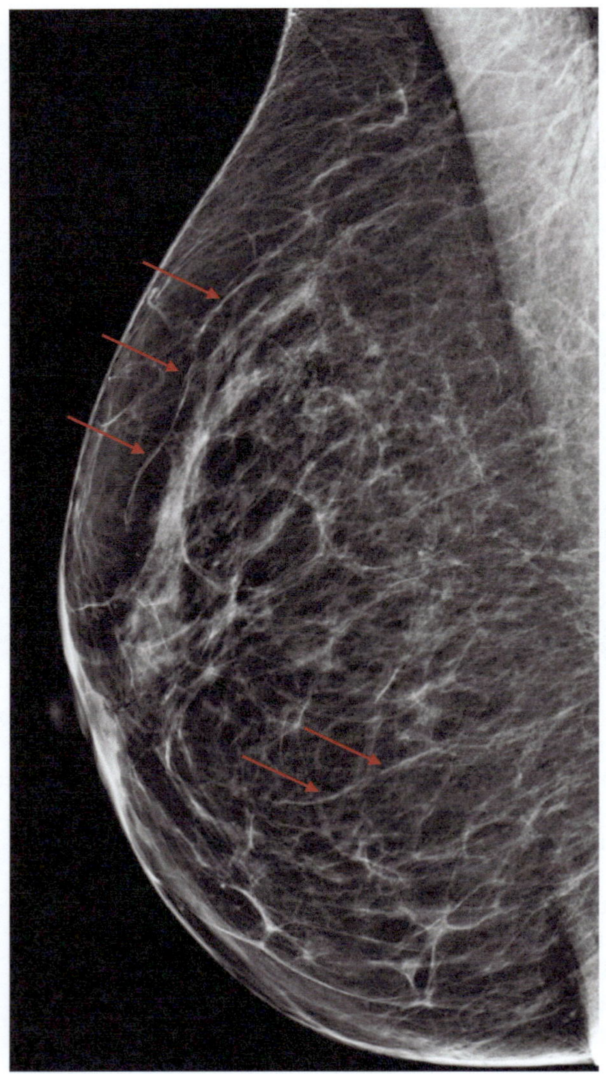

    (a) On ultrasound, they can create posterior acoustic shadowing which could appear suspicious.
    (b) Force on these ligaments can create skin retraction.
    (c) They are absent in the male breast.
    (d) They decrease with age.

19. The nipple areolar complex contains all of the following except:
    (a) Montgomery glands.
    (b) Acini.
    (c) Morgagni tubercles.
    (d) Lactiferous sinuses.

20. What is the appropriate BI-RADS designation for this screening ultrasound?
    The remainder of the study is negative.

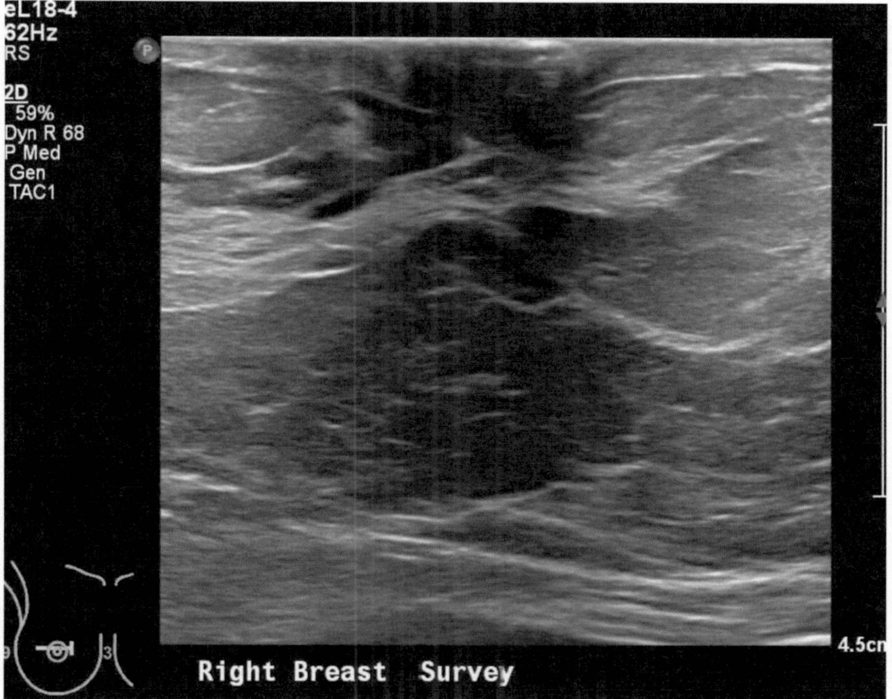

    (a) BI-RADS Category 0.
    (b) BI-RADS Category 1.
    (c) BI-RADS Category 2.
    (d) BI-RADS Category 3.
    (e) BI-RADS Category 4.

21. What structure is responsible for the majority of milk production?
    (a) Lactiferous sinus.
    (b) Lobular acini.
    (c) Terminal ducts.
    (d) Segmental ducts.

22. Where do most ductal breast cancers begin?
    (a) Terminal ducts.
    (b) Lactiferous sinus.
    (c) Segmental ducts.
    (d) Collecting ducts.

23a. What is the appropriate management of this axillary lymph node detected on ultrasound?

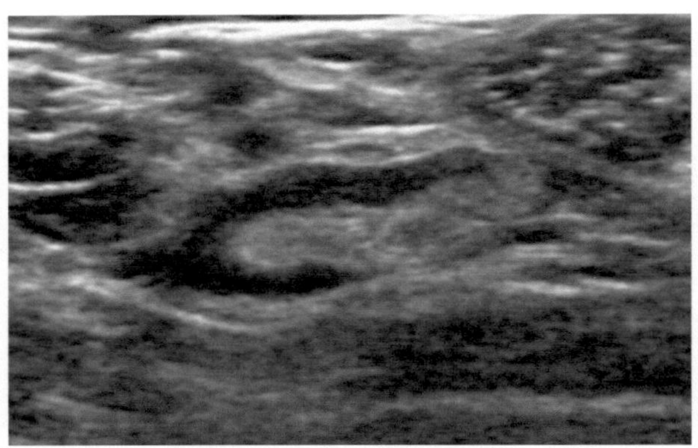

    (a) Nothing; recommend a return to normal screening.
    (b) Recommend short-term follow-up ultrasound.
    (c) Call the patient back for additional imaging.
    (d) Call the patient back for biopsy.

24a.   How would you describe the abnormality on this baseline screening
       mammogram

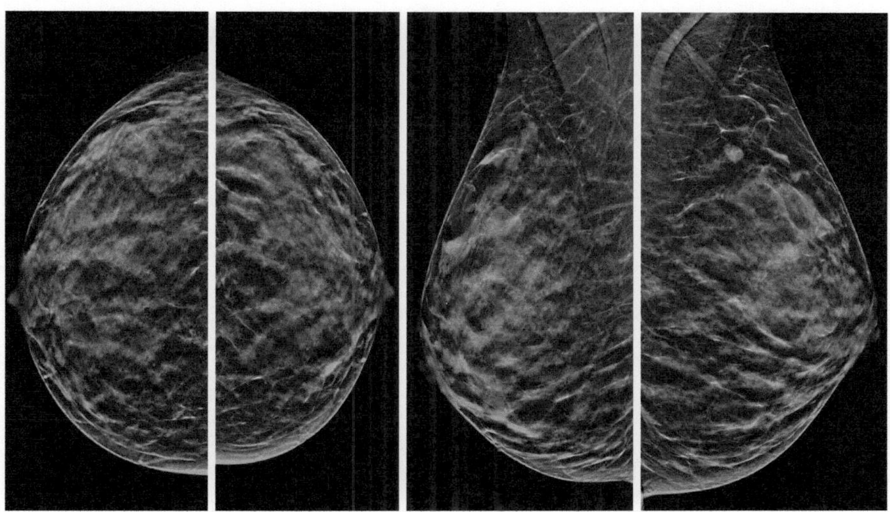

   (a) There is a round mass in the left upper outer quadrant.
   (b) There is an asymmetry in the left upper outer quadrant.
   (c) There is an asymmetry in the left superior breast.
   (d) There is a focal asymmetry in the left superior breast.

24b.   The above single view finding can be localized using the methods except:
   (a) Use relative information from tomosynthesis.
   (b) Perform a 90-degree lateral view.
   (c) Perform medial and lateral exaggerated craniocaudal views.
   (d) Perform a rolled craniocaudal view.

24c.   Why is this lesion seen on left MLO, and not seen on CC view?
   (a) There is inadequate compression on the CC view.
   (b) Nipple is not in profile on the CC view.
   (c) The posterior nipple line (PNL) is too short on the CC view.
   (d) There is motion on the CC view.

25a. A 65-year-old female presents for screening mammogram. What is the best management?

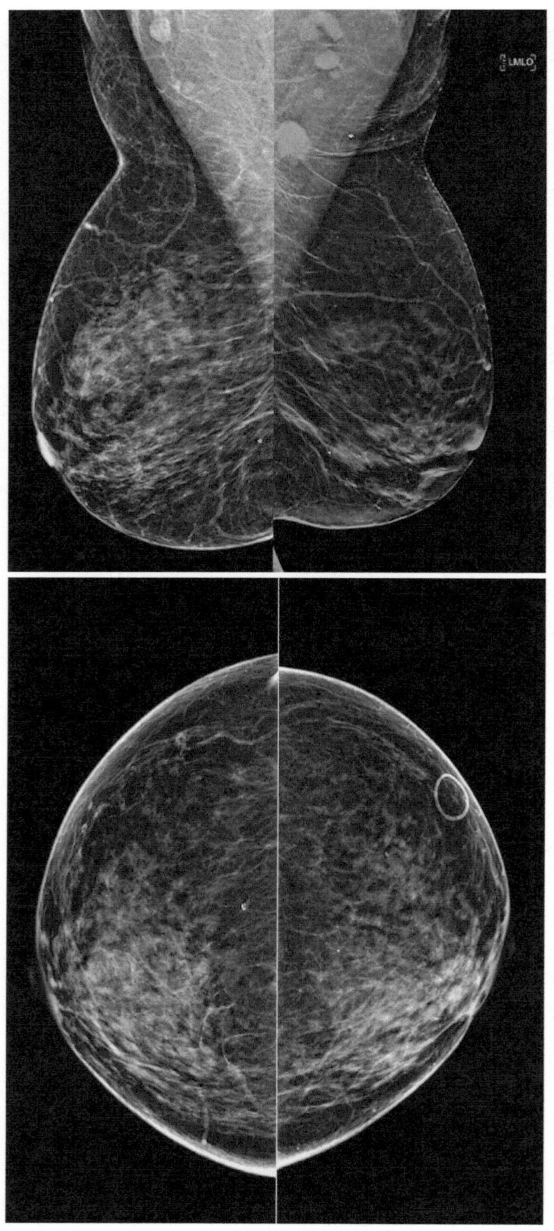

(a) BI-RADS Category 2: Benign. Routine annual follow up is suggested.
(b) BI-RADS Category 4: Suspicious. Tissue diagnosis is suggested.
(c) BI-RADS Category 0: Incomplete. Additional workup is recommended.
(d) BI-RADS Category 0: Incomplete. MRI is recommended.

25b. The mammogram from the previous year is now uploaded and the asymmetry noted on the current screening mammogram is partly seen in the old study. What is your BI-RADS assessment now?

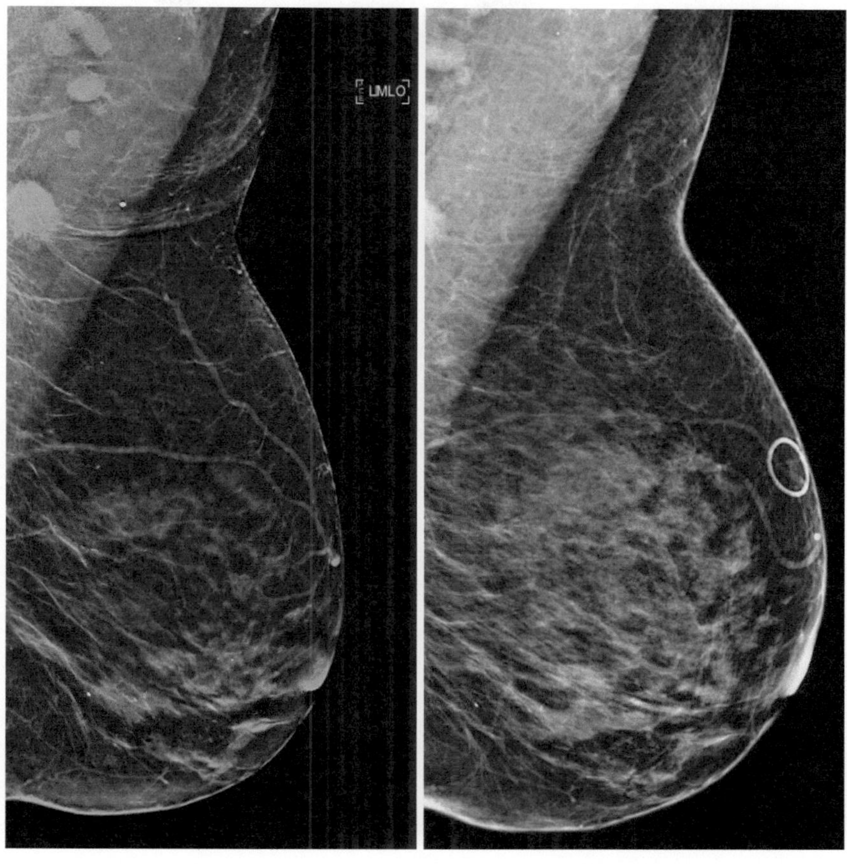

Current   13 months ago

(a) BI-RADS Category 2: Benign. Routine annual follow-up is recommended.
(b) BI-RADS Category 3: Probably Benign. Return for follow-up mammogram in 6 months.
(c) BI-RADS Category 4: Suspicious. Tissue diagnosis is recommended.
(d) BI-RADS Category 0: Incomplete. Additional workup is recommended.

26. The following are all factors that can cause a false NEGATIVE screening mammogram except:
(a) Improper positioning.
(b) Breast density.
(c) Stable mass.
(d) Interrupted workflow.
(e) Scattered bilateral calcifications.

27. What is the BI-RADS assessment for the calcifications?

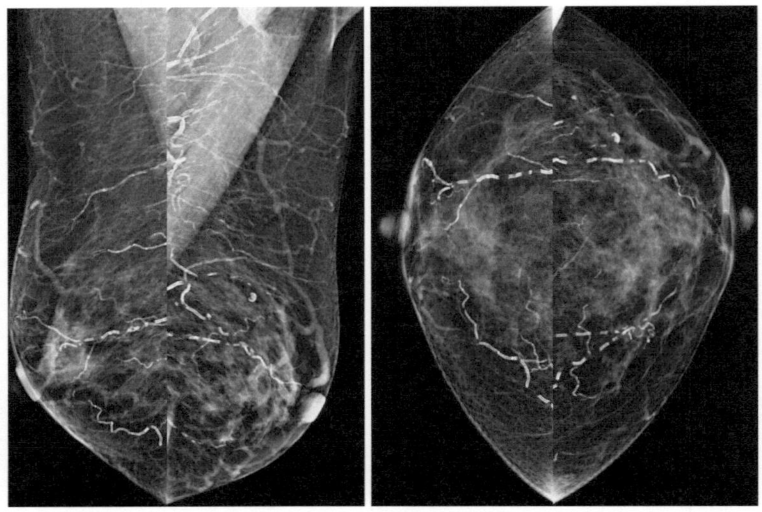

(a) BI-RADS Category 0.
(b) BI-RADS Category 2.
(c) BI-RADS Category 3.
(d) BI-RADS Category 4.

28. A 54-year old presents for a baseline screening mammogram. Based on the below images what is your assessment?

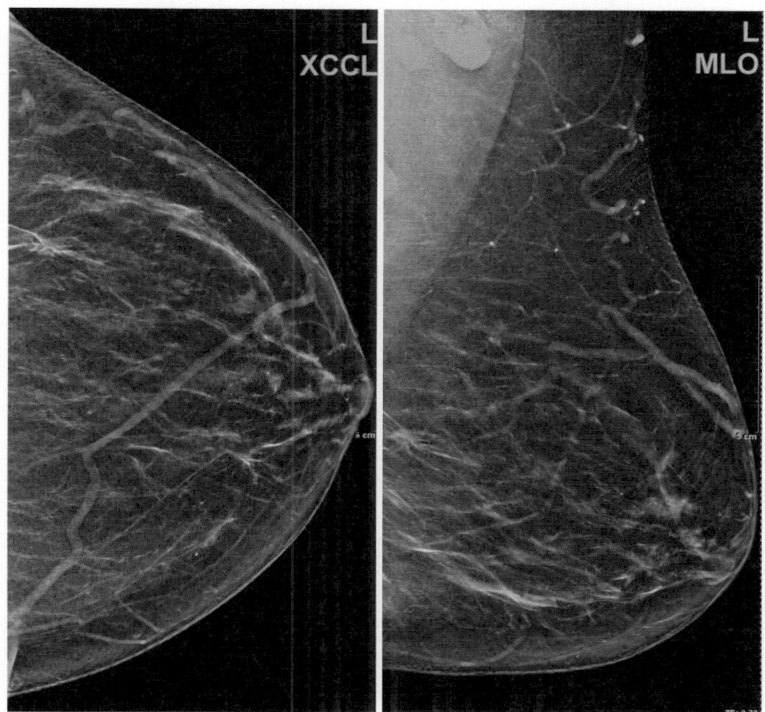

(a) BI-RADS Category 1: Negative.
(b) BI-RADS Category 0: There are abnormal nodes in the left axilla.
(c) BI-RADS Category 0: There is an asymmetry in the left lateral breast.
(d) BI-RADS Category 0: There is a mass and abnormal nodes in the left breast.

29. What is the best management for the findings on this screening mammogram?

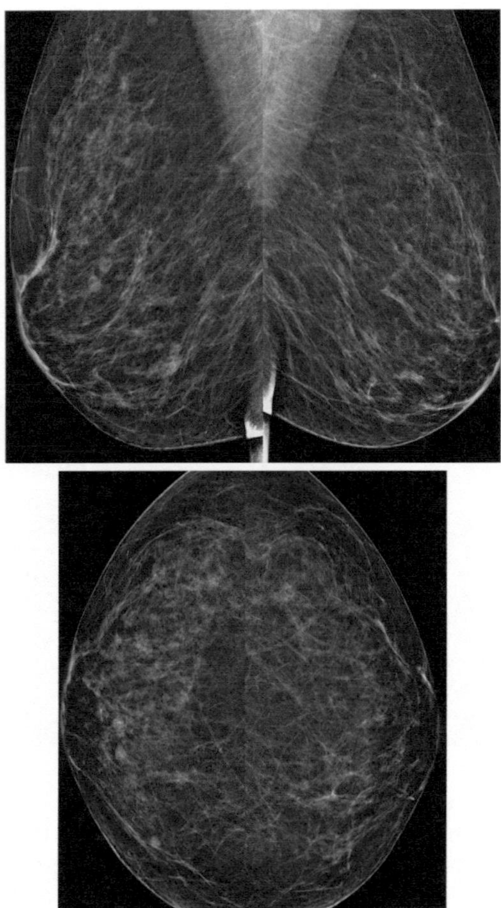

(a) BI-RADS Category 2: Benign findings.
(b) BI-RADS Category 3: Probably benign findings. Short-term follow-up is suggested.
(c) BI-RADS Category 0: Incomplete. Recommend bilateral ultrasound.
(d) BI-RADS Category 0: Incomplete. Recommend additional mammographic views and ultrasound.

30. Left-sided screening mammogram in a 55-year-old female with a history of right mastectomy 10 years ago in Europe recently immigrated to the USA. What is your assessment?

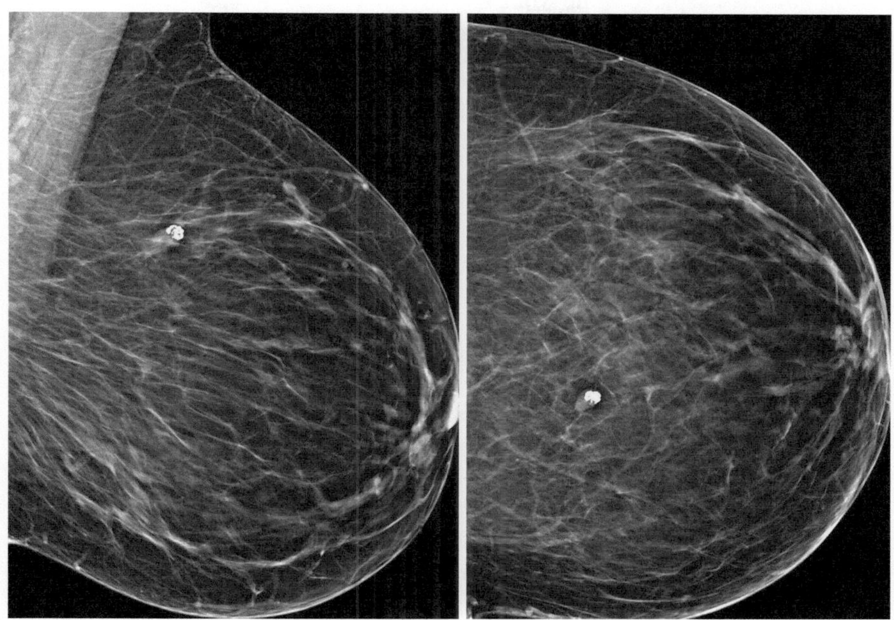

(a) BI-RADS Category 0: Incomplete. Recommend comparison with old films.
(b) BI-RADS Category 0: Incomplete. Recommend ultrasound.
(c) BI-RADS Category 2: Benign. Routine follow-up suggested.
(d) BI-RADS Category 3: Probably Benign. Recommend short-term follow-up mammography in 6 months.

31. The new ACR/SBI guidelines recognize African-American women at high risk for breast cancer secondary to which of the following factors:
    (a) The incidence of breast cancer is higher in African-American women than in non-Hispanic white women.
    (b) African-American women are more likely to die from breast cancer than non-Hispanic white women.
    (c) African-American women are more likely to be diagnosed with stage I breast cancer.
    (d) African-American women have a lower risk of aggressive tumors.

32. Which of the following is true for breast cancers caused by the BRCA1 and BRCA2 mutations?
    (a) Approximately 20% of breast cancers are caused by the BRCA1 and BRCA2 mutations.
    (b) The average age of breast cancer onset is 60 years in patients who are BRCA mutation carriers.
    (c) Cancers in patients with the BRCA1 mutation tend to be of higher grade with an overall poorer prognosis than cancers in the general population.
    (d) The sensitivity of mammography for the detection of cancer in patients with a BRCA mutation is higher than that in the general population.

33. Which breast screening modality has been shown to have a mortality benefit?
    (a) Breast MRI.
    (b) Breast Ultrasound.
    (c) Mammography.
    (d) FDG-PET.

34. This screening mammogram was considered technically inadequate. Standard views as well as magnified views of the left breast are provided. What is the technical issue?

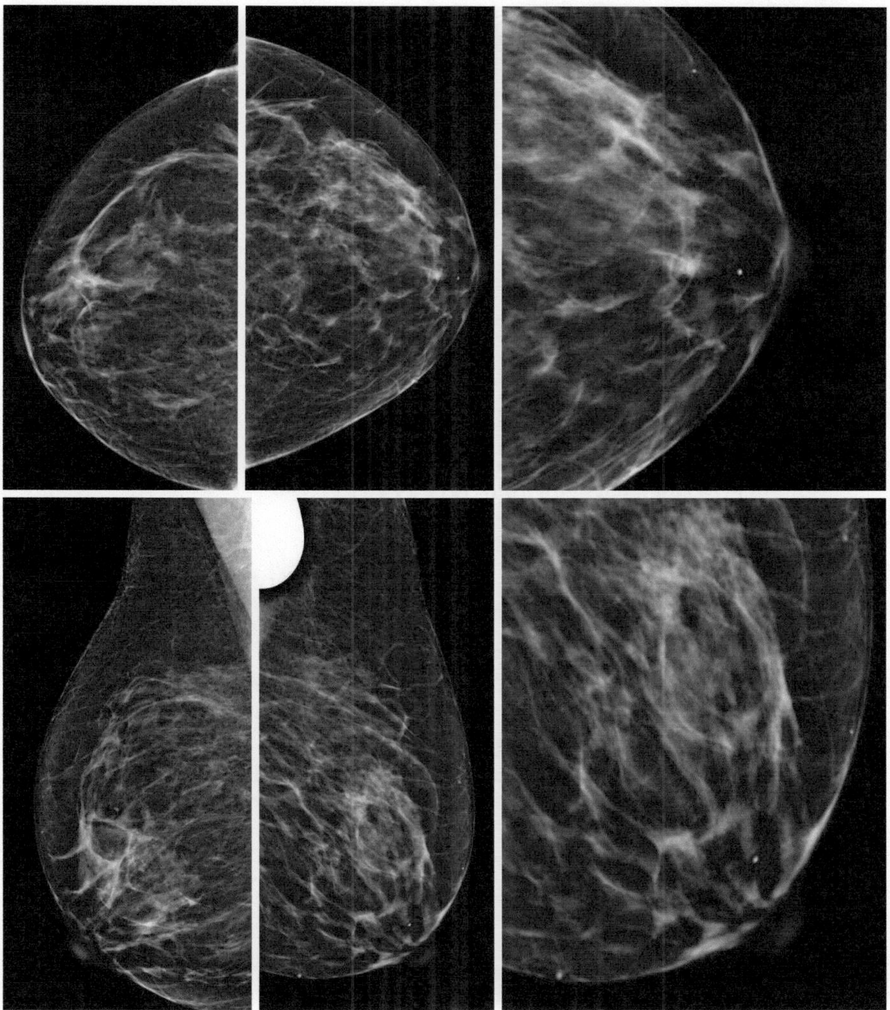

(a) Pacemaker left chest.
(b) Motion left MLO.
(c) Skin folds.
(d) Inadequate visualization of posterior tissues on right CC.

35a. How would you describe the abnormality in the screening mammogram?

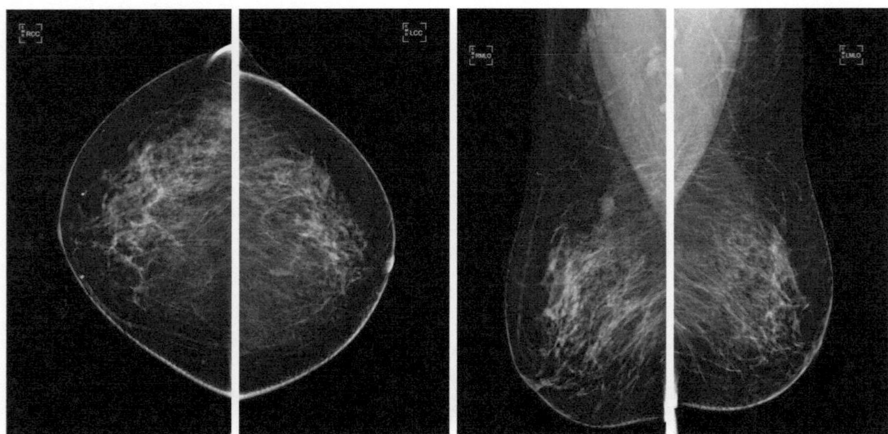

    (a) Asymmetry in the left upper breast.
    (b) Mass in the right upper outer breast.
    (c) Focal asymmetry in the right lower outer breast.
    (d) Bilateral axillary lymphadenopathy.

35b. What is the correct BI-RADS Final Assessment for this screening mammogram, and what is the correct recommendation?
    (a) BI-RADS Category 4. Recommend biopsy.
    (b) BI-RADS Category 0. Recommend additional evaluation with MRI.
    (c) BI-RADS Category 0. Recommend additional evaluation with diagnostic mammography and ultrasound.
    (d) BI-RADS Category 3. Recommend short-term follow-up.

36. Representative images at the same level of a screening breast MRI are shown. Regarding MRI technique for this study, which is true?

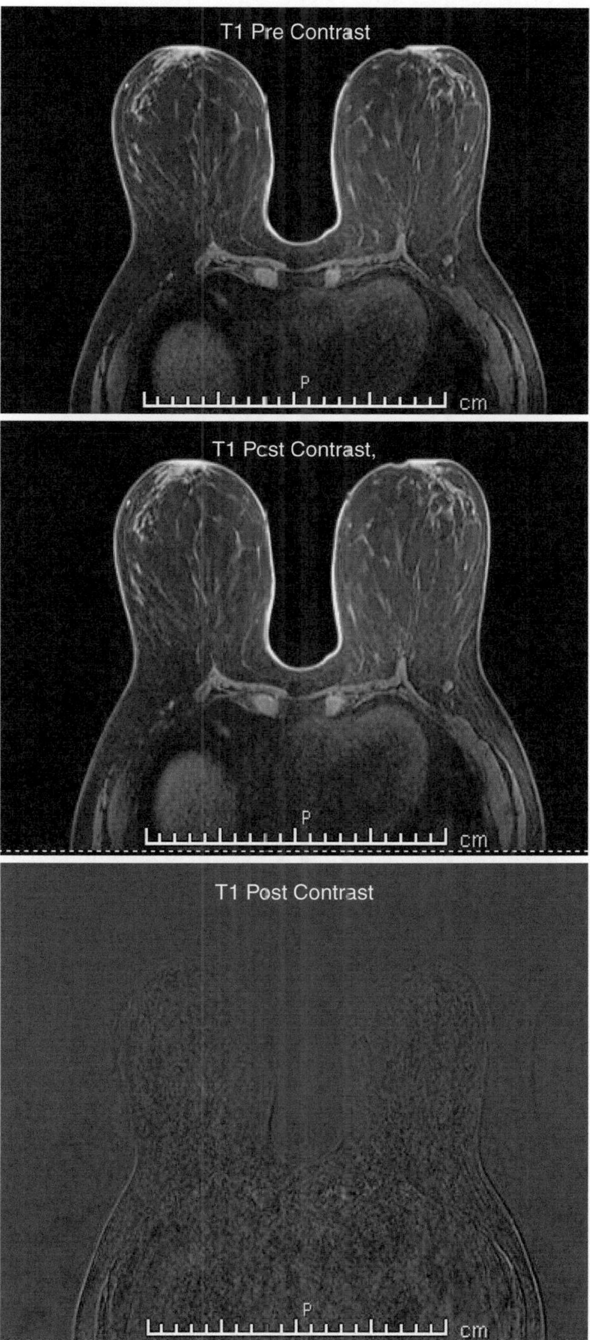

(a) Inadequate technique, motion.
(b) Adequate technique.
(c) Inadequate technique, insufficient field of view.
(d) Inadequate technique, insufficient contrast enhancement.

37. The advantages of Digital Breast Tomosynthesis versus Full Field Digital Mammography include:
    (a) Improved Cancer Detection Rate.
    (b) Reduced Screening Recall rate.
    (c) Improved Screening Specificity.
    (d) All of the above.

38. Digital Breast Tomosynthesis (DBT) reduces screening recall rates as compared to Full Field Digital Mammography (FFDM). Which type of finding is mostly responsible for false positives seen on FFDM?
    (a) Asymmetries.
    (b) Masses.
    (c) Architectural Distortions.
    (d) None of the above.

39. The advantages of the use of commercially available Computer-Aided Detection (CAD software) in the interpretation of screening mammography include:
    (a) Improved Cancer Detection Rate.
    (b) Improved Screening Mammography Specificity.
    (c) Both of the above.
    (d) None of the above.

40. Regarding screening with whole breast ultrasound, which of the following are true?
    (a) Screening ultrasound is a supplemental test to mammography, and does not replace screening mammography.
    (b) Whole breast ultrasound can detect cancers, which would have been missed by mammography in dense breast tissue.
    (c) The addition of screening ultrasound to screening mammography can reduce advanced breast cancer.
    (d) All of the above.

41. Which of the following are true regarding automated breast ultrasound versus handheld ultrasound?
    (a) Studies have shown no significant differences in sensitivity, specificity, and predictive values between automated breast ultrasound and handheld ultrasound.
    (b) Automated breast ultrasound requires recall for targeted handheld ultrasound of lesions.
    (c) False-positive rates are the most significant criticism of both techniques, but this can be reduced with experience.
    (d) All of the above.

Answers

1. b. 40.

   Various organizations recommend beginning screening mammography at different ages. The ACR recommends annual screening beginning at 40 years of age, based on the benefits of life years gained which is higher for women with screen-detected breast cancer in their 40s than in the 50–70 year-old population [1]. Per ACR guidelines, annual screening should continue as long as a woman's life expectancy exceeds 5–7 years [1]. Table 3.1 summarizes age and frequency recommendations for breast cancer screening with mammography in average-risk women [2].

2. b. <15%.

   Average-risk women have a < 15% lifetime risk of breast cancer. A lifetime risk of 15–20% is considered intermediate-risk. A lifetime risk of >20% is considered high-risk [1].

Table 3.1 Screening age and frequency recommendations for breast cancer screening with mammography in average-risk women by organization [3]

Organization	Start age	End age	Frequency
U.S. Preventive Services Task Force	50 years Choice to start at age 40–49 years	74 years	Every 2 years
American Cancer Society	45 years Choice to start at age 40–44 years	No upper limit; continue as long as life expectancy is ≥10 years	Age 45–54 years: Every year Age 55 years and older: Every year or every 2 years
American College of Obstetricians and Gynecologists	50 years Choice to start age 40–49 years	No upper limit; continue based on woman's health status and longevity	Every year or every 2 years
International Agency for Research on Cancer	50 years	74 years	Not addressed
American College of Radiology	40 years	No upper limit; continue based on woman's health status and life expectancy of at least 5–7 years	Every year
American College of Physicians	50 years Choice to start age 40–49 years	No upper limit; continue as long as life expectancy is ≥10 years	Every 2 years
American Academy of Family Physicians	50 years Choice to start age 40–49 years	74 years	Every 2 years

3. a. A 50-year-old asymptomatic female with a history of one first-degree relative with breast cancer diagnosed in her 50s.

The purpose of screening mammography is to detect early, unsuspected breast cancer in asymptomatic women. The individual described in answer choice A is most appropriate for screening mammography. Answer choices b and e require diagnostic mammography and/or ultrasound for further evaluation, regardless of symptoms. Answer choices c and d require diagnostic mammography and ultrasound to further evaluate symptoms and clinical findings [1, 3].

4. d. A 31-year-old untested daughter whose mother has a BRCA gene mutation.

High-risk breast cancer screening recommendations should be followed for women with a BRCA gene mutation and their untested first-degree relatives, history of chest irradiation between 10 and 30 years of age, and 20% or greater lifetime risk of breast cancer due to family history. Intermediate-risk factors include personal history of breast cancer, lobular neoplasia, atypical ductal hyperplasia, or 15–20% lifetime risk of breast cancer [1].

5. a. 38 years of age.

Women with biopsy-proven lobular neoplasia or atypical ductal hyperplasia should undergo annual breast cancer screening with mammography beginning at age of diagnosis, but not younger than 30 years of age [1].

6a. d. High-risk.

Based on this patient's history, she would be considered at high-risk for breast cancer. Table 3.2 outlines the American College of Radiology designations of each risk group. Low-risk is not a risk category.

6b. b. At age 30.

Women with genetics-based increased risk and their untested first-degree relatives should begin breast cancer screening with mammogram at the age of 30 years [1, 4].

Table 3.2 Risk-based categories for breast cancer screening [1]

Risk category	Description
Average-risk	• Less than 15% lifetime risk of breast cancer.
Intermediate-risk	• Personal history of breast cancer. • Personal history of lobular neoplasia. • Personal history of atypical ductal hyperplasia. • 15–20% lifetime risk of breast cancer.
High-risk	• Patients with BRCA gene mutation and their untested first-degree relatives. • History of chest irradiation between 10 and 30 years of age. • 20% or greater lifetime risk of breast cancer.

6c. c. Mammography with breast MRI or ultrasound.

The American College of Radiology, American Cancer Society, and Society of Breast Imaging recommend high-risk screening with digital mammography with or without digital breast tomosynthesis, in addition to annual supplemental screening with breast MRI. For those unable to undergo MRI, screening ultrasound is indicated. The combination of mammography and supplemental screening has the highest sensitivity for breast cancer detection in high-risk women, especially those with a genetic predisposition, than mammography alone [1, 4]. There is a lack of evidence in large screening populations to support supplemental screening with molecular breast imaging or FDG-PET [1].

7. b. High-risk and unable to tolerate MRI.

Screening ultrasound is indicated as an adjunct to mammography for high-risk patients who cannot tolerate MRI [1]. A woman presenting with a palpable mass should undergo diagnostic ultrasound rather than a screening ultrasound, with or without diagnostic mammography depending on her age. Breast cancer screening during pregnancy at the age of 40 years is usually performed with mammography, as the dose to the fetus is negligible and lead shielding can be done safely [5]. Screening whole-breast ultrasound during pregnancy has not been well evaluated, but may be used as a screening adjunct while keeping in mind the possibility of increased false-positive rates prompting additional biopsies [5]. In women with dense breasts, such as the patient described in the question stem, screening ultrasound may be considered in addition to screening mammography but is not clearly recommended [1]. For women with dense breasts, the benefit of increased cancer detection with adjunct screening ultrasound should be balanced with the increased risk of a false-positive result [1].

8. a. Dense breast tissue lowers the sensitivity of mammography and increases breast cancer risk compared to patients with fatty breast tissue.

Answer choice a is true. Answer choice b is false because dense breast notification laws mandate, not suggest, that mammogram reports include information regarding the risks related to dense breast tissue. Answer choice c is false because screening ultrasound in women with dense breasts increases the false-positive rate of breast cancer as well as a number of short-interval follow-up and biopsy recommendations, with decreased positive predictive value of biopsies [1]. Answer choice d is false as a blanket statement; however, screening breast MRI in women with dense breast tissue is recommended for women with a personal history of breast cancer and dense breast tissue [4].

9. c. Based on her history, she should start breast cancer screening 6–12 months post-radiation.

Women with a personal history of breast cancer should start screening with mammography 6–12 months post-radiation if the breast is conserved; otherwise mammography every 12 months is indicated. Women with a personal history of breast cancer diagnosed before the age of 50 years, or who also have increased lifetime risk greater than 20% are recommended to undergo screening with mammography supplemented with contrast-enhanced MRI [1, 4].

10. a. A 35-year-old pregnant female with high-risk of breast cancer.

Screening mammography remains indicated in pregnant women at high-risk under the age of 30 years, and at elevated risk (intermediate or high risk) between the ages 30 and 39 years. At age 40 years or older, breast cancer screening during pregnancy is recommended for all levels of risk. The fetal radiation dose from a 4-view mammogram is <0.03 mGy, which is well below the 50 mGy threshold below which no teratogenic effects have been demonstrated. Lead shielding can also be safely used with pregnant women undergoing mammography [4]. Answer choices b and c require diagnostic imaging due to symptoms. There is no indication for screening mammography with answer choice d.

11. b. 25 years old.

For BRCA gene mutation carriers, annual breast cancer screening with contrast-enhanced MRI is recommended to start as early as age 25 years [4, 6]. Most societies recommend starting annual screening with contrast-enhanced MRI between the ages of 25 and 30 years [6]. Annual MRI breast cancer screening should be obtained in addition to annual screening mammography at and beyond age 30 years. In practice, these two modalities are often alternated every 6 months starting at age 30 years.

12. c. Fatty breasts.

Dense breasts, not fatty breasts, are considered a risk factor for breast cancer because the increased amount of connective tissue can make it harder to see tumors on a mammogram. General risk factors for breast cancer include:
- Age (most breast cancers are diagnosed after age 50 years).
- Genetic mutations (e.g., BRCA1 and BRCA 2).
- Reproductive history with longer exposure to hormones (e.g., early menses before age 12 years, menopause after age 55 years, first pregnancy after age 30 years, never breastfeeding, never having a full-term pregnancy).
- Dense breasts.
- Personal history of breast cancer or high-risk lesion.
- Family history of breast or ovarian cancer.
- Prior radiation therapy to the chest or breasts before age 30 years.
- Prior exposure to diethylstilbestrol (DES).
- Sedentary lifestyle/obesity.
- Hormone replacement therapy after menopause for greater than 5 years.
- Alcohol consumption [7].

13. b. Represents a normal anatomical variant.

The sternalis muscle is a normal anatomical variant of the chest wall musculature present in approximately 8% of the general population. When present, it is
twice as often unilateral as bilateral. It is important to be aware of this variant
as it can often be seen on screening mammography and should not be confused
for a suspicious mass. It appears as a mass-like density in the medial aspect of
the breast at posterior depth on the craniocaudal view (indicated by the red
arrow below). It is essentially never seen in the MLO projection due to its far
medial and posterior location on the chest wall [8].

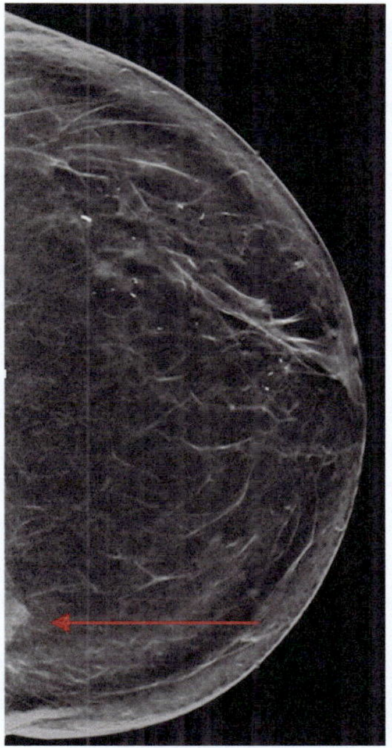

14. d. If unilateral, additional diagnostic workup is indicated.

The breast is composed of fibroglandular tissue as well as fatty elements. The ratio
of these two components determines the fibroglandular density of a breast on
screening mammogram, which is reported in every screening mammography report
as "almost entirely fatty (A)," "scattered areas of fibroglandular density (B)," "heterogeneously dense (C)," and "extremely dense (D)." Common factors affecting
breast density are detailed in the table below. Bilateral increase in density detected
at screening mammogram typically does not warrant further workup, but a unilateral increase could suggest lymphatic obstruction and could be malignant [10–12].

Common causes for changes in breast density [10–12]	
Increased density	Decreased density
Hormonal stimulation (e.g., hormone replacement therapy and pregnancy)	Tamoxifen
	Increasing age
Systemic conditions causing edema (e.g., congestive heart failure)	Weight gain

15. b. It most commonly occurs in the axilla, but may be present anywhere along the "milk line".

Accessory breast tissue, also known as ectopic breast tissue, refers to any breast tissue outside of the expected location of the breast. While the precise etiology of accessory breast tissue is not definitively understood, one theory purports that the mammary ridges, derived from the ectoderm, migrate along the "milk line" on the ventral surface of the fetus and regress everywhere except at the breasts. If the ridges do not regress, accessory breast tissue is left behind along the pathway of normal migration which extends from the anterior axilla to the medial thigh, most commonly in the axilla. Incidence of accessory breast tissue is approximately 6% and is frequently bilateral. Just like breast tissue within the breast, accessory breast tissue responds to hormonal stimulation and may thus display the same benign/physiologic and malignant processes as the breast [11, 12].

16. a. Reassure the patient that the mass she is feeling is a normal anatomical structure.

It is important to be familiar with the normal sonographic appearance of the breast and surrounding structures. The breast parenchyma demonstrates varying echogenicity based on its composition of fat (hypoechoic), fibrous (hyperechoic), and glandular (intermediate echogenicity) tissue. The structures of the chest wall, including the pectoralis muscle (which appears as a longitudinally oriented structure with linear bands of alternating hyper- and hypoechoic lines), the ribs, and the costal cartilage are often seen. In this case, the patient's palpable abnormality corresponds to a rib (indicated by the circle on the image below), which can be easily identified by its thin echogenic rim with dense posterior acoustic shadowing and location posterior to the pectoralis and anterior to the lung [13, 14].

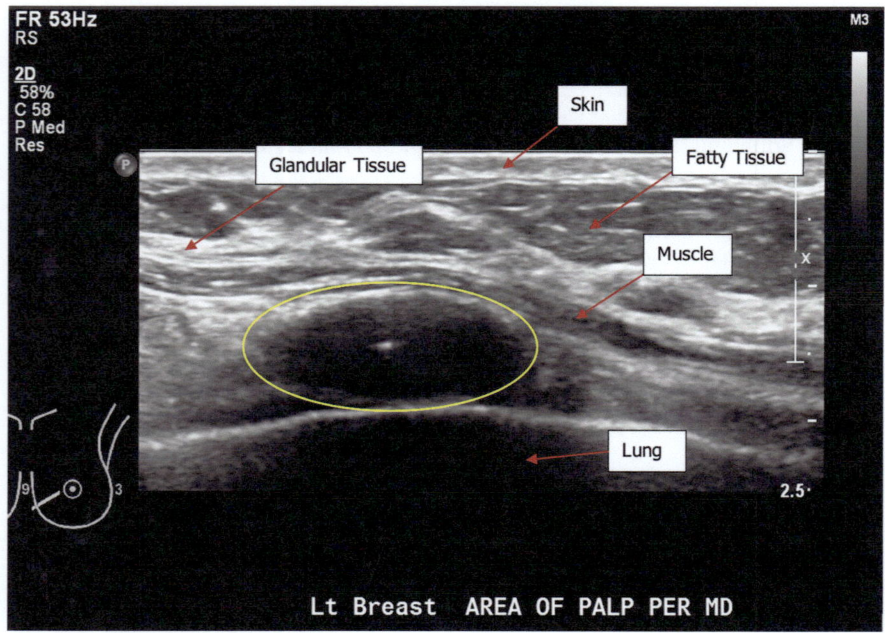

17. b. Week 2 (days 7–14).

Background parenchymal enhancement is highest during days 1–6 and 21–28 of the menstrual cycle. A breast MRI is ideally performed during the second week of the menstrual cycle (days 7–14) to maximize the sensitivity of lesion detection [15, 16].

18. d. They decrease with age.

Cooper's ligaments, which make up the underlying ligamentous supporting structure of the breast, are seen as fine white lines on mammography. Any straightening or distortion of Cooper's ligaments should be viewed with suspicion as an indication of underlying malignancy. Similarly, a mass that is exerting force on Cooper's ligaments can create skin or nipple retraction, a suspicious physical exam finding. On ultrasound, Cooper's ligaments are seen as thin hyperechoic lines that can create acoustic shadows. These shadows are typically thin and hypoechoic, but have the potential to mimic malignancy if the shadow is wider. Differentiating features include the lack of an associated mass and the disappearance of the shadow with increased transducer pressure and changes in the angle of insonation. Cooper's ligaments are stable over a women's lifetime and are not present in the male breast [18–20].

19. b. Acini.

The breast is composed of approximately 15–20 segments, each of which has a corresponding mammary duct that converges at the nipple. These draining ducts come together in the subareolar breast to form lactiferous sinuses, which each measure approximately 5–8 mm. Occasionally, a palpable normal lactiferous sinus will bring in a woman for a diagnostic exam. The nipple-areolar complex also contains the Montgomery glands, which secrete milk into the Morgagni tubercles. The Morgagni tubercles are seen as tiny (1–2 mm) raised lesions on the surface of the areolar skin [20].

20. b. BI-RADS Category 1.

The image above demonstrates the normal sonographic appearance of the nipple. On ultrasound, the nipple produces severe attenuation of the sound beam from whirled smooth muscle bundles. When seen on static images, the nipple can be occasionally misinterpreted as a shadowing breast mass. Thus, it is important to interpret images knowing the relative position of the nipple and to interrogate the subareolar parenchyma using different angles of insonation [17]. In this case, the body marker to the left of the image demonstrates that the sonographer is imaging directly over the nipple, and this study should be given a BI-RADS 1: Negative.

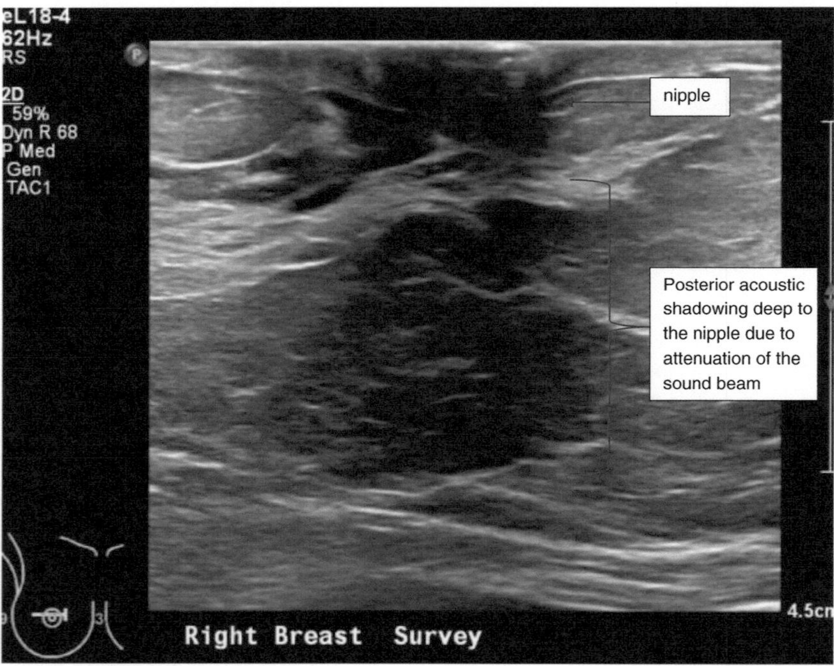

21. b. Lobular acini.

The terminal duct lobular unit (TDLU) is considered a "functional unit" of the breast (see image below) and contains the lobular acini which are responsible for milk production. The epithelial cells lining the acini produce milk which is then transferred through the terminal ducts to segmental ducts to the lactiferous sinus. The outer lining of the acini is formed by myoepithelial cells which help excrete the milk into the terminal ducts [21].

22. a. Terminal ducts.

Most cancers in the breast begin in the terminal duct-lobular unit (TDLU), the functional unit of the breast. The two most common types of breast cancer, which account for approximately 90% of breast cancers are ductal carcinoma and lobular carcinoma. The majority of ductal carcinomas begin in the terminal ducts. The lobular carcinomas begin in the lobules of the TDLU. Invasive ductal carcinoma is the most common breast cancer, accounting for 70–80% of invasive breast cancers [22–24].

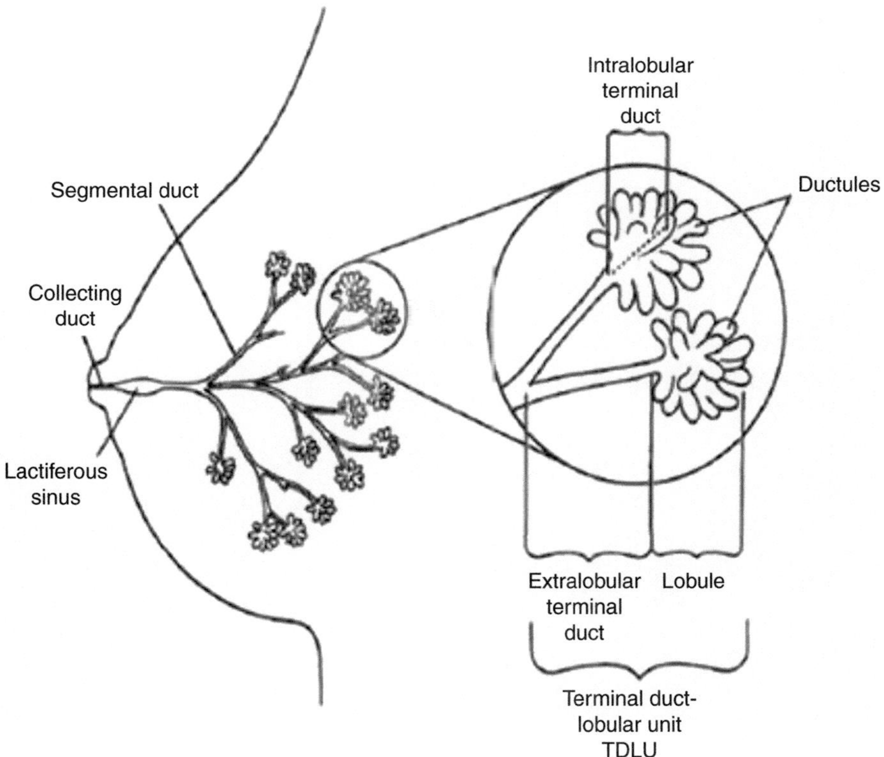

(Image from Hindle W.H. (1999) Breast Disease for Primary Health Care Providers for Women: An Overview. In: Hindle W.H. (eds) Breast Care. Springer, New York, NY. https://doi.org/10.1007/978-1-4612-2144-9_1; Reprinted with permission)

23.   a. Nothing; recommend return to normal screening.

This ultrasound depicts a morphologically normal axillary lymph node, which is commonly imaged as part of breast screening ultrasound. Normal lymph nodes are oval in shape with thin, uniform hypoechoic cortices measuring 3 mm or less (image A below). There is preservation of a fatty hilum, where a feeding vessel can often be seen. Suspicious features include focal or diffuse cortical thickening (image B), loss of the fatty hilum, round shape, and non-hilar cortical blood flow (image C). Since this lymph node lacks any suspicious feature, no further imaging is required and the patient should return to routine screening [24, 25].

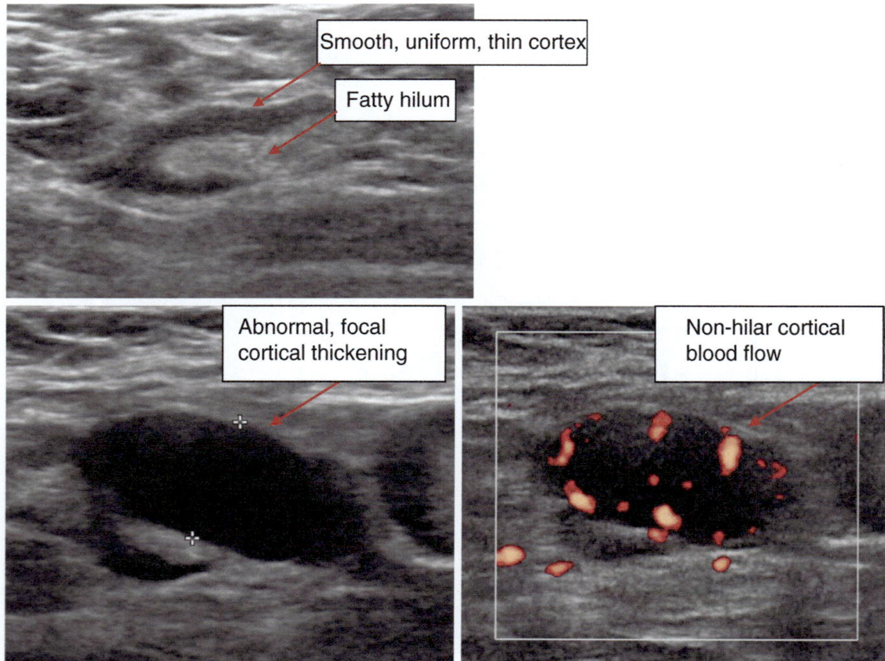

24a. c. There is an asymmetry in the left superior breast.

The lesion is a single view finding only seen on the left MLO view superiorly and hence labeled an "asymmetry." An asymmetry is a planar finding seen on only one of the two mammographic views, usually lacking convex margins, and with or without interspersed fat. It is different from a focal asymmetry, which is defined as a finding having a similar appearance on two orthogonal views, lacking convex margins, with or without interspersed fat, and occupying less than one quadrant of the breast. It also differs from a mass, which is defined as a three-dimensional (3D) structure with convex margins that is visible on two orthogonal views. According to the BI-RADS lexicon, an apparent mass (round or oval shape with convex margins) seen on only one mammographic view is termed an asymmetry until it is localized in 3D space [26, 27].

Answer choices a and d are incorrect as the finding is not seen on craniocaudal view and cannot be labeled as a mass or focal asymmetry both of which are two view findings.

Answer choice b is incorrect as an asymmetry is a single view finding and hence without 3D data can only be localized to a hemisphere of breast (i.e., lateral, medial, superior, or inferior) but not to a quadrant.

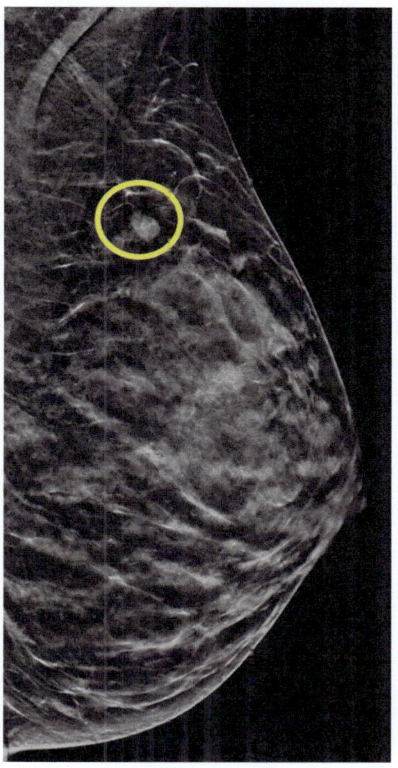

24b. d. Perform a rolled craniocaudal view.

  a. The relative 3D information from breast tomosynthesis can be used to esti-
      mate whether the lesion is lateral or medial and guide additional views.

  b. If a lesion shifts inferiorly relative to the nipple from the MLO view to the
      ML view, then it is *L*ateral in location (*L*ead drops). If a lesion shifts supe-
      riorly relative to the nipple from the MLO view to the ML view, then it is
      *M*edial in location (*M*uffins rise). If a lesion does not move significantly, it
      is likely more central/retroareolar in location.

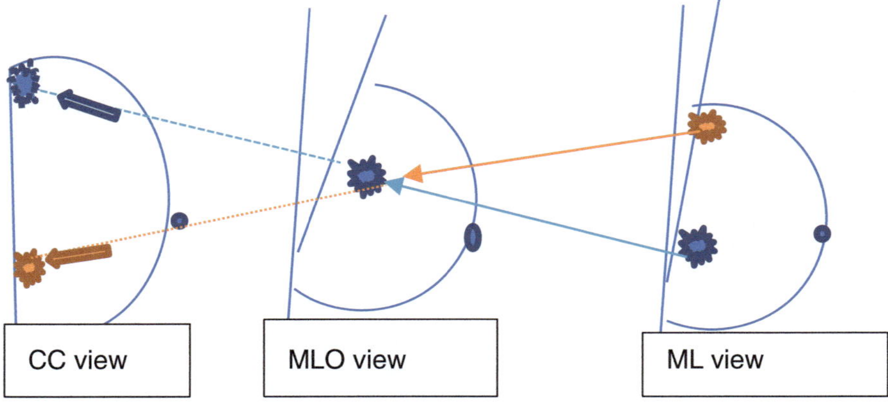

  c. Exaggerated lateral and medial CC views can be performed to visualize
      the deeper portions of the relative hemispheres of the breast.

  d. Rolled CC views can be used to assess whether an asymmetry seen on CC
      view is real or localize a finding only seen on CC view to the superior or
      inferior breast depending upon the relative movement of the lesion. For
      example, if a lesion on a "rolled lateral CC view" (meaning superior breast
      is rolled laterally as the inferior breast is rolled medially) moves medially
      relative to a routine CC view, that lesion is in the inferior breast. In our
      case, the finding is not seen on the original CC view and rolled views are
      of no additional value.

24c. c. Posterior nipple line (PNL) is too short on the CC view.

Proper positioning criteria exist for breast imaging modalities aimed to ensure greatest amount of tissue has been included in the examination.

On the MLO view:

– Pectoralis muscle should be visible down to at least the PNL (line drawn from the nipple, perpendicular to surface of pectoralis muscle).
– Anterior margin of pectoralis should be convex (relaxed muscle to allow maximum pulling of tissue).
– Inframammary fold should be included and open.
– Nipple should point anterior and not inferior to allow spreading of tissue and uniform compression (avoid sagging tissue with a "Camel nose" appearance).

On CC view:

– PNL should be within 1 cm of the length of the line on MLO view.
– Try to include as much posteromedial tissue without exaggerating as this part of the breast may be excluded on MLO [28, 29].

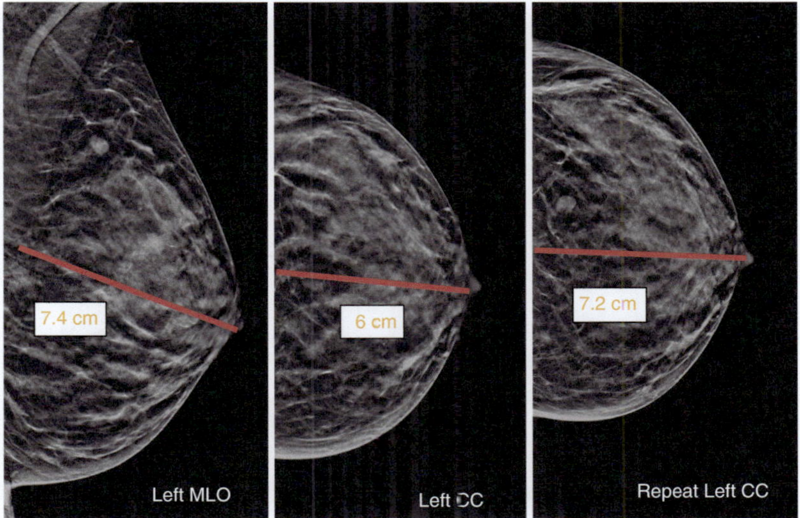

Left MLO and CC views show that the PNL on the left CC view is not within 1 cm from that on the left MLO view. The patient was called back, and a repeat left CC view was performed with improved positioning. Now, the PNL line on the left CC view is within 1 cm of the PNL line on the MLO view

25a. c. BI-RADS Category 0: Incomplete. Additional workup is recommended.

There is an asymmetry with convex somewhat spiculated margins overlying the left pectoralis muscle only seen on the left MLO view that needs further evaluation. Hence, assignment of "Benign" to this mammogram is inaccurate.

Category 4 can only be assigned after a diagnostic workup and not from a screening mammogram. The asymmetry requires verification (whether it is a true lesion versus overlapping tissue), localization and further characterization (either with additional mammographic views and/or ultrasound) and workup to assess how the biopsy is to be performed.

MRI is not used for diagnostic workup from a screening mammogram.

25b. d. BI-RADS Category 0: Incomplete. Additional workup is recommended.

A suspicious finding, whether it has been stable or increasing, warrants additional workup and potential biopsy.

Comparison should preferably be made to multiple older mammograms to detect slowly growing tumors. Women taking tamoxifen may have breast lesions that appear stable or even decreasing.

Any abnormality noted on screening mammography needs to be worked up before a BI-RADS 3, 4, or 5 can be assigned [30].

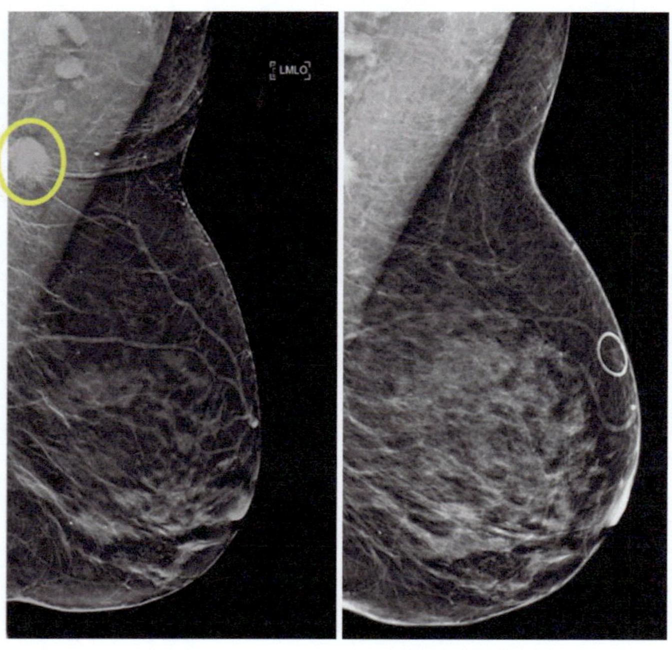

Current   13 months ago

26. e. Scattered bilateral calcifications.

Causes of missed breast cancer:

1. Technical factors (improper positioning, suboptimal exposure, motion, etc.).
2. Patient factors (breast size and breast density).
3. Lesion factors (one view finding, developing asymmetry, slow-growing mass, malignancy with benign features, subtle calcifications/architectural distortion).
4. Reader factors (distractions, interruptions and cognitive bias such as difficult location of an obvious mass, blind spots, and satisfaction of search).

In order to reduce Cognitive bias, the reader should:

- Be strict about technical factors to ensure optimal quality.
- Follow a systematic review of the screening mammogram and check the common blind spots which are located overlying and anterior to the pectoralis muscle, inferior and medial breast, retroareolar region, and the retroglandular fat).
- Compare the current mammogram to multiple prior mammograms 5–7 years old if possible (slowly changing lesions or relatively stable lesions with suspicious or indeterminate features still require workup and biopsy) [31].

Causes of missed breast cancer and potential strategies to improve

Type	Example	Potential remedies
Technical factors	Positioning Motion Exposure	Provide proper training and continuous feedback to technologists and repeat the image when needed
Patient factors	Breast size Tissue density	Ensure appropriate positioning and technique
Lesion factors	One view finding or developing asymmetry Subtle calcifications or architectural distortion Stable or benign appearing masses	• Be aware of interval changes and suspicious features • Be aware if the finding is in an area of palpable concern • Be careful of areas in the breast that are only seen in one view • Compare current mammograms to older mammograms up to 5–7 years old • Do appropriate workup with additional views • Be aware of stable calcifications with suspicious features • Be aware of new or slowly increasing calcifications • Do not trust negative ultrasound, especially when an architectural distortion is suspected on the mammogram, proceed with biopsy • Be aware of stable lesions with suspicious features • Be sure all features of a benign mass are present • Have a low threshold for biopsy in high-risk patients

Causes of missed breast cancer and potential strategies to improve		
Type	Example	Potential remedies
Reader factors (most common)	1. Cognitive bias: – Satisfaction of search – Inattention blindness – Difficult location 2. Distraction and interruptions	• Systematic search method and secondary search • Careful when correlating findings on different modalities • Check blind spots and "forbidden zones" • Pay attention to areas of clinical concern • Be vigilant on positioning and triangulation • Try to read in a quiet place when possible • Dedicated screening time when feasible • Focus and double check

27. b. BI-RADS Category 2.

Prominent bilateral "tram-track" calcifications are seen, consistent with vascular calcifications. This type of calcifications can be seen in older patients or patients with chronic diseases such as diabetes, cardiovascular disease, or renal failure [32]. Early calcifications can mimic cancer if only one edge of the artery is calcified [33].

28. d. BI-RADS Category 0: There is a mass and abnormal nodes in the left breast.

There is a spiculated mass in the left 3 o'clock as well as prominent nodes in the left axilla. An additional asymmetry with architectural distortion in the left superior breast was also noted on tomosynthesis images. Patient was called back and an additional workup was performed confirming two masses with distortion at the left 2 and 3 o'clock posteriorly

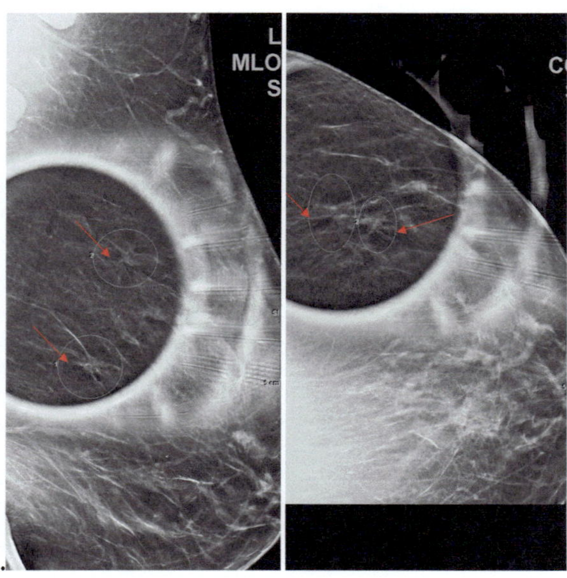

There was a sonographic correlate for the 3 o'clock mass but the 2 o'clock lesion could not be seen sonographically. Multiple axillary nodes showed borderline cortical thickening with preservation of fatty hila.

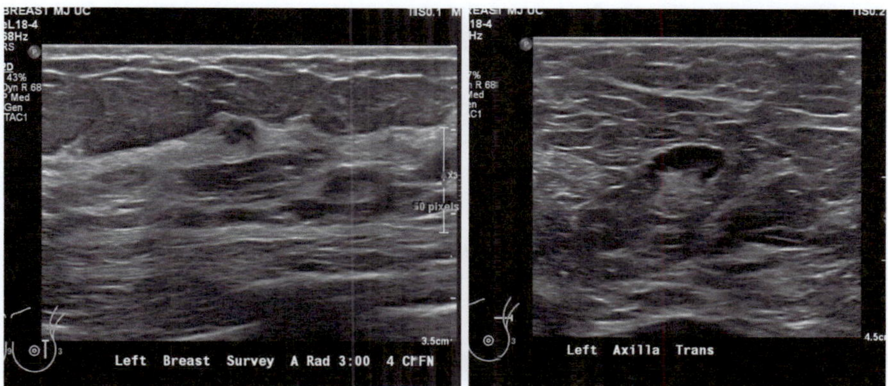

Stereotactic core needle biopsy of both masses showed invasive carcinoma with ductal and lobular features.

"Satisfaction of search" is defined as decreased vigilance regarding and/or decreased awareness of additional abnormalities after the first abnormality has been identified. This form of cognitive bias, has been reported to account for 22% of missed radiologic finding, and can result in missed breast cancers [31]. Once an obvious (benign or malignant appearing) finding is seen (in this case spiculated 3 o'clock mass), make sure to search for additional sites of potential disease or associated findings (such as calcifications outside of a suspicious mass or more than one mass or groups of calcification) on the image(s).

29. a. BI-RADS Category 2, benign findings.

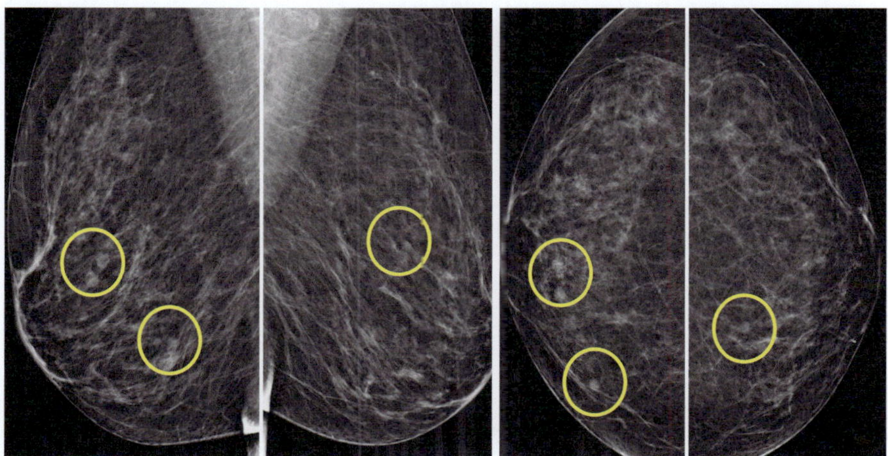

Multiple bilateral benign-appearing masses are defined as at least three circumscribed or mostly circumscribed masses, with at least one mass in each breast. To be considered partially circumscribed, at least 75% of the margins of a mass should be circumscribed, with the remaining margins obscured by adjacent fibroglandular tissue. No part of the margins may be indistinct or spiculated. The multiple masses must have a similar appearance in that not one of them can be substantially different from the others in terms of size, margin characteristics, or density. Studies have suggested that interval cancer rate for patients with multiple benign-appearing masses as described above, was similar to that reported for the general population undergoing routine mammography in various screening studies and hence no further workup is necessary [34].

b. BI-RADS Category 3 should not be assigned based on screening mammography and is not indicated based upon low rate of cancer development as mentioned.

c and d. Again based on the above no additional workup is necessary. Furthermore, correlation of sonographic with mammographic findings in case of multiple bilateral masses may be confusing and ultrasound may yield findings other than simple cysts requiring follow-up and or aspirations with no apparent benefit given no increased risk of interval cancers.

30. c. BI-RADS Category 2—Benign. Routine follow-up suggested.

The oval mass with mostly circumscribed margins containing coarse popcorn-like calcification in the left 11–12 o'clock is a classic appearance of a calcified/degenerating fibroadenoma. Once these classic calcifications appear, no further workup is necessary. Earlier calcifications however can appear more pleomorphic, mimicking a malignant mass with calcifications, necessitating a biopsy.

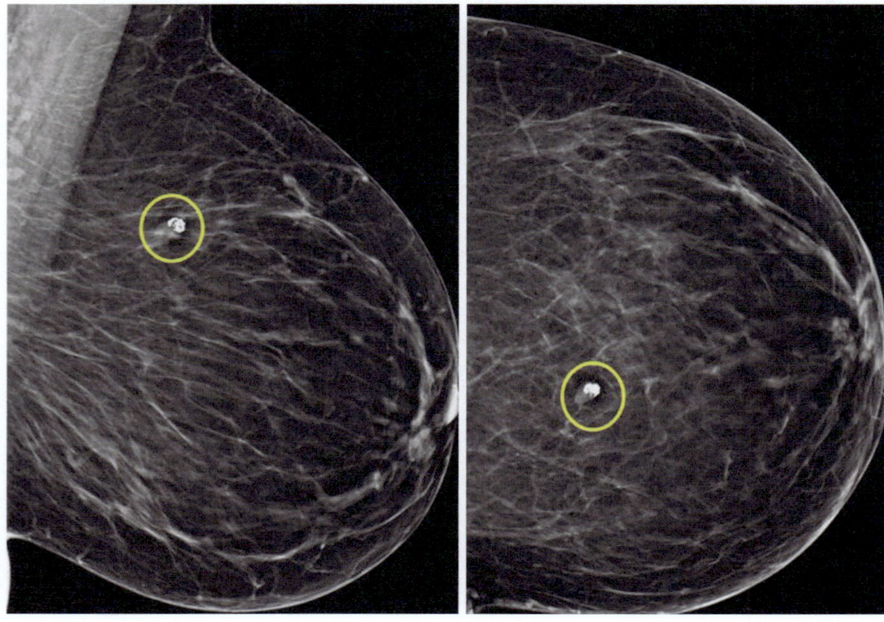

31. b. African-American women are more likely to die from breast cancer than non-Hispanic white women.

Although the incidence of breast cancer is not higher in African-American women, they have higher mortality.

Factors that contributed to the ACR/SBI reclassification of African-American women include that:
- African-American women are 42 percent more likely to die from breast cancer than non-Hispanic white women despite similar incidence rates.
- African-American women have a two-fold higher risk of aggressive breast cancer, including the triple-negative breast tumors.
- African-American women are less likely to be diagnosed with stage I breast cancer, but twice as likely to die of early breast cancers.
- African-American women have a higher risk of BRCA1 and BRCA2 genetic mutations than women of Western European ancestry [4].

32. c. Cancers in patients with the BRCA1 mutation tend to be of higher grade with an overall poorer prognosis than cancers in the general population.

Answer choice a is incorrect. The vast majority of breast cancers occur sporadically, and only approximately 6% of breast cancer cases are caused by BRCA1 and BRCA2 mutations.

Answer choice b is incorrect. The age at breast cancer onset is much younger in BRCA1 and BRCA2 mutation carriers than in the general population. The average age of breast cancer onset is 40 years in patients who are BRCA mutation carriers, but 61 years in the general population. Approximately 55%–65% of women with BRCA1 mutation and 45% of women with BRCA2 mutation will develop breast cancer by 70 years.

Answer choice c is correct. Breast cancers in patients with BRCA1 mutation tend to be of a higher grade, are negative for hormone receptors, and are larger in size, with an overall poorer prognosis than those in the general population.

Answer choice d is incorrect. The sensitivity of mammography for the detection of breast cancer in patients with a BRCA mutation is significantly lower than that in the general population. This is likely due to the fact that patients with a BRCA mutation are younger at diagnosis and tend to have denser breast tissue [35].

33. c. Mammography.

Screening mammography is the only breast imaging modality that has been evaluated in case controlled studies and shown to reduce the death rate from breast cancer. In the late 1970s, a Swedish trial of over 130,000 women, showed a 30% reduction in breast cancer mortality with invitation to screening. Since then, numerous observational trials and follow-up of these patients have also shown mortality benefit. No other breast screening modality has been evaluated with such extensive case controlled studies [36].

34. b. Motion left MLO.

The left MLO view is degraded by motion. This is visualized as blurring of the lines in the left MLO view. Also, the round calcification in the left subareolar breast is much sharper on the left CC view than the left MLO view.

A is incorrect. The pacemaker does not make the study inadequate. It limits visualization of the axilla, and should be mentioned in the report.

C is incorrect. There are no significant skin folds.

D is incorrect. The right CC view includes adequate tissue as the retroglandular fat is visualized and the posterior nipple line on the right CC views measures within expected limits.

35a. b. Mass in the right upper outer breast.

Answer choice b is correct. There is a space-occupying mass visualized on two views in the right upper outer breast. The pertinent finding is a mass, not an asymmetry or a focal asymmetry. There are lymph nodes in the axilla bilaterally, which are of normal size and appearance.

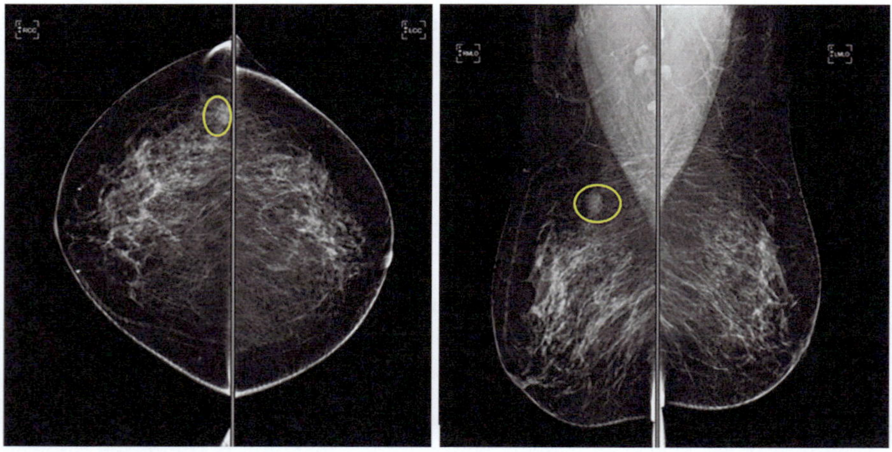

35b. c. BI-RADS 0.

Recommend additional evaluation with diagnostic mammography and ultrasound. Additional evaluation of the mass must be obtained to further characterize the mass.

A is incorrect. Although the abnormality is suspicious, the choices for BI-RADS assessment from screening mammography include 1,2, or 0. Additional evaluation must be obtained for further evaluation before any other BI-RADS category can be assigned.

B is incorrect. Breast MRI is not indicated in the evaluation of this lesion at this point. Breast MRI can be used for equivocal mammographic lesions, including one-view findings with no US correlate. It is not the first-line evaluation of breast masses. Breast MRI should never be used as a substitute for complete imaging evaluation (with mammography or ultrasound) or for biopsy [37].

d is incorrect. This mass requires further evaluation before a decision can be made if it is probably benign or requires biopsy. BI-RADS 3 cannot be assigned to a screening mammogram.

36. d. Inadequate technique, insufficient contrast enhancement.

There is no contrast in the study. There is a lack of contrast enhancement in the vessels, heart, and breast. The technologist did not notice that the contrast had not been injected and inadvertently obtained the post-contrast images.

a is incorrect. There is minimal, but not significant motion.

b is incorrect. This study is non-diagnostic. Breast MRI for detection of breast cancer must be performed following contrast administration. The most sensitive sequences for detection of breast abnormalities are dynamic T1-weighted contrast-enhanced series.

c is incorrect. The positioning of the breast is adequate. The nipples are in profile and centered and the entire breast is in the field of view.

Breast MRIs should be obtained on a scanner with a field strength of at least 1.5 T, to allow for adequate spatial resolution. Breast MRI must be obtained with a dedicated breast coil, with at least four channels. Newer coils have over 16 channels (increasing the number of channels improves the signal-to-noise ratio). Protocols can vary, and many centers include T2-weighted and Diffusion-Weighted imaging, however, the basis of the study are the dynamic T1-weighted post-contrast series. A pre-contrast T1-weighted sequence (most commonly axial) is followed by contrast infusion at a rate of approximately 2 mL/sec, followed by 2–5 post-contrast series. The use of dynamic series allows for evaluation of the rate of contrast enhancement and washout. This evaluation can be expedited with the use of commercially available CAD software. Abbreviated MRI protocols have recently been developed allowing reduction in cost and duration of breast MRI and increasing accessibility [38].

37. d. All of the above.

Multiple large studies have shown Digital Breast Tomosynthesis (DBT) detecting more cancers while reducing the screening call back rate as compared to Full Field Digital Mammography (FFDM). This leads to improved sensitivity and specificity of screening mammography. The improved cancer detection rate is mostly due to improved detection of invasive breast cancers. The detection of DCIS (Ductal Carcinoma in Situ) appears to be similar between DBT and FFDM [39, 40].

38. a. Asymmetries.

Asymmetries are responsible for a large number of false-positive screening mammograms. Asymmetries are often caused by overlapping breast tissue on

FFDM. DBT reduces the overlapping breast tissue as the breast can be visualized through a series of slices. Therefore, there are fewer unnecessary callbacks for asymmetries with DBT. Architectural distortions are much better visualized with DBT, and many times are caused by radial scars or other benign processes. So, DBT recall rates for distortions are actually higher than that of FFDM. Masses are better detected by DBT, but these are often cancers and lead to improvement in cancer detection rates [41].

39. d. None of the above.

The FDA approved computer-aided detection (CAD) for mammography in 1998, and the Centers for Medicare and Medicaid Services (CMS) provided increased payment in 2002 for mammograms interpreted with the use of CAD. Since then, CAD technology disseminated rapidly. Even though there has been little evidence that CAD improves the accuracy of mammographic interpretations, CAD is currently used by a large percentage of breast imaging centers in the USA. A very large-scale study for the Breast Cancer Surveillance Consortium published in 2015 showed no significant improvement with the use of CAD in interpreting screening mammograms. However, there are new investigational artificial intelligence-based computer-aided detection (AI-CAD) systems that have shown improved accuracy and sensitivity for detection of breast cancer in small trials. As of the time of this publication, these are not yet fully evaluated and are not widely commercially available [42, 43].

40. d. All of the above.

Whole breast ultrasound can be used as a supplementary screening tool, in conjunction with screening mammography, especially in women with dense breast tissue. Ultrasound can detect some lesions missed by mammography, especially in dense breast tissue. In women with dense breast tissue, screening mammography alone reduced advanced breast cancer by 31% over no screening mammography, while the combination of screening mammography and ultrasound reduced advanced breast cancer by 40% [44].

41. d. All of the above.

Whole breast screening by ultrasound can be performed by Automated Breast Volume Scanning (ABVS) or handheld ultrasound. Handheld ultrasound is the technique used in the diagnostic evaluation of the breast. These two techniques have been shown to have similar specificity and sensitivity. The advantage of the automated device is time saving. However, this will require eventual review by a radiologist who will bring the patient back for re-evaluation of any indeterminate lesion, similar to screening mammography.

The major criticism of screening ultrasound (as with screening mammography) is the relatively high false-positive rate (identification of lesions that are eventually shown to be benign). However, the false-positive rate can be reduced with long-term experience [45].

References

1. Breast Cancer Screening. In: ACR Appropriateness Criteria. American College of Radiology. 2017. https://acsearch.acr.org/docs/70910/Narrative/. Accessed 21 Dec 2020.
2. Breast Cancer Screening Guidelines for Women. In: What is Breast Cancer Screening? Centers for Disease Control and Prevention. https://www.cdc.gov/cancer/breast/pdf/breast-cancer-screening-guidelines-508.pdf. Accessed 21 Dec 2020.
3. ACR Practice Parameter for the Performance of Screening and Diagnostic Mammography. In: Practice Parameters and Technical Standards. American College of Radiology. 2018. https://www.acr.org/-/media/ACR/Files/Practice-Parameters/screen-diag-mammo.pdf. Accessed 27 Dec 2020.
4. Monticciolo DL, Newell MS, Moy L, Niell B, Monsees B, Sickles EA. Breast cancer screening in women at higher-than-average risk: recommendations from the ACR. J Am Coll Radiol. 2018;15:408–14.
5. Breast Imaging of Pregnant and Lactating Women. In: ACR Appropriateness Criteria. American College of Radiology. 2018. https://acsearch.acr.org/docs/3102382/Narrative/. Accessed 22 Dec 2020.
6. Elezaby M, Lees B, Maturen K, et al. BRCA mutation carriers: breast and ovarian cancer screening guidelines and imaging considerations. Radiology. 2019;291:554–69.
7. Breast Cancer: What are the Risk Factors? Centers for Disease Control and Prevention. https://www.cdc.gov/cancer/breast/basic_info/risk_factors.htm. Accessed 19 Apr 2021.
8. Bradley F, Hoover H, Hulka C, et al. The Sternalis muscle: an unusual Normal finding seen on mammography. AJR. 1996;166:33–6.
9. Freer P. Mammographic breast density: impact on breast cancer risk and implications for screening. Radiographics. 2015;35:302–15.
10. Winkler N, Raza S, Mackesy M, et al. Breast density: clinical implications and assessment methods. Radiographics. 2015;35:316–24.
11. Andolina V, Lille S. Mammographic imaging: a practical guide. 3rd ed. Baltimore, MD and Philadelphia, PA: Wolters Kluwer Health / Lippincott Williams & Wilkins; 2011.
12. DeFillippis E, Arleo E. The ABCs of accessory breast tissue: basic information every radiologist should know. AJR. 2014;202:1157–62.
13. Venta L, Dudiak C, Salomon C, et al. Sonographic evaluation of the breast. Radiographics. 1994;14:29–50.
14. Oliff M, Birdwell R, Raza S, et al. The breast Imager's approach to nonmammary masses at breast and axillary US: imaging technique, clues to origin, and management. Radiographics. 2016;36:7–18.
15. Dontchos B, Rahbar H, Partridge S, et al. Influence of menstrual cycle timing on screening breast MRI background parenchymal enhancement and diagnostic performance in premenopausal women. J Breast Imaging. 2019;1(3):205–11.
16. Giess C, Yeh E, Raza S, et al. Background parenchymal enhancement at breast MR imaging: Normal patterns, diagnostic challenges, and potential for false-positive and false-negative interpretation. Radiographics. 2014;34:234–47.
17. Baker J, Soo M, Rosen E. Artifacts and pitfalls in sonographic imaging of the breast. AJR. 2001;176:1261–6.
18. Charlot M, Beatrix O, Chateau F, et al. Pathologies of the male breast. Diagn Interv Imaging. 2013;94:26–37.
19. Ikeda D. Breast imaging: the requisites. 2nd ed. St. Louis, MO: Elsevier; 2011.
20. Nicholson B, Harvey J, Cohen M. Nipple-areolar complex: Normal anatomy and benign and malignant processes. Radiographics. 2009;29:509–23.
21. Ferris-James D, Iuanow E, Mehta T, et al. Imaging approaches to diagnosis and Management of Common Ductal Abnormalities. Radiographics. 2012;32:1009–30.
22. Kopans D. Breast imaging. 2nd ed. Philadelphia, PA: Lippincott-Raven; 1998.
23. Li C, Uribe D, Daling J. Clinical characteristics of different histologic types of breast cancer. Br J Cancer. 2005;93:1046–52.

24. Ecanow J, Abe H, Newstead G, et al. Axillary staging of breast cancer: what the radiologist should know. Radiographics. 2013;33(6):1589–612.
25. Dialani V, James D, Slanetz P. A practical approach to imaging the axilla. Insights Imaging. 2015;6(2):217–29.
26. Giess CS, Frost EP, Birdwell RL. Interpreting one-view mammographic findings: minimizing callbacks while maximizing cancer detection. Radiographics. 2014;34:928–94.
27. D'Orsi CJ, Bassett LW, Berg WA, et al. Mammography. In: Breast imaging reporting and data system (BI-RADS). 4th ed. Reston, Va: American College of Radiology; 2003.
28. Bassett L, Hirbawi I, DeBruhl N, et al. Mammographic positioning: evaluation from the view box. Radiology. 1993;188:803–6.
29. Hendrick RE, Bassett L, Botsco MA, et al. Mammography Quality Control Manual. American College of Radiology. 1999. https://www.acr.org/-/media/ACRAccreditation/Documents/Mammography/1999_Mammo_QCManual_Book_final.pdf. Accessed 21 Aug 2021.
30. Korhonen KE, Weinstein SP, McDonald ES, Conant EF. Strategies to increase cancer detection: review of true-positive and false-negative results at digital breast Tomosynthesis screening. Radiographics. 2016;36:1954–196.
31. Lamb LR, Mohallem Fonseca M, Verma R, Seely JM. Missed breast cancer: effects of subconscious bias and lesion characteristics. Radiographics. 2020;40:941–96.
32. Oliveira ELC, Freitas-Junior R, Afiune-Neto A, Murta EFC, Ferro JE, Melo AFB. Vascular calcifications seen on mammography: an independent factor indicating coronary artery disease. Clinics (Sao Paulo). 2009;64(3):763–7.
33. Ikeda DM, Miyake KK. The requisites: breast imaging. 3rd ed. St. Louis, Missouri: Elsevier; 2017.
34. Leung JWT, Sickles EA. Multiple bilateral masses detected on screening mammography assessment of need for recall imaging. AJR. 2000;175:23–9.
35. Bharucha P, Chiu K, François F, Scott J, Khorjekar G, Tirada N. Genetic testing and screening recommendations for patients with hereditary breast cancer. Radiographics. 2020;40(4):913–36.
36. Laszlo T, Vitak B, Chen H, et al. The Swedish Two-County trial twenty years later: updated mortality results and new insights from long-term follow-up. Radiol Clin N Am. 2000;38(4):625–51.
37. Giess C, Chikarmane S, Sippo D, Birdwell R. Breast MR imaging for equivocal mammographic findings: help or hindrance? Radiographics. 2016;36:943–58.
38. Mann R, Cho N, Moy L. Breast MRI: state of the art. Radiology. 2019;292:520–36.
39. Alsheikh N, Dabbous F, Pohlman S, et al. Comparison of resource utilization and clinical outcomes following screening with digital breast Tomosynthesis versus digital mammography: findings from a learning health system. Acad Radiol. 2019;26(5):597–605.
40. Friedewald S, Rafferty E, Rose S, et al. Breast cancer screening using Tomosynthesis in combination with digital mammography. JAMA. 2014;311(24):2499–507.
41. Durand M, Haas B, Yao X, et al. Early clinical experience with digital breast Tomosynthesis for screening mammography. Radiology. 2015;274(1):85–92.
42. Lehman C, Wellman R, Buist D, Kerlikowske K, Tosteson A, Miglioretti D. Diagnostic accuracy of digital screening mammography with and without computer-aided detection. JAMA Intern Med. 2015;175(11):1828–37.
43. Watanabe A, Lim V, Vu H, et al. Improved cancer detection using artificial intelligence: a retrospective evaluation of missed cancers on mammography. J Digit Imaging. 2019;32:625–37.
44. Grady I, Chanisheva N, Vasquez T. The addition of automated breast ultrasound to mammography in breast cancer screening decreases stage at diagnosis. Acad Radiol. 2017;24(12):1570–4.
45. Wang L, Qi Z. Automatic breast volume scanner versus handheld ultrasound in differentiation of benign and malignant breast lesions: a systematic review and meta-analysis. Ultrasound Med Biol. 2019;45(8):1874–81.

Diagnostic Mammogram and Ultrasound

Tiffany L. Chan, Tiffany Yu, and Irene Tsai

T. L. Chan (✉) · T. Yu
Department of Radiology, David Geffen School of Medicine at UCLA, Los Angeles, CA, USA
e-mail: tlchan@mednet.ucla.edu; TTYu@mednet.ucla.edu

I. Tsai
Breast Imaging, UCI Department of Radiological Sciences, Orange, CA, USA
e-mail: itsai@hs.uci.edu

© The Author(s), under exclusive license to Springer Nature Switzerland AG 2022
L. Chow, B. Li (eds.), *Absolute Breast Imaging Review*,
https://doi.org/10.1007/978-3-031-08274-0_4

1a. A 60-year-old female presents with a left breast palpable abnormality. What is the finding of the mammogram?

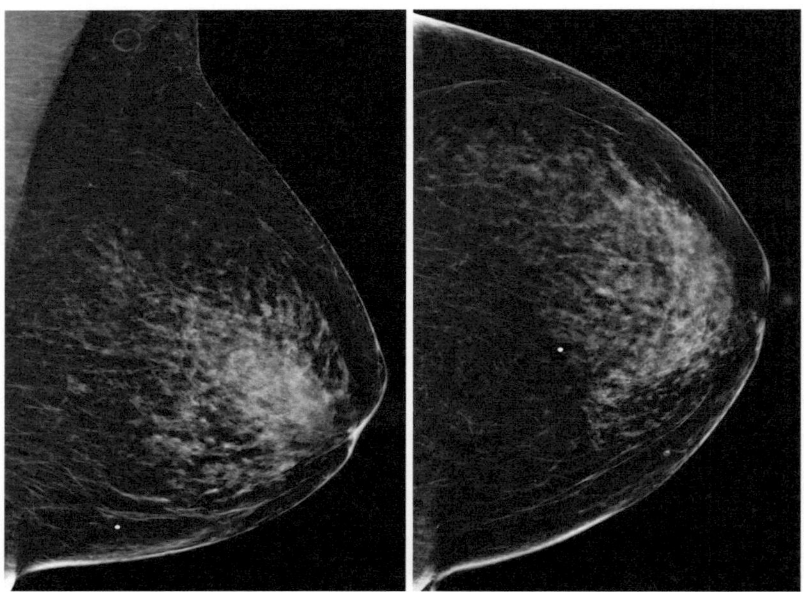

   (a) Fat-containing mass adjacent to the BB marker.
   (b) Architectural distortion in the area of the BB marker.
   (c) Fine pleomorphic calcifications in a linear distribution.
   (d) Irregular mass with spiculated margins.

1b. What is the next best step?
   (a) Magnification view.
   (b) Exaggerated craniocaudal view.
   (c) True lateral view.
   (d) Spot compression view.

1c. Spot compression views are obtained. What is the most likely diagnosis?

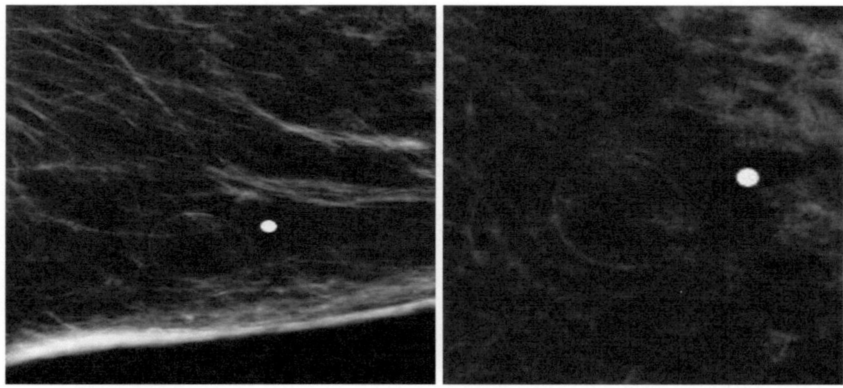

   (a) Hamartoma.
   (b) Fibroadenoma.
   (c) Lymph node.
   (d) Oil cyst.

1d. Which disorder is associated with multiple and extensive intradermal oil cysts?
   (a) Cowden disease.
   (b) Neurofibromatosis type 1.
   (c) Poland syndrome.
   (d) Steatocystoma multiplex.

2a. A 45-year-old female presents with a right breast palpable abnormality. Diagnostic ultrasound is performed. What is a key feature to diagnosing this finding?

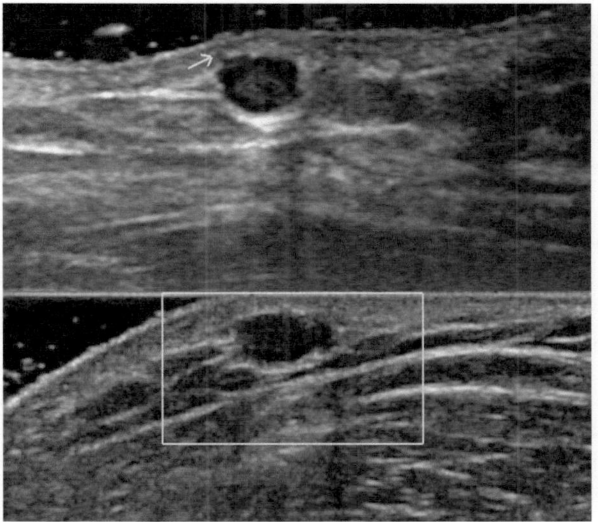

   (a) Hypoechoic.
   (b) Parallel.
   (c) Skin tract.
   (d) Avascular.

2b. What is the next best step?
   (a) Biopsy.
   (b) Aspiration.
   (c) Follow-up with ultrasound in 6 months.
   (d) No follow-up is needed.

3a. A 45-year-old female presents with a two-month history of left bloody nipple discharge. Diagnostic ultrasound demonstrates an intraductal mass that extends toward the nipple. What is the most common type of mass that produces bloody nipple discharge?

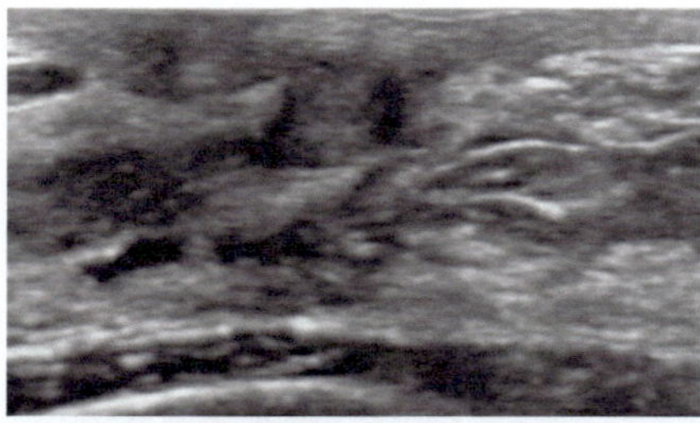 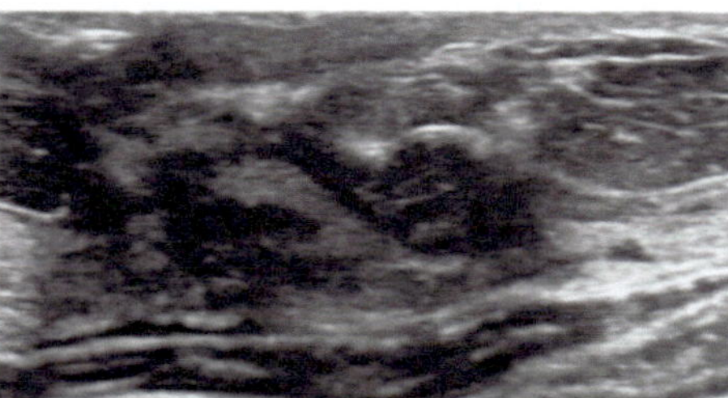

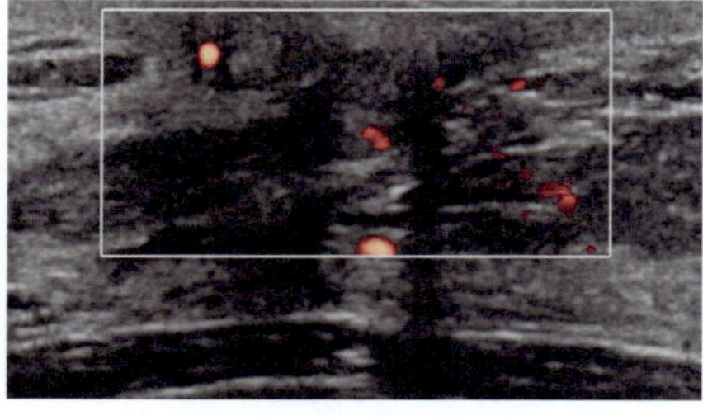

   (a) Prolactinoma.
   (b) Cyst.
   (c) Intraductal papilloma.
   (d) Ductal carcinoma in situ.

3b. Which of the following statements regarding papillomas is TRUE?
   (a) Peripheral papilloma presents as a solitary lesion.
   (b) Peripheral papillomas are more associated with malignancy than central papillomas.
   (c) Spontaneous nipple discharge is an atypical feature of papillomas.
   (d) Central papillomas almost always arise in the terminal ductal lobular unit.

3c. Which of the following features of nipple discharge is concerning for malignancy?
   (a) Spontaneous.
   (b) Arises from multiple ducts.
   (c) Bilateral.
   (d) Milky.

3d. What is the most appropriate management of suspicious nipple discharge if diagnostic mammogram and ultrasound are negative?
(a) FDG-PET.
(b) Molecular breast imaging.
(c) MRI.
(d) Follow-up with diagnostic mammogram and ultrasound in six months.

4a. A 47-year-old female presents for screening mammogram. What is the abnormality?

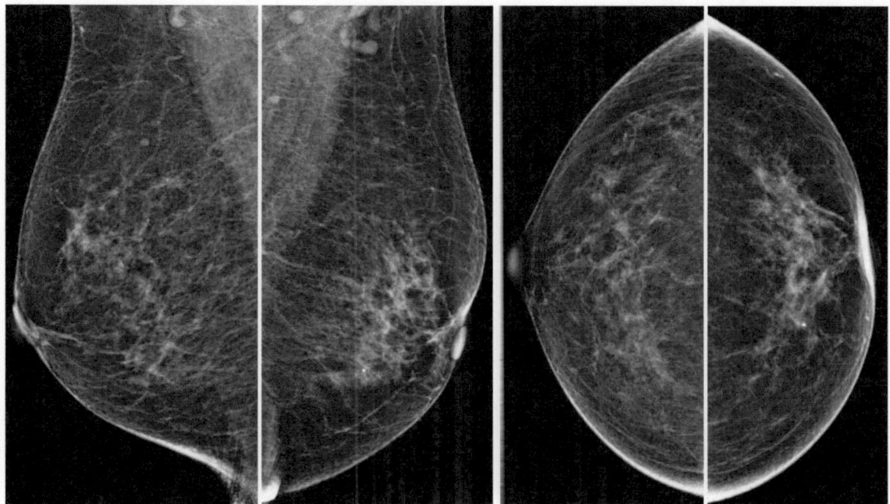

(a) Axillary lymphadenopathy.
(b) Calcifications.
(c) Irregular Mass.
(d) Nipple retraction.

4b. Biopsy results revealed invasive lobular carcinoma of the breast. What is the next best step?
(a) Contrast-enhanced MRI.
(b) Radiation Therapy.
(c) Molecular Breast Imaging.
(d) PET-CT.

5a. A 59-year-old female presents for two-month history of left breast redness, swelling, pain and low-grade fevers despite the use of antibiotics. Diagnostic mammogram and ultrasound are performed. What is the finding seen on the mammogram?

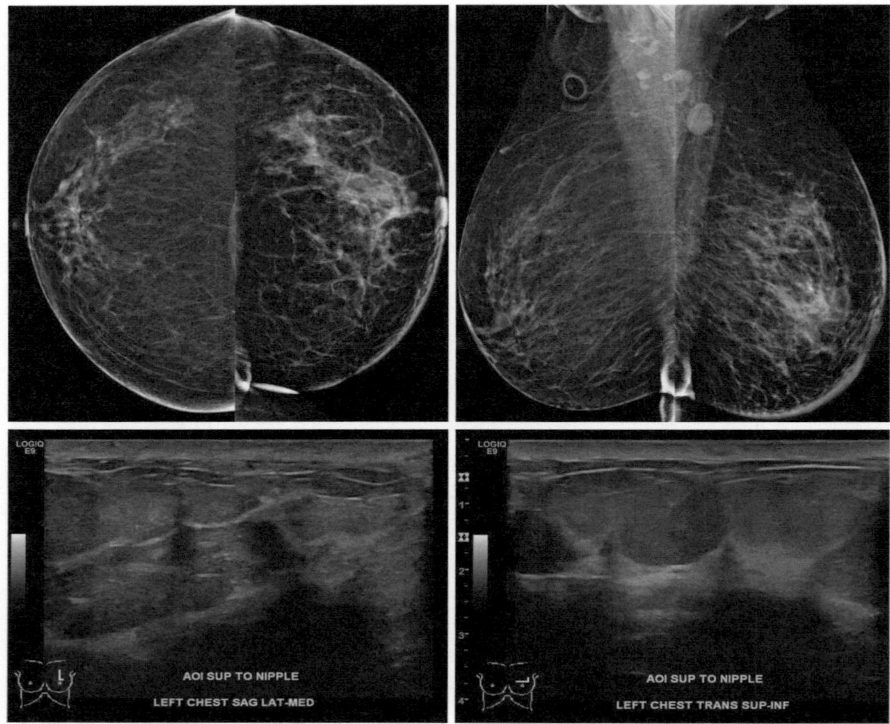

   (a) Architectural distortion.
   (b) Asymmetry.
   (c) Mass.
   (d) Skin thickening and increased trabeculation.

5b. Based on her presentation, what is the most likely diagnosis?
   (a) Congestive heart failure.
   (b) Inflammatory breast cancer.
   (c) Mastitis.
   (d) Post-radiation change.

5c. What is the next best step for t1his patient?
   (a) Skin punch biopsy.
   (b) Stereotactic core needle biopsy.
   (c) Ultrasound-guided core needle biopsy.
   (d) MRI-guided core needle biopsy.

5d. For patients presenting with mastitis and/or breast abscess, what is the most appropriate management after antibiotics?
  (a) Clinical follow-up.
  (b) Reassurance.
  (c) Follow-up imaging.
  (d) Self-breast exam.

6a. Magnification views are obtained on a diagnostic mammogram study to further evaluate calcifications seen on screening mammogram. Calcifications span above and below the nipple. Which of the following descriptions best describes the morphology and distribution of these calcifications?

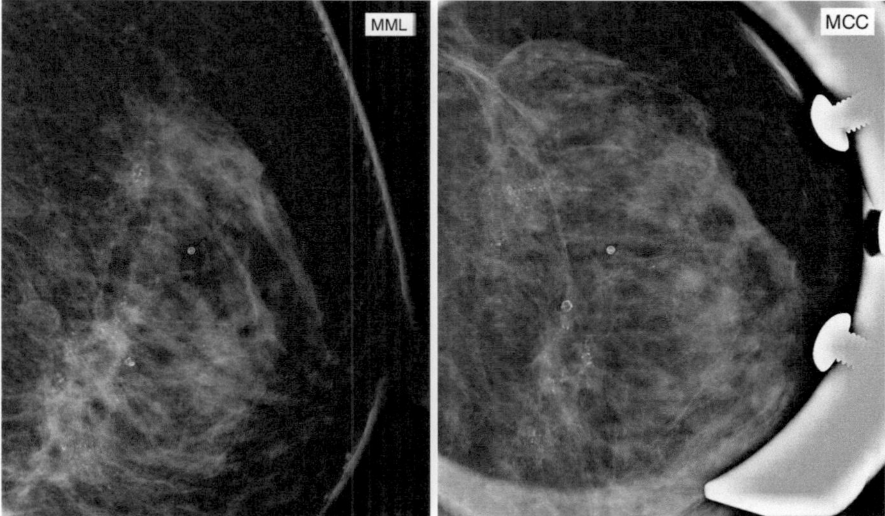

  (a) Round, regional.
  (b) Fine pleomorphic, segmental.
  (c) Fine pleomorphic, regional.
  (d) Rod-like, regional.

6b. What is the most appropriate BI-RADS classification for these calcifications?
  (a) BI-RADS 4A.
  (b) BI-RADS 4B.
  (c) BI-RADS 4C.
  (d) BI-RADS 5.

7a. A 70-year-old female presents for a callback of left breast calcifications. What is the best descriptor for these calcifications?

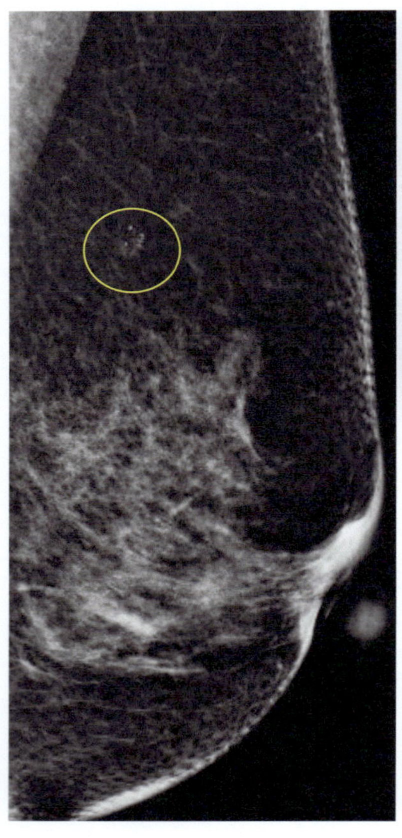

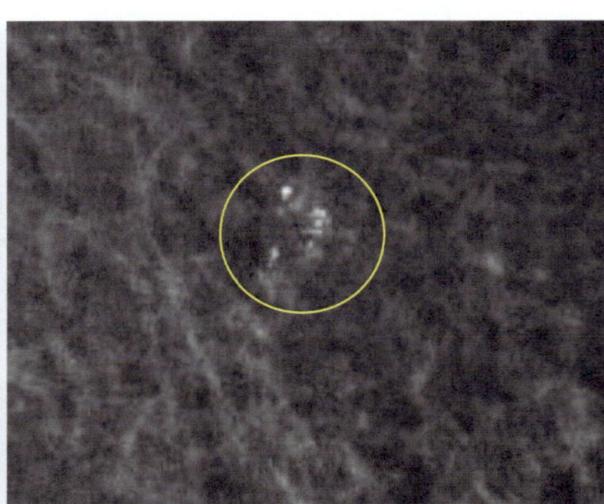

(a) Grouped punctate calcifications.
(b) Regional coarse heterogeneous calcifications.
(c) Grouped coarse heterogeneous calcifications.
(d) Grouped round calcifications.

7b. What is the most appropriate BI-RADS category for these calcifications?
(a) BI-RADS 3.
(b) BI-RADS 4A.
(c) BI-RADS 4B.
(d) BI-RADS 4C.

8a. A 45-year-old female presents with a right breast palpable abnormality. Diagnostic mammogram is obtained. What is the next best step?

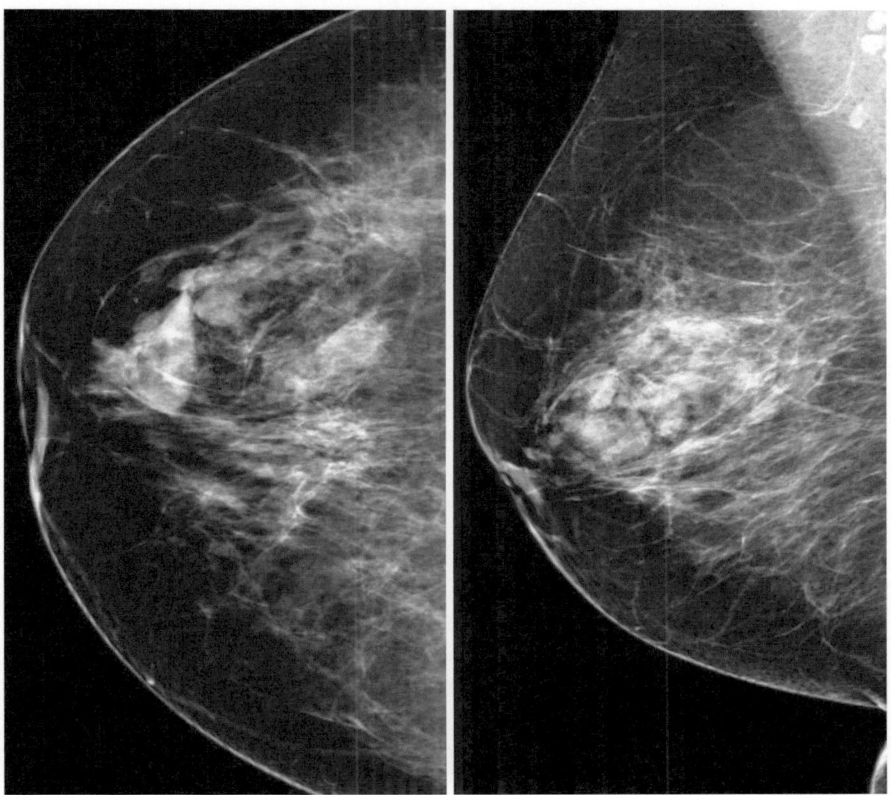

(a) Rolled views.
(b) True lateral view.
(c) Spot compression.
(d) Magnification.

8b. Spot compression images are obtained. What is the BI-RADS assessment?

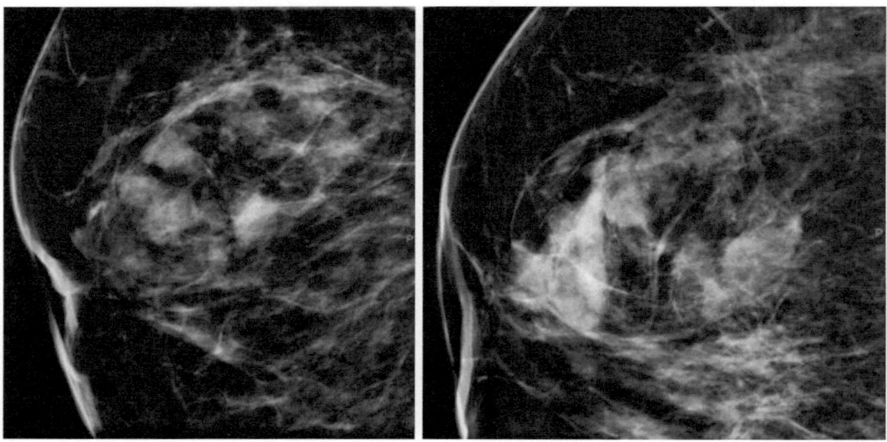

   (a) BI-RADS 2.
   (b) BI-RADS 3.
   (c) BI-RADS 4.
   (d) Needs diagnostic ultrasound prior to making a BI-RADS assessment.

8c. If ultrasound imaging was obtained for the above hamartoma, what is the expected typical sonographic appearance?
   (a) Oval, circumscribed, parallel mass with uniformly hypoechoic echogenicity.
   (b) Oval, circumscribed, parallel mass with mixed hypo- and hyperechoic echogenicity.
   (c) Oval, parallel mass with indistinct margins and isoechoic echogenicity.
   (d) Irregular, parallel mass with indistinct margins and mixed hypo- and hyperechoic echogenicity.

9. A 80-year-old female taking anticoagulation medications presents with the following diagnostic mammography and ultrasound findings. What is on the differential diagnosis?

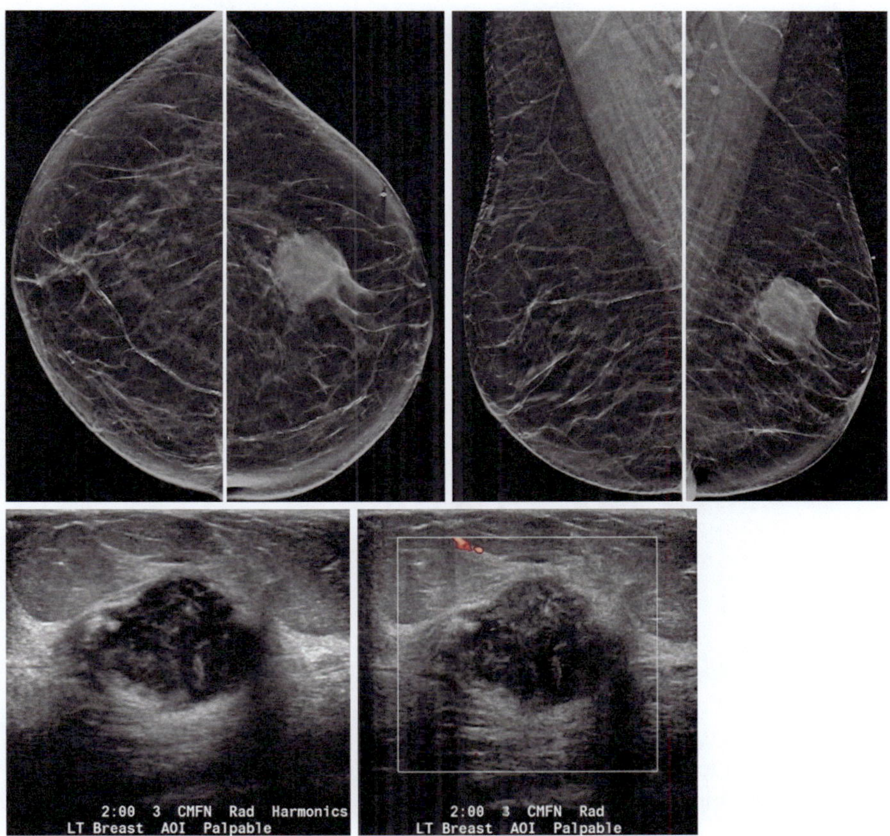

(a) Malignancy.
(b) Hematoma.
(c) Abscess.
(d) All of the above.

10a. A 68-year-old female presents with a palpable abnormality. Diagnostic mammogram and ultrasound images are below. Where is the finding on mammographic views?

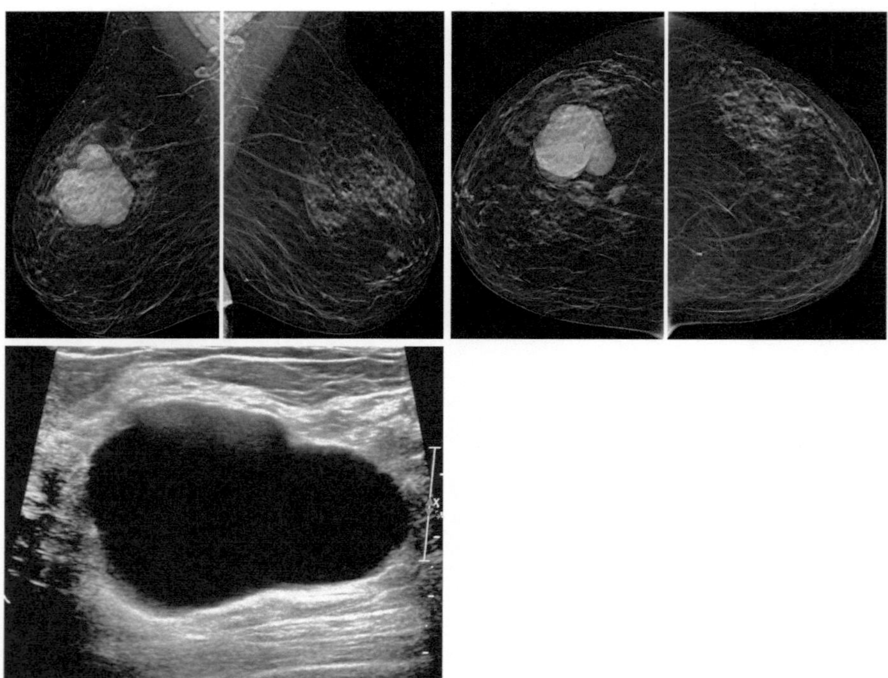

    (a) Right upper outer quadrant.
    (b) Right lower outer quadrant.
    (c) Left upper outer quadrant.
    (d) Left lower outer quadrant.

10b. Based on the mammogram and ultrasound findings, what is the BI-RADS assessment?
    (a) BI-RADS 2.
    (b) BI-RADS 3.
    (c) BI-RADS 4.
    (d) BI-RADS 5.

10c. What BI-RADS assessment should be given for a simple cyst for which a patient desires aspiration?
    (a) BI-RADS 2.
    (b) BI-RADS 3.
    (c) BI-RADS 4.
    (d) BI-RADS 0.

10d. Which of the following types of fluid aspirated from a simple cyst should be sent to cytology for further evaluation?
 (a) Clear.
 (b) Green.
 (c) Bloody.
 (d) Blue.

11a. A 35-year-old female, currently breastfeeding, presents with a palpable breast lump. Diagnostic ultrasound is performed. What is the most characteristic feature of this finding?

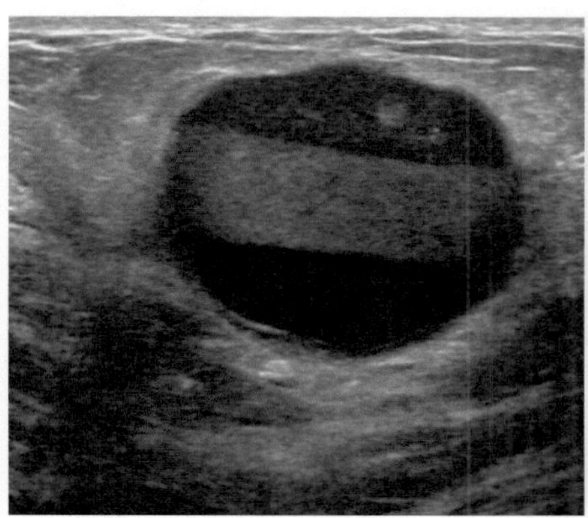 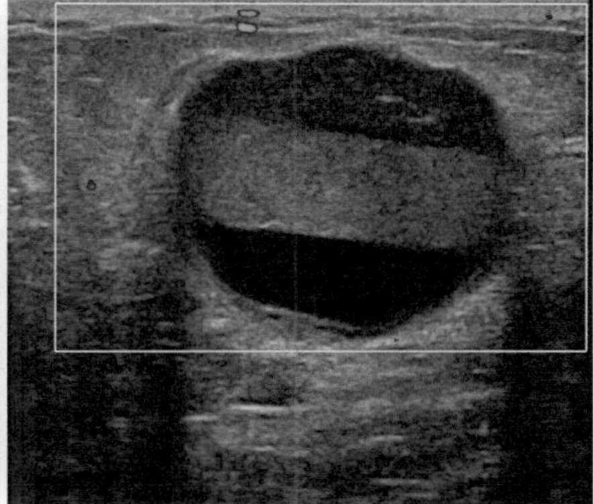

 (a) Retracting mural clot.
 (b) Fat-fluid level.
 (c) Posterior acoustic enhancement.
 (d) Circumscribed margins.

11b. Which of the following is a complication of galactocele?
 (a) Malignancy.
 (b) Infection.
 (c) Malignancy and infection.
 (d) Hematoma.

12a. A 35-year-old female who is 12 weeks postpartum and breastfeeding present with a right breast palpable abnormality for six weeks. What is the most appropriate initial diagnostic imaging modality for this patient?
 (a) Bilateral diagnostic mammogram and right breast ultrasound.
 (b) Right diagnostic mammogram and right breast ultrasound.
 (c) Bilateral diagnostic mammogram and bilateral breast ultrasound.
 (d) Right breast ultrasound.
 (e) Bilateral breast ultrasound.

12b. Targeted right breast ultrasound is performed. Based on the findings, what area, if any, should be scanned next?

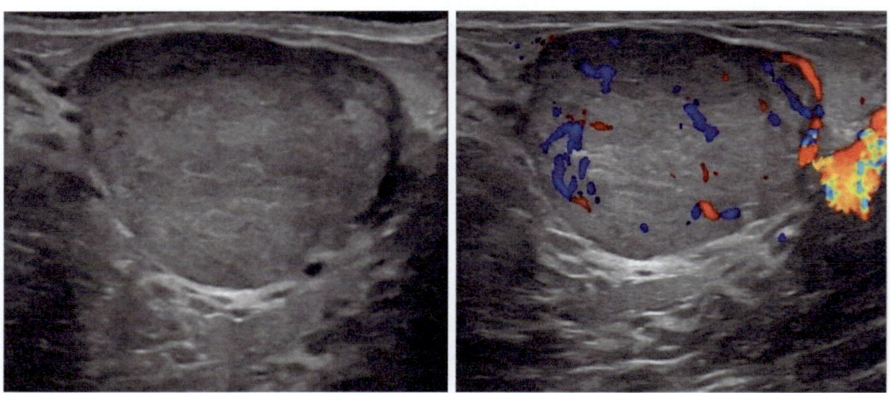

    (a) No further images are necessary.
    (b) Ultrasound of the ipsilateral axilla.
    (c) Ultrasound of contralateral breast.
    (d) Ultrasound of the contralateral breast and bilateral axillae.

12c. The right axilla is scanned. Based on the breast and axilla findings, what is the most appropriate BI-RADS assignment?

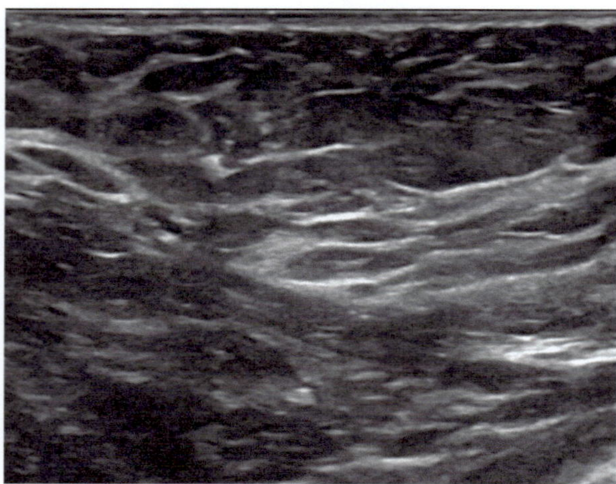

    (a) BI-RADS 3, follow-up with right breast ultrasound in 3 months.
    (b) BI-RADS 3, follow-up with right breast ultrasound in 6 months.
    (c) BI-RADS 4, ultrasound-guided core needle biopsy.
    (d) BI-RADS 4, breast surgical consultation.

12d. What is a specific complication unique to this situation that the patient must be consented for prior to biopsy?

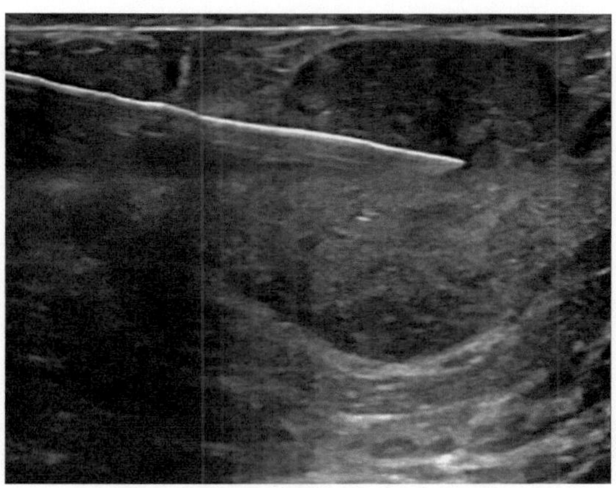

   (a) Milk fistula.
   (b) Hematoma.
   (c) Infection/abscess.
   (d) Vasovagal reaction.

12e. The patient undergoes ultrasound-guided core needle biopsy. Pathology reveals a lactating adenoma. What radiological pathology correlation and recommendation is most appropriate?
   (a) Discordant, breast surgical consultation recommended.
   (b) Concordant, routine annual mammography at age 40 years.
   (c) Concordant, follow-up right breast ultrasound in 6 months.
   (d) Concordant, clinical follow up to ensure resolution after cessation of breastfeeding.

13a. A 61-year-old female with known gastric cancer presents for evaluation of a right breast palpable abnormality. What is the finding on the initial diagnostic MLO and CC mammographic views?

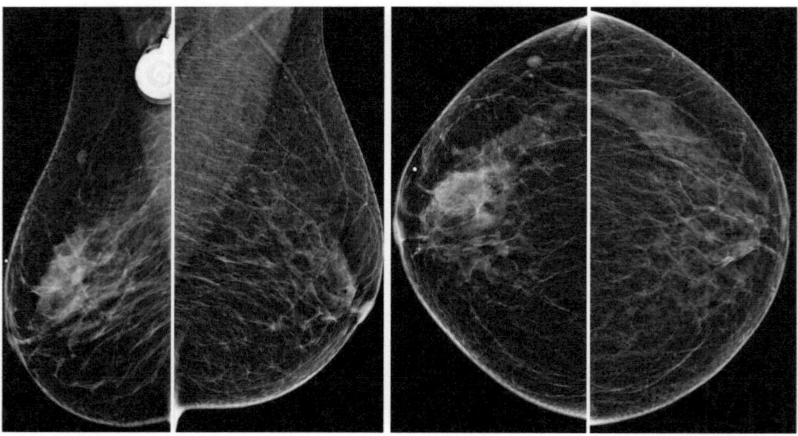

    (a) Mixed-density fat-containing mass.
    (b) Hypodense mass with microlobulated margins.
    (c) Unilateral increased skin thickening.
    (d) Focal asymmetry.

13b. What is the most appropriate next step?
    (a) Spot compression mammographic views and ultrasound.
    (b) Rolled mammographic views and ultrasound.
    (c) XCCL views and ultrasound.
    (d) Magnification mammographic views and ultrasound.

13c. Spot compression mammographic views and ultrasound are obtained. What is
the appropriate management recommendation?

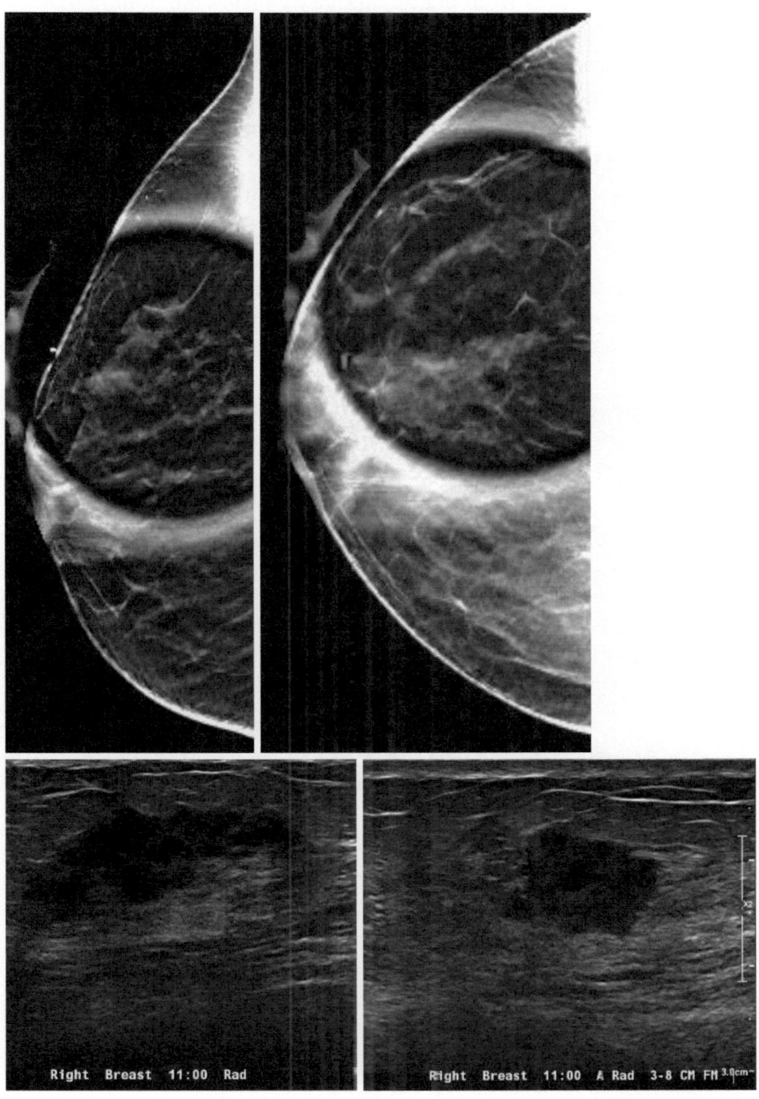

(a) Antibiotics with short-term interval follow-up with ultrasound.
(b) Ultrasound-guided core needle biopsy.
(c) Stereotactic core needle biopsy.
(d) Breast MRI.

13d. Which of the following statements is true regarding breast metastases from extramammary malignancies?
- (a) Breast metastases from extramammary cancers are common and usually represent poor prognosis.
- (b) The most common location for extramammary metastases to the breast is the upper-outer quadrant.
- (c) Colon cancer is the most common extramammary malignancy to metastasize to the breast.
- (d) The most common mammographic appearance of any extramammary metastasis is a spiculated mass.

14a. A 31-year-old female presents with a right breast palpable abnormality which she has felt for many years, but it has significantly increased in size over the last 3 months. What is the most appropriate management for the sonographic finding?

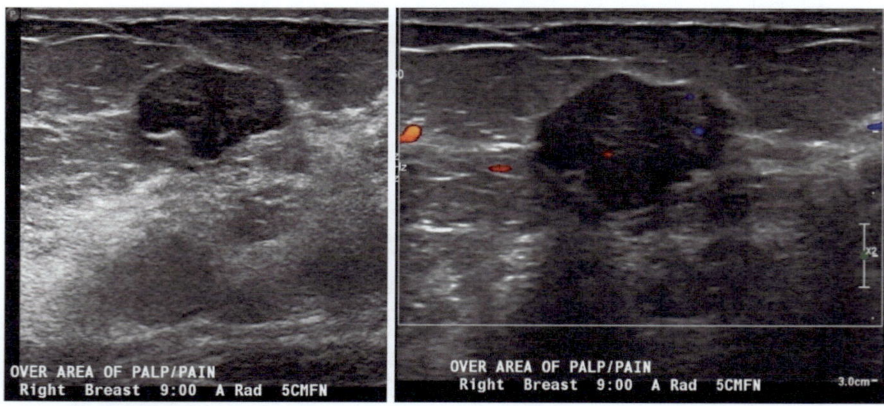

- (a) No imaging follow-up; clinical follow-up as indicated.
- (b) Short-term follow-up with sonography in 6 months.
- (c) Ultrasound-guided core needle biopsy.
- (d) Referral for surgical consultation.

14b. Which of the following is an atypical imaging feature for fibroadenoma?
- (a) Internal vascularity.
- (b) Posterior acoustic shadowing.
- (c) Microlobulated margins.
- (d) Hypoechoic echotexture.

14c. What amount of interval growth of a probable fibroadenoma warrants biopsy?
- (a) >10%.
- (b) >20%.
- (c) >30%.
- (d) >50%.

15a. A 65-year-old asymptomatic female presents for screening mammogram with no prior exams. What is the BI-RADS assessment and recommendation?

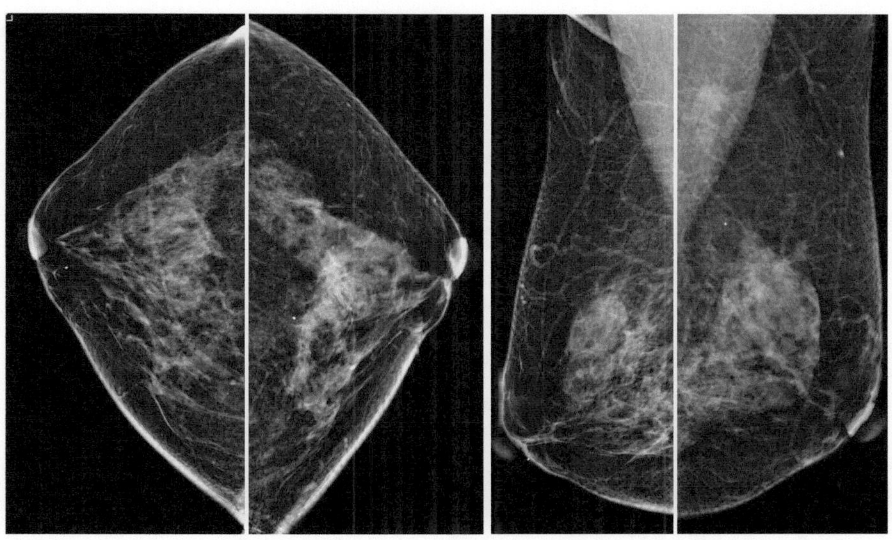

   (a) BI-RADS 1, routine annual mammography recommended.
   (b) BI-RADS 0, left breast spot compression views and ultrasound recommended.
   (c) BI-RADS 0, left breast magnification views and ultrasound recommended.
   (d) BI-RADS 0, left breast ultrasound recommended.

15b. How many abnormalities are seen in the left breast?
   (a) 1.
   (b) 2.
   (c) 3.
   (d) 4.

15c. Spot compression views and targeted ultrasound are performed. What is the most appropriate BI-RADS category for this exam?

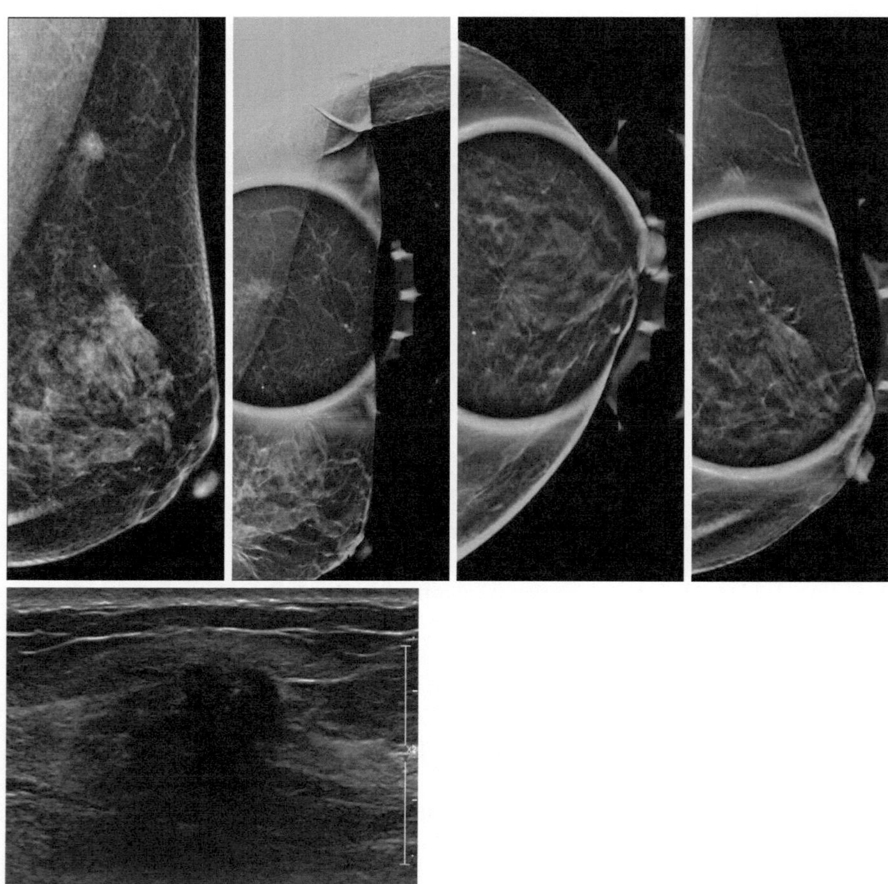

(a) BI-RADS 1.
(b) BI-RADS 2.
(c) BI-RADS 3.
(d) BI-RADS 4.

16a. A 70-year-old female is recalled from screening mammogram for a developing finding in the right medial breast compared to prior imaging. What is the most appropriate descriptor of this finding?

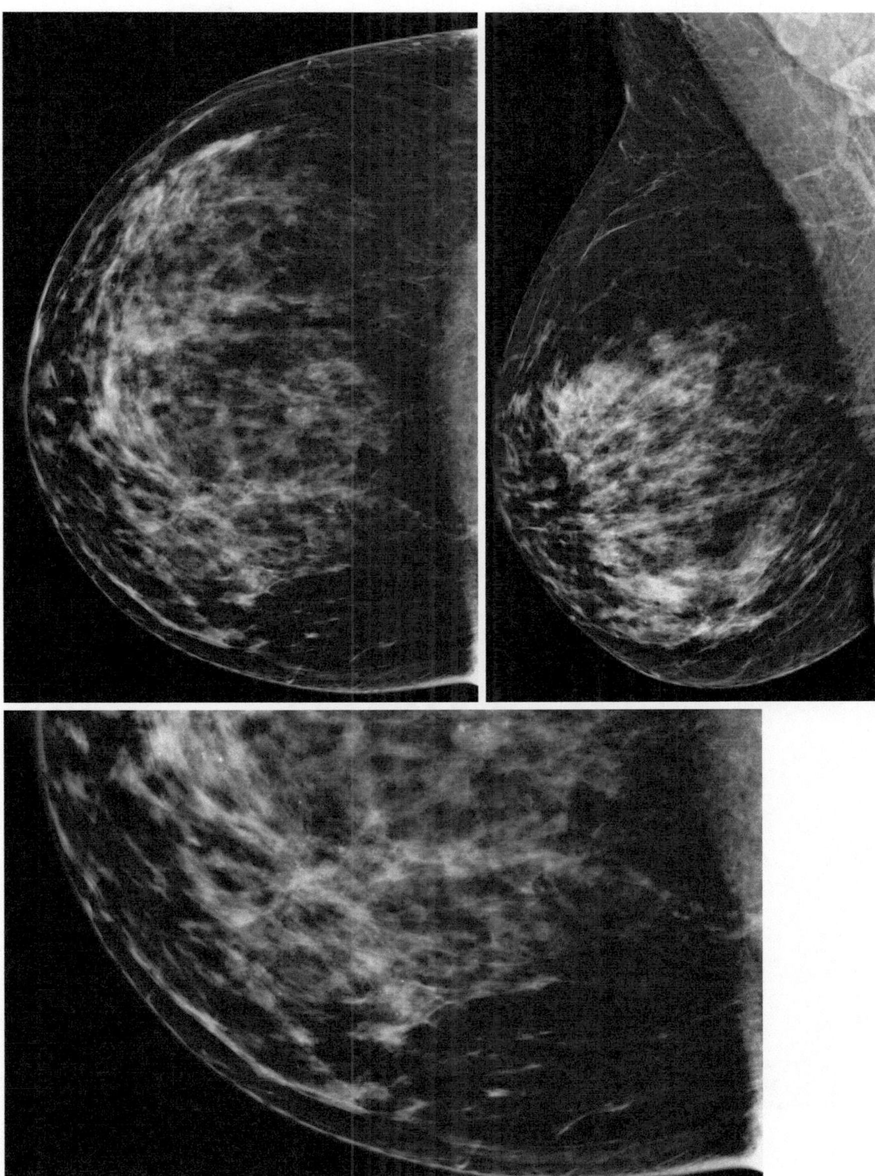

    (a) Architectural distortion.
    (b) Focal asymmetry.
    (c) Oil cyst.
    (d) Nipple retraction.

16b. Diagnostic mammogram and ultrasound are performed. Spot compression demonstrates persistence of the architectural distortion. No sonographic correlate is seen on ultrasound. What is the most appropriate BI-RADS assignment and management?
(a) BI-RADS 1, return to routine annual mammography.
(b) BI-RADS 2, return to routine annual mammography.
(c) BI-RADS 3, follow-up diagnostic mammogram in 6 months.
(d) BI-RADS 4, ultrasound-guided core needle biopsy.
(e) BI-RADS 4, stereotactic core needle biopsy.

16c. This finding underwent stereotactic core needle biopsy with pathology demonstrating tubular carcinoma, grade 1. What radiologic pathologic correlation should be assigned?
(a) Malignant concordant.
(b) Benign concordant.
(c) Benign discordant.
(d) Malignant discordant.

17a. A 50-year-old female presents for screening mammogram. Prior year screening mammogram is also provided for reference. MLO views of (a) current screening mammogram and (b) prior year screening mammogram for the same female patient. What is the abnormality?

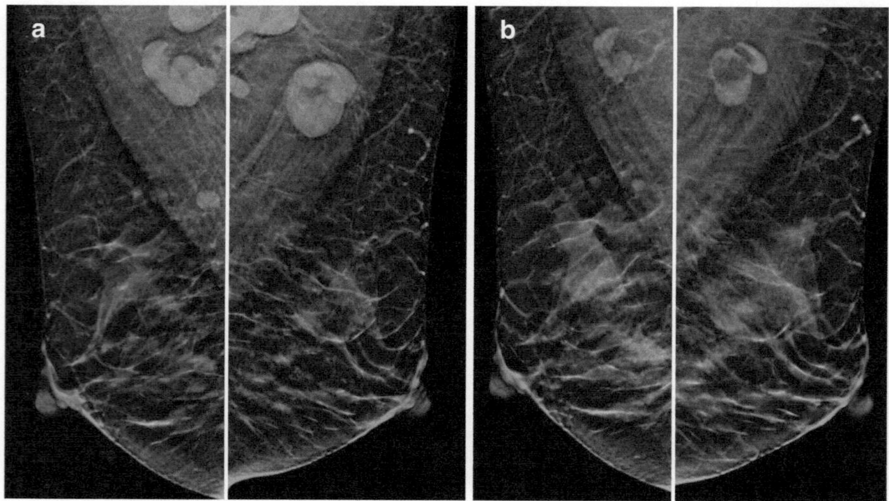

(a) New breast masses.
(b) Increased fatty breast density.
(c) Bilateral axillary lymphadenopathy.
(d) No abnormality.

17b. What is the best next step?
  (a) Clinical follow-up as indicated.
  (b) Diagnostic MRI.
  (c) Diagnostic ultrasound.
  (d) No imaging or clinical follow-up needed.

17c. Diagnostic ultrasound confirms abnormal lymph nodes with loss of the normal central fatty hilum. What is the size criteria of cortical thickening for axillary lymphadenopathy?

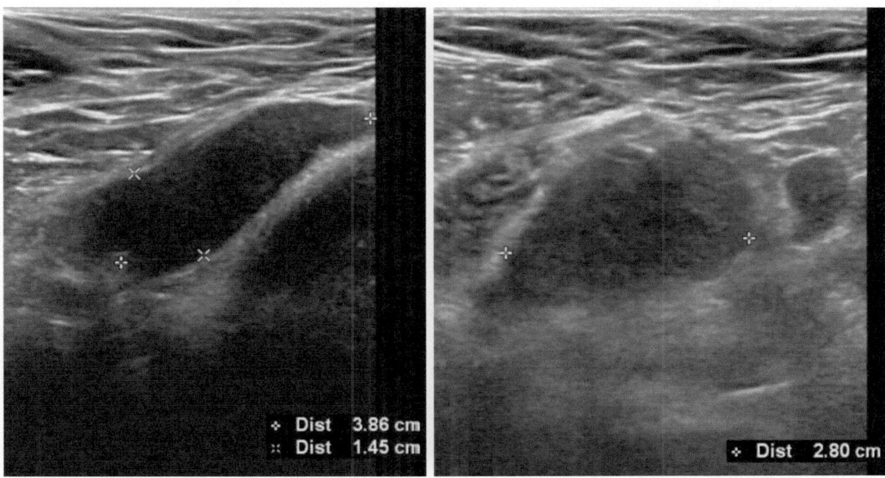

  (a) Cortical thickness greater than 3 mm.
  (b) Cortical thickness greater than 10 mm.
  (c) Cortical thickness greater than 15 mm.
  (d) Long-axis greater than 10 mm.

17d. What is the best next step?
  (a) Biopsy the right axillary lymph nodes.
  (b) Recommend follow-up ultrasound in 6 months.
  (c) Question the patient about her medical history, including underlying systemic diseases and concurrent illnesses.
  (d) Assign these lymph nodes a BI-RADS 2 and instruct the patient to follow up with her ordering clinician.

17e. The patient denies any known systemic, autoimmune diseases, or current illnesses. Given this history, what is the most appropriate BI-RADS assignment and management?
   (a) BI-RADS 2, recommend clinical follow-up for causes of bilateral axillary lymphadenopathy.
   (b) BI-RADS 3, recommend follow-up bilateral axillary ultrasound in 6 months.
   (c) BI-RADS 4, recommend ultrasound-guided core needle biopsy of both axillae.
   (d) BI-RADS 4, recommend ultrasound-guided core needle biopsy of the largest axillary lymph node in either the right or left axilla.

18a. A 25-year-old female with a left nipple ring presents with a fever, focal left subareolar erythema and a palpable abnormality. What is the most appropriate initial imaging study for this patient?
   (a) Mammogram.
   (b) Ultrasound.
   (c) MRI.
   (d) Image-guided core needle biopsy.

18b. Targeted ultrasound of the left breast is performed. What is the most likely diagnosis?

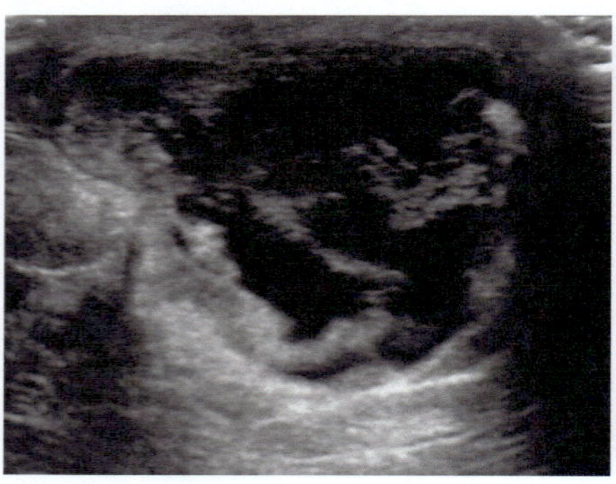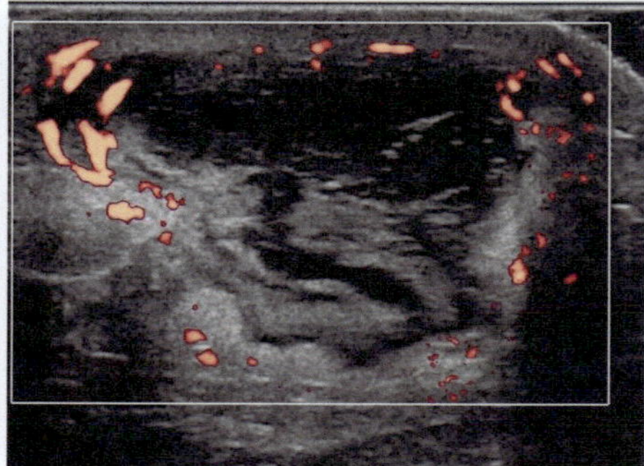

   (a) Malignancy.
   (b) Abscess.
   (c) Seroma.
   (d) Sebaceous cyst.

19a. A 49-year-old female presents with a palpable lump in the left breast, and has associated overlying erythema. What is the most appropriate initial imaging study?
   (a) Mammogram.
   (b) Ultrasound.
   (c) MRI.
   (d) Image-guided core needle biopsy.

19b. A mammogram is performed. What is the most suspicious feature of the primary abnormal finding?

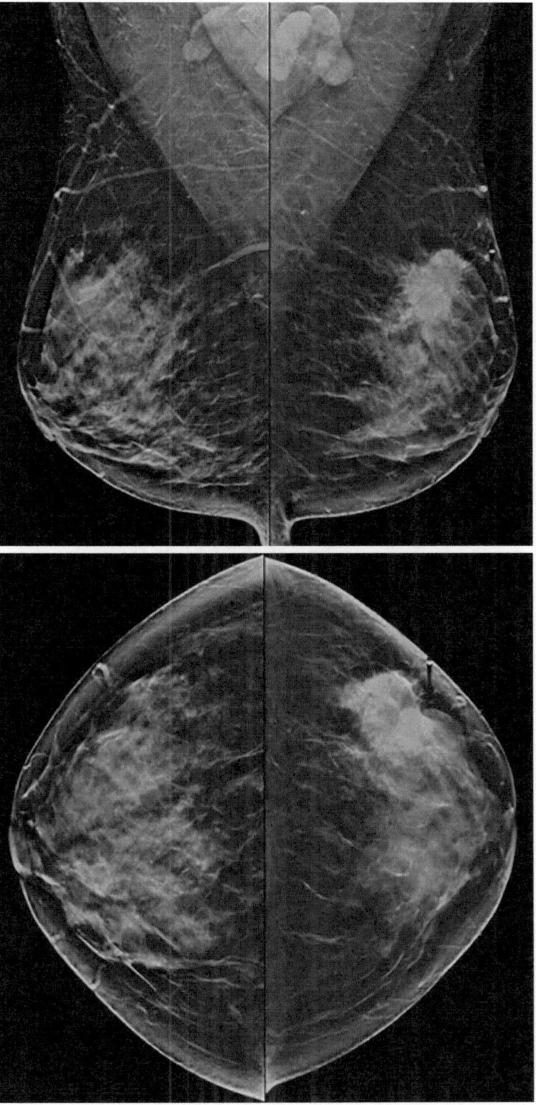

(a) Margins.
(b) Nipple retraction.
(c) Size.
(d) Extensive calcifications.

19c. What is the most likely diagnosis for this spiculated breast mass?
  (a) Ductal carcinoma in situ.
  (b) Invasive ductal carcinoma.
  (c) Metastatic extramammary malignancy.
  (d) Post-biopsy scar.

20a. A 29-year-old female presents with a left breast abnormality. Diagnostic ultrasound is performed. What is the next best step?

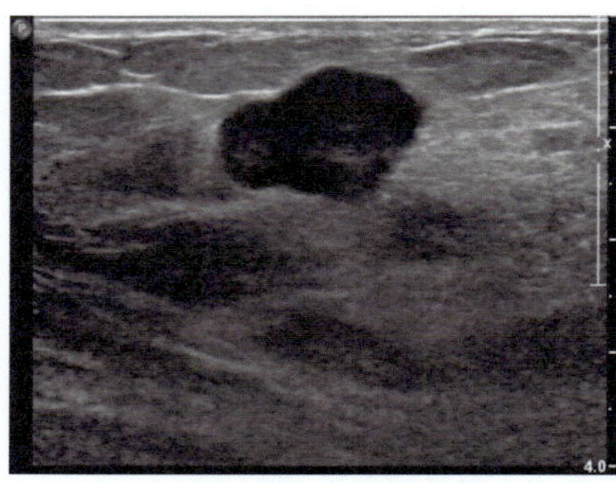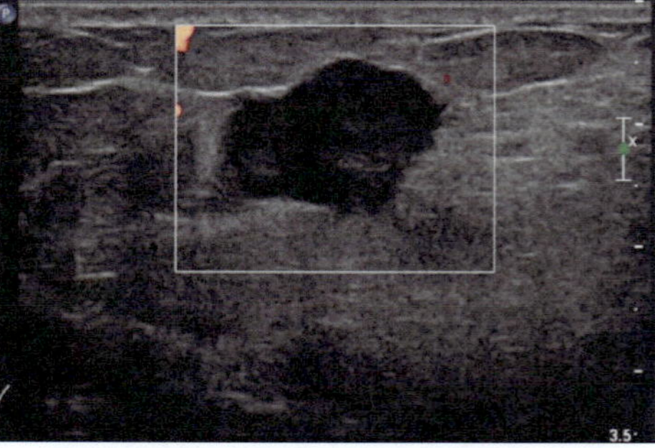

  (a) Clinical follow-up as indicated.
  (b) Breast MRI for further evaluation.
  (c) Ultrasound-guided core needle biopsy.
  (d) Genetic testing.

20b. Which of the following statements regarding triple-negative invasive ductal carcinoma (IDC) is true?
  (a) Triple-negative IDC tends to affect younger women.
  (b) Triple-negative IDC is often associated with ductal carcinoma in situ.
  (c) Triple-negative IDC has the best prognosis of all breast cancer subtypes.
  (d) Triple-negative IDC typically has spiculated margins.

21a. A 43-year-old female is called back for a new right breast mass seen on routine screening mammography. Targeted left breast sonography demonstrates a well-circumscribed, parallel, hypoechoic mass with internal anechoic foci. The patient underwent ultrasound-guided core needle biopsy revealing pseudoangiomatous stromal hyperplasia (PASH). What is the mammographic appearance of PASH?

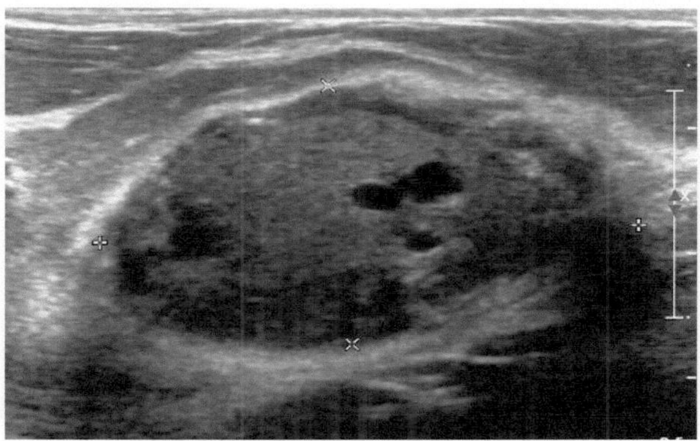

(a) Circumscribed, homogeneous mass.
(b) Focal asymmetry.
(c) Mammographically occult.
(d) All of the above.

21b. Which of the following statements is FALSE regarding PASH?
(a) PASH is characterized by a complex network of slit-like spaces lined by slender spindle cells within a background of stromal hyperplasia.
(b) PASH is more commonly seen in premenopausal women.
(c) PASH is a high-risk lesion with malignant potential.
(d) PASH can be mistaken for a low-grade angiosarcoma.

22a. A 35-year-old female presents for evaluation of a right breast palpable abnormality with pain for two months. She has been previously treated with two courses of antibiotics in the past for the same issue, with minimal improvement. She reports no family history of breast cancer. What are the pertinent imaging findings on diagnostic mammogram?

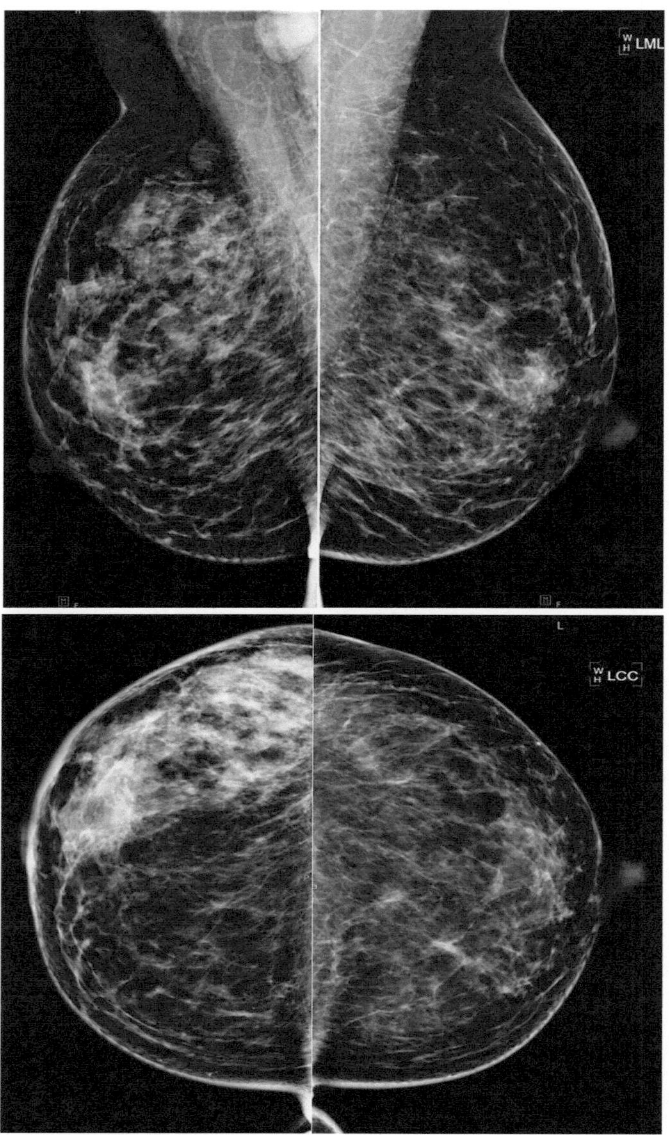

(a) Increased trabeculation and skin thickening involving the entire right upper outer breast and enlarged right axillary lymph node.
(b) Large asymmetry in the left lateral breast.
(c) Normal mammogram.
(d) Large mass in the right upper outer breast.

22b. Diagnostic ultrasound of the upper outer quadrant of the right breast (images a–c), axillary tail (image d), and axilla (image e) was performed. What is the most appropriate BI-RADS assessment?

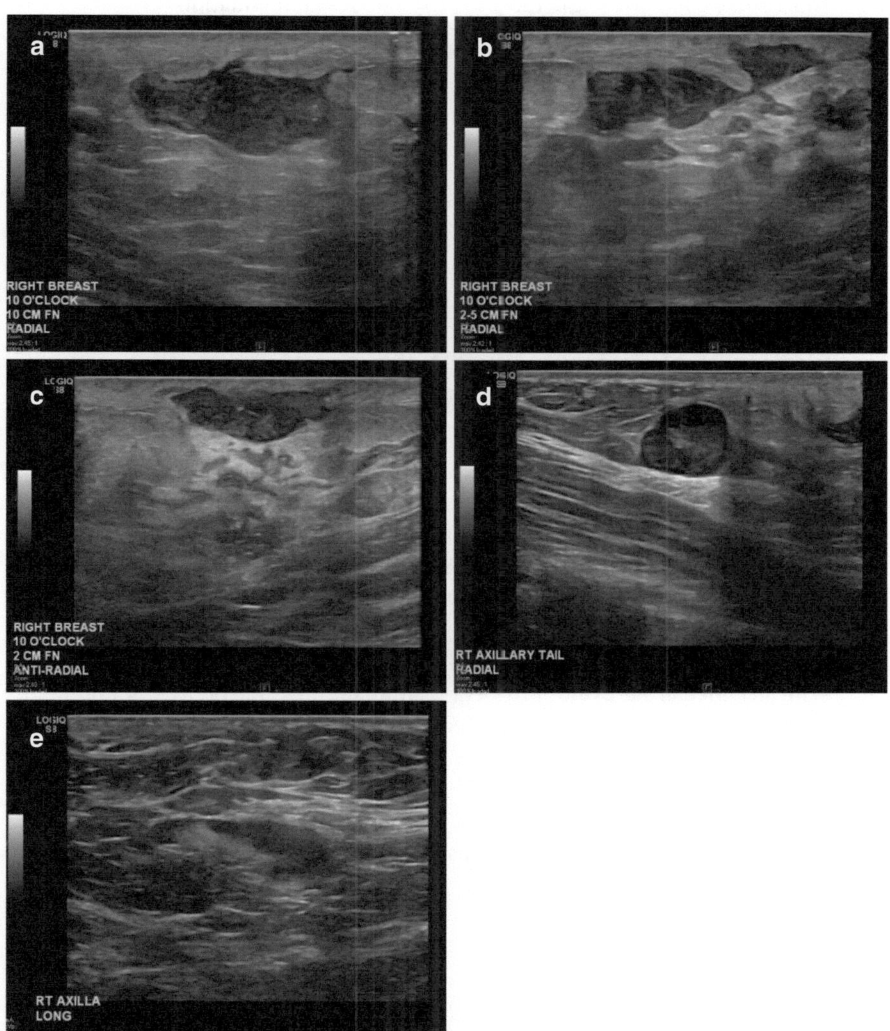

(a) BI-RADS 2, recommends clinical follow-up.
(b) BI-RADS 3, recommends clinical follow-up and antibiotic treatment.
(c) BI-RADS 4, recommends surgical consultation.
(d) BI-RADS 4, recommends ultrasound-guided core needle biopsy of the largest hypoechoic area.

22c. Ultrasound-guided core needle biopsy is performed. Pathology returns as "acute and chronic granulomatous inflammation, several well-formed non-necrotizing granulomas." What is the radiologic-pathologic concordance of this result, and what is the most appropriate recommendation?

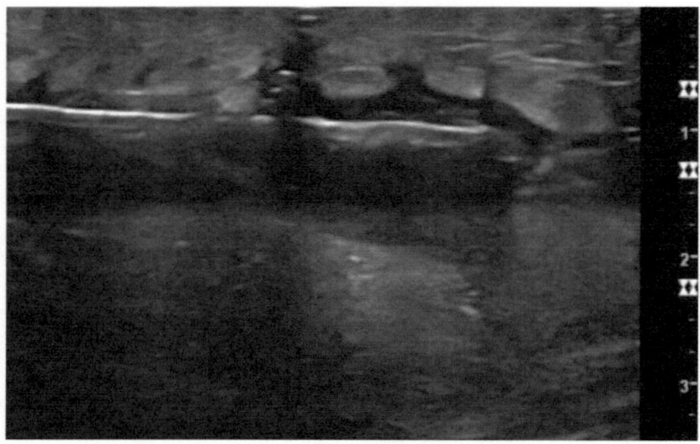

    (a) Benign and Discordant, surgical consultation for excision.
    (b) Benign and Concordant, return for mammogram at age 40 years.
    (c) Benign and Discordant, repeat ultrasound-guided biopsy.
    (d) Benign and Discordant, repeat stereotactic biopsy.
    (e) Benign and Concordant, surgical consultation for further management

23a. A 25-year-old female presents with diffuse bilateral breast pain that occurs with her menstrual cycle. Physical examination of her breasts is unremarkable. Which of the following is a feature of clinically significant breast pain?
    (a) Diffuse breast pain.
    (b) Cyclical breast pain.
    (c) Focal breast pain.
    (d) Any breast pain in a woman under age 30.

23b. What is the most appropriate initial imaging study for this patient?
    (a) No imaging needed.
    (b) Ultrasound.
    (c) Mammography.
    (d) MRI.

23c. A patient with focal, nonpalpable, and noncyclic breast pain undergoes further evaluation with mammogram and ultrasound which are both negative. What is the next best step?
    (a) Breast MRI.
    (b) PET-CT.
    (c) Biopsy.
    (d) Clinical follow-up.

24a. A large area of fine pleomorphic calcifications spanning the 9:00 axis from anterior to posterior depth in a segmental distribution measuring up to 7.3 cm in maximal superior-inferior dimension is noted on diagnostic mammogram. What BI-RADS assignment should be given to these calcifications?

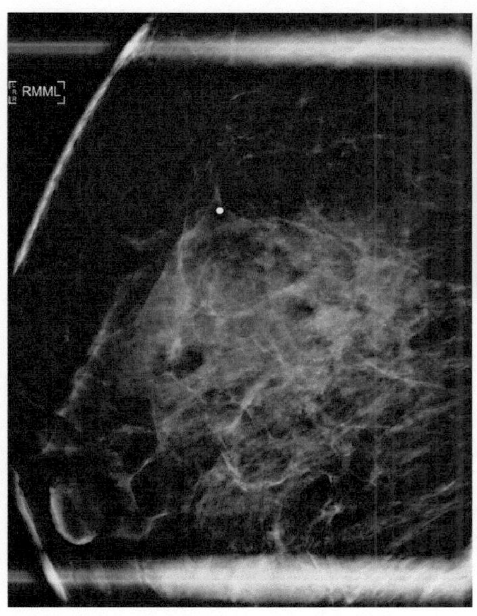
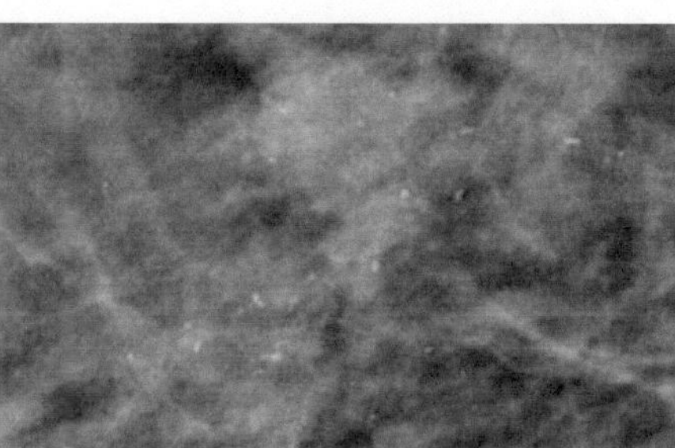

    (a) BI-RADS 2.
    (b) BI-RADS 3.
    (c) BI-RADS 4.
    (d) BI-RADS 5.

24b. Biopsy of the anterior portion of the segmental calcifications is performed. The surgeon requests that an additional site should be biopsied to evaluate for the extent of disease. What is the most appropriate site?
    (a) Biopsy a different part of the anterior region of calcifications.
    (b) Biopsy the middle aspect of the calcifications.
    (c) Biopsy the posterior aspect of the region of calcifications.
    (d) Look for an abnormal axillary lymph node to biopsy.

25a. A 47-year-old female presents for further evaluation of calcifications seen in the right breast on baseline screening mammogram. What is the morphology of these calcifications?

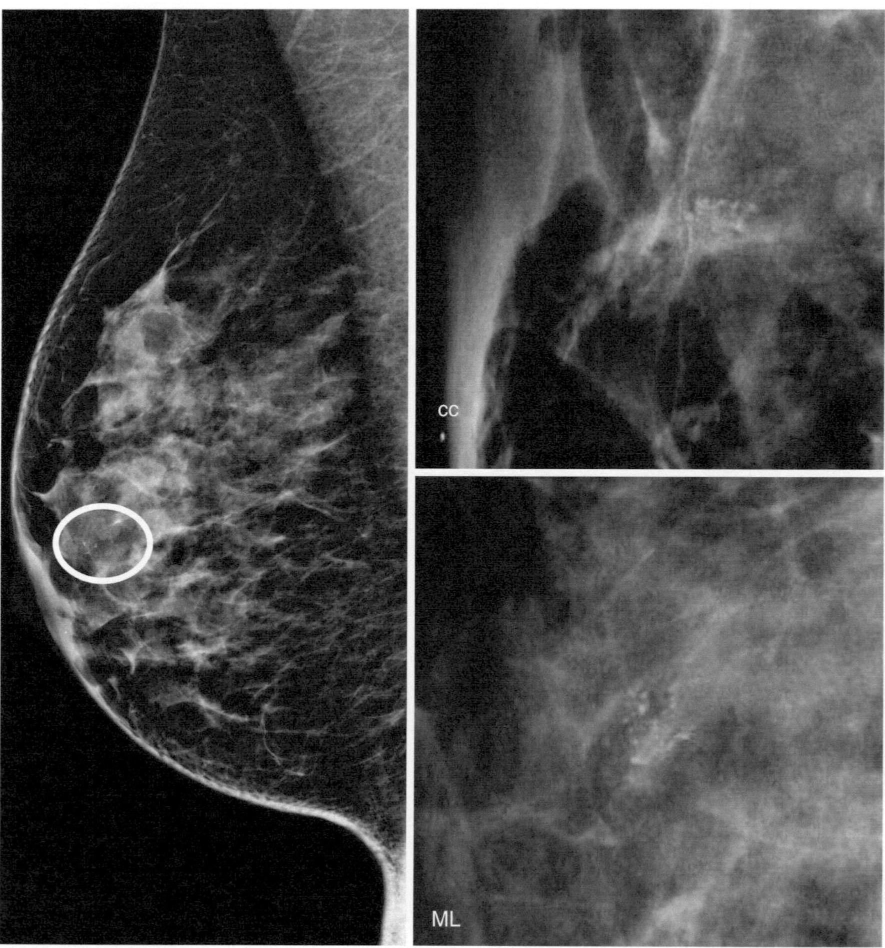

(a) Faint amorphous.
(b) Fine pleomorphic.
(c) Smudgy on ML view and layering on CC view.
(d) Smudgy on CC view and layering on ML view.

25b. Diagnostic ultrasound was performed and demonstrated multiple benign simple and complicated cysts seen scattered throughout the right breast. What would be the most appropriate BI-RADS category and recommendation for this case?

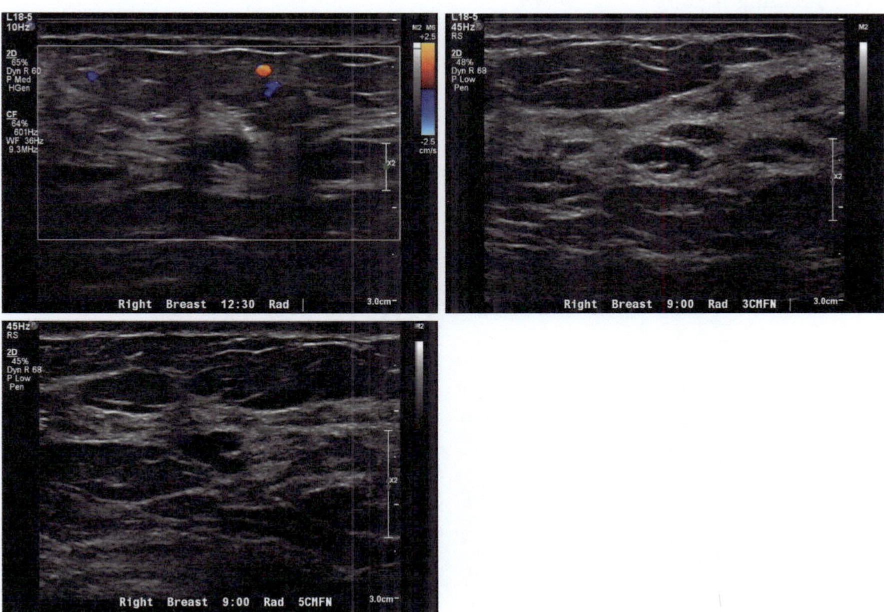

(a) BI-RADS 2: Recommends routine annual mammography.
(b) BI-RADS 3: Recommends right breast follow-up diagnostic mammogram in 6 months.
(c) BI-RADS 4: Recommends stereotactic core needle biopsy.
(d) BI-RADS 4: Recommends ultrasound-guided core needle biopsy.

26. Which type of asymmetry can be assigned BI-RADS 3 after a complete diagnostic work-up demonstrate a persistent finding but no associated sonographic correlate?
(a) Unilateral asymmetry.
(b) Developing asymmetry.
(c) Focal asymmetry.
(d) Suspicious asymmetry.

27. A patient presents with an enlarging palpable mass. Diagnostic mammogram and ultrasound show no imaging correlate. All of the following are acceptable options for management EXCEPT:
(a) Return to screening.
(b) Further evaluation with breast MRI.
(c) Obtain surgical consultation.
(d) Re-evaluation of the lump by ultrasound.

28a. A patient with a history of systemic skin lesions presents for diagnostic evaluation of bilateral palpable breast abnormalities. The skin lesions in this patient can be differentiated from intraparenchymal breast masses by what associated imaging finding?

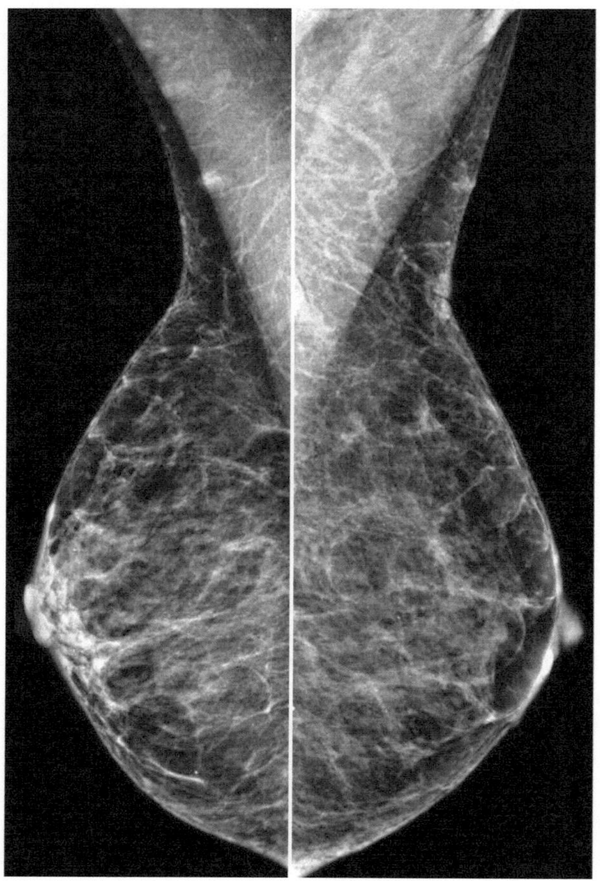

(a) Calcifications.
(b) Air.
(c) Axillary lymphadenopathy.
(d) Skin thickening.

28b. What is the inheritance pattern of NF1?
   (a) Autosomal dominant.
   (b) Autosomal recessive.
   (c) X-linked dominant.
   (d) X-linked recessive.

29. Patient presents for diagnostic evaluation of intermittent breast pain. What clinical disorder does the patient have?

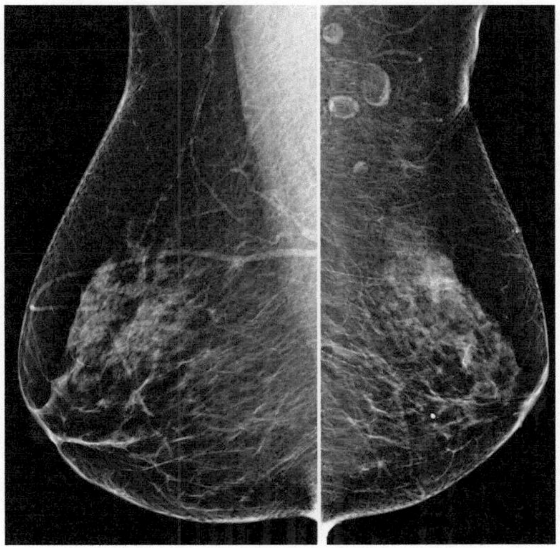

   (a) Neurofibromatosis 1.
   (b) Steatocystoma multiplex.
   (c) Cowden syndrome.
   (d) Poland syndrome.

30. A 48-year-old female is called back from screening for further evaluation of a possible right subareolar mass. Diagnostic mammogram demonstrates persistence of this finding. Diagnostic ultrasound images are presented below. What is the diagnosis?

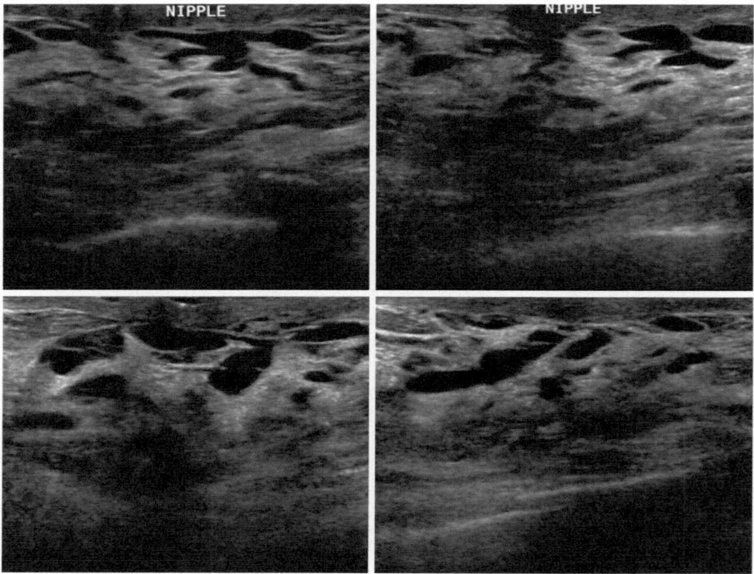

(a) Duct ectasia.
(b) Mixed cystic and solid mass.
(c) Cluster of simple cysts.
(d) Intraductal papilloma.

31. A patient presents with acute onset right breast pain and tenderness associated with a palpable cord-like mass. Diagnostic mammogram and ultrasound images are obtained. What is the appropriate next step?

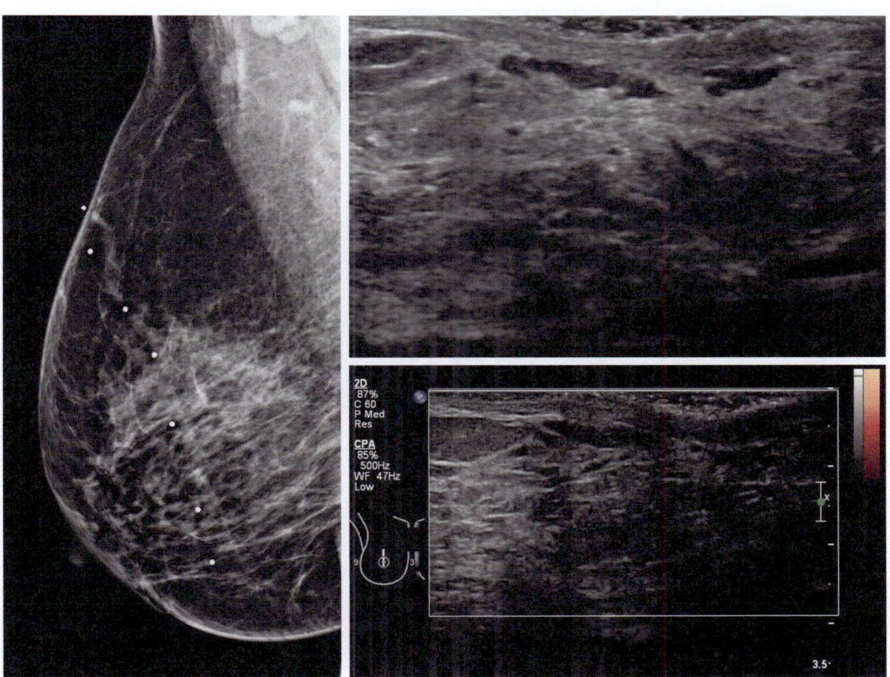

    (a) Ultrasound-guided biopsy.
    (b) Supportive care.
    (c) Surgical consultation.
    (d) Antibiotics.

32. Which of the following statements about Paget's disease of the nipple is true?
    (a) It is always a benign entity.
    (b) It most often coexists with breast ductal carcinoma.
    (c) Mammogram findings are always abnormal.
    (d) It is not associated with invasive disease.

33. A 56-year-old patient is called back from screening for further evaluation of new possible calcifications seen in a left axillary lymph node. Lateral mammographic magnification views of the left axilla and targeted ultrasound are shown below. What is the next best step?

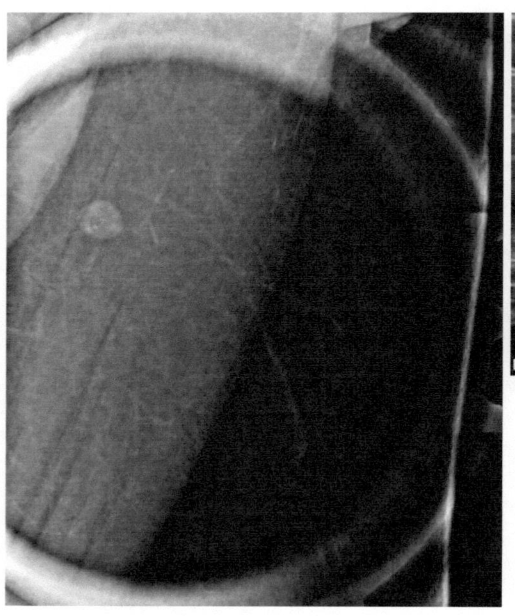
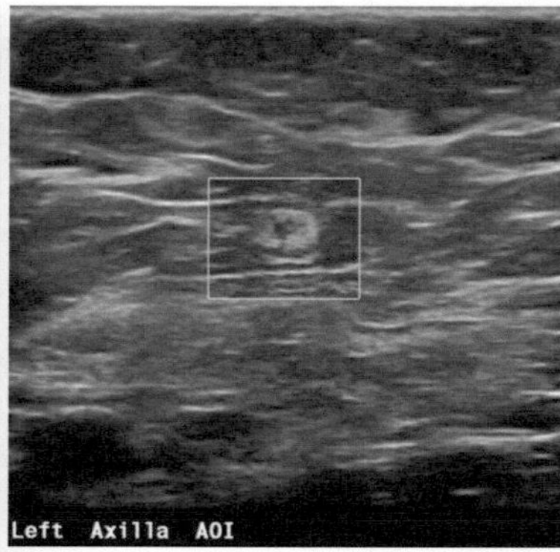

(a) Ultrasound-guided biopsy.
(b) Surgical consultation.
(c) Fine needle aspiration.
(d) Obtain more history from the patient.

Answers

1a. a. Fat-containing mass adjacent to the BB marker.

A subtle fat-containing mass with rim calcification is seen adjacent to the BB marker (circles).

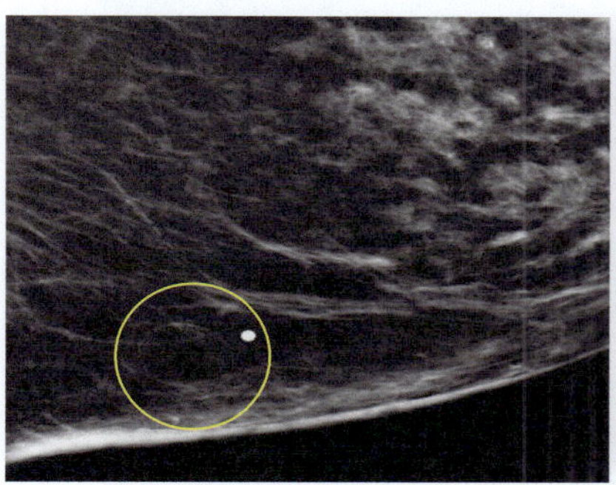 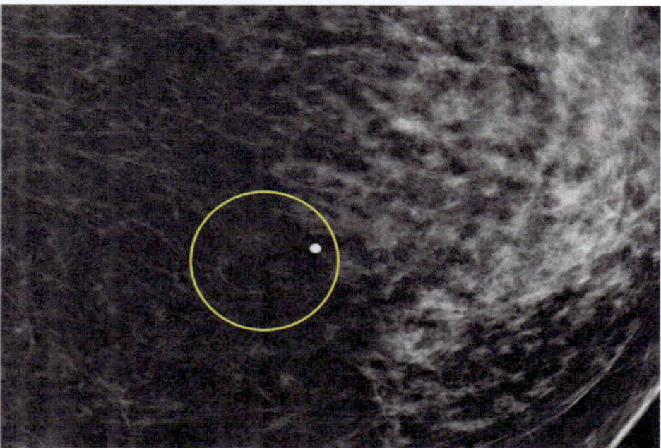

1b. d. Spot compression view.

Spot compression is the best next step for suspected masses. It allows the best characterization of margins and differentiates true lesions from overlapping tissue. A magnification view can be obtained with spot compression but is usually helpful for calcifications, which are already clearly evaluated on the initial views. Exaggerated craniocaudal (CC) views pull either lateral or medial breast tissue into the detector, which is not as helpful for this mass. True lateral views, also known as mediolateral view, are useful for triangulating findings seen on MLO view that is not seen on the CC view, which is not the case here [1].

1c. d. Oil cyst.

Oil cysts initially appear as a fat density on mammography and subsequently develop rim calcifications from saponification. Radiolucent or fat density mass with a thin rim-calcified or eggshell-type calcified wall is a classic mammographic appearance of a benign oil cyst secondary to fat necrosis [2]. Oil cysts are benign.

In a patient with a history of breast cancer, new oil cyst rim calcifications may be difficult to discern from malignant recurrent calcifications. Comparison to prior images to evaluate for prior non-calcified oil cyst is essential. Fibroadenomas do not usually contain fat. Differential considerations of fat-containing masses include hamartoma, lymph node, fat-containing invasive breast cancer, liposarcoma, and galactocele [3].

Oil cysts have variable sonographic appearances, ranging from hypoechoic to complex cystic or solid masses, echogenic bands, and posterior acoustic shadowing [4].

1d. d. Steatocystoma multiplex.

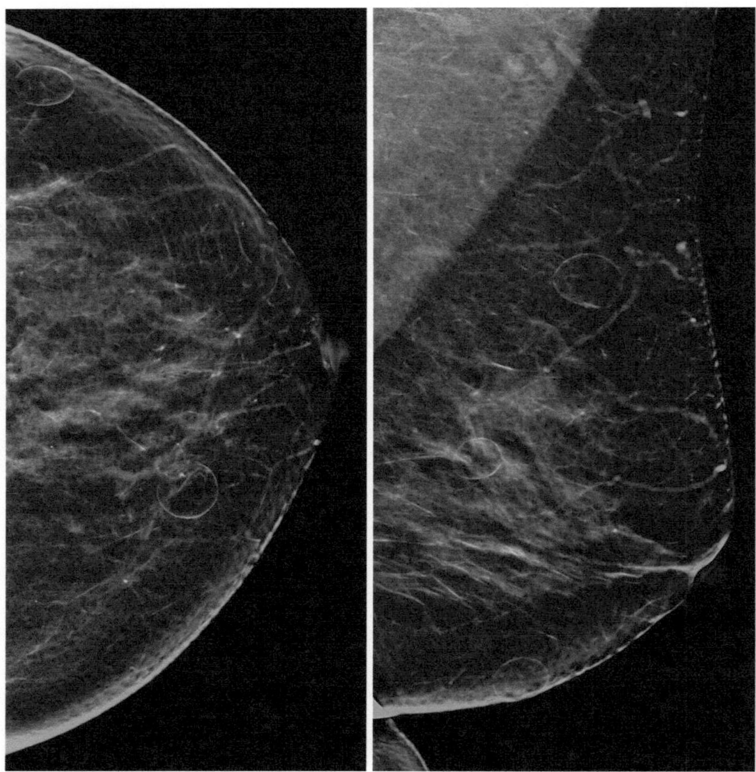

Steatocystoma multiplex is a rare, autosomal dominant disorder of multiple and extensive bilateral superficial intradermal rim-calcified fat-containing oil cysts (see provided image). The key to differentiating steatocystoma multiplex oil cysts from posttraumatic intraparenchymal oil cysts is the intradermal location, bilaterality, lack of trauma or surgery history, and innumerable quantity. Cowden disease, also called multiple hamartoma syndrome, is characterized by multiple hamartomas, not intradermal oil cysts. Neurofibromatosis type 1 lesions are intradermal, however, present as tissue masses outlined by air, indicating that they are skin lesions rather than intraparenchymal masses. Poland syndrome is characterized by unilateral absence of the pectoralis muscle [3].

2a. c. Skin tract.

The abnormal finding seen on ultrasound is a sebaceous or epidermal inclusion cyst. The arrow is pointing to a skin tract arising from the lesion, confirming its intradermal origin. Ultrasound may demonstrate this hypoechoic tract extending into the skin, which represents a dilated hair follicle [5]. Sebaceous cysts can be subdermal or intradermal in location (cannot be differentiated on imaging as both the dermis and the epidermis are seen together as a 0.5–2 mm hyperechoic layer) [5]. Sebaceous cysts result from keratin accumulation in plugged ducts and have an epithelial cell lining from the sebaceous gland, whereas epidermal cysts have a true epidermal cell lining and no sebaceous glands. On mammogram, they appear as subcutaneous oval or round circumscribed masses near the skin surface. On ultrasound, they appear as oval, circumscribed hypoechoic or anechoic masses [3]. Epidermal inclusion cysts may occasionally occur in breast parenchyma deep to the dermis due to epidermal displacement during breast biopsy or surgery [3]. The below image provides an example of an intradermal sebaceous or epidermal inclusion cyst.

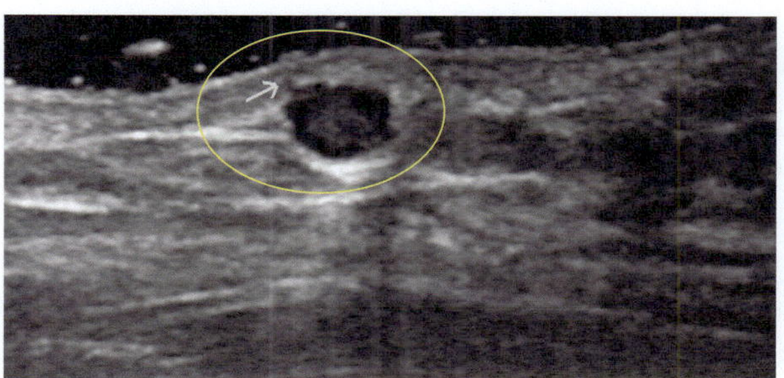

2b. d. No follow-up is needed.

Sebaceous or epidermal inclusion cysts are benign lesions. Dermatology consult can be obtained if findings are equivocal or concerning for malignancy, but a classic appearance with an intradermal location and skin tract is diagnostic. Aspiration and biopsy of epidermal inclusion cysts should be avoided because the cyst may rupture and cause an inflammatory reaction or infection in the surrounding tissue [5].

3a. c. Intraductal papilloma.

Biopsy of this patient's mass resulted as an intraductal papilloma. Benign intraductal papilloma is the most common mass that causes bloody nipple discharge; approximately 5% of women are found to have malignancy at biopsy. Papillomas consist of a fibrovascular stalk attached to the breast duct wall and epithelium. The bloody nipple discharge is caused by the papilloma twisting on its fibrovascular stalk, with subsequent infarction and bleeding. Intraductal papilloma can be single or multiple, extend along the ducts for a long distance, and appear cystic or multilobulated [3]. The differential diagnosis for an intraductal mass includes intraductal debris, papilloma (benign or atypical), or cancer [3]. Management with surgical excision versus imaging follow-up remains controversial [6].

Ductal carcinoma in situ can also cause bloody nipple discharge but less commonly than intraductal papilloma. Prolactinoma, is a cause of milky discharge and often will affect both breasts. Cysts may cause green or white nipple discharge if connected to a duct [3].

3b. b. Peripheral papillomas are more associated with malignancy than central papillomas.

Papillomas can be central or peripheral, with peripheral papillomas considered a risk factor for breast cancer [3]. Spontaneous nipple discharge is associated with central papillomas, which tend to be solitary lesions arising in the main lactiferous ducts. Peripheral papillomas tend to be multiple and arise in terminal ductal lobular units beyond the subareolar region. Papillomatosis, a type of usual ductal hyperplasia, is papillary hyperplasia lacking fibrovascular stalks [6].

3c. a. Spontaneous.

Nipple discharge is concerning if it is spontaneous, unilateral, arises from a single duct, or appears bloody or clear [3].

3d. c. MRI.

MRI, or less commonly performed ductography (not given as an answer choice), should be considered following negative mammographic and ultrasound evaluation of suspicious nipple discharge [6]. If imaging workup is still negative, referral to a breast surgeon can be considered.

4a. d. Nipple retraction.

Left nipple retraction is seen on the MLO and CC views. There is no axillary lymphadenopathy, calcification, or discrete mass seen on the screening mammogram. Nipple retraction or inversion may be congenital or acquired and unilateral or bilateral. Acquired unilateral nipple retraction or inversion may be caused by an underlying malignancy or inflammatory condition and requires further evaluation [7].

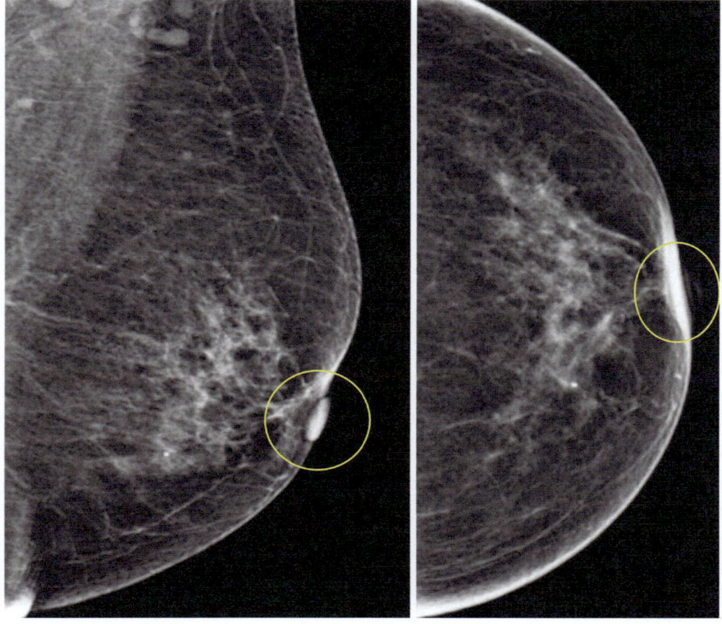

4b. a. Contrast-enhanced MRI.

Contrast-enhanced MRI is recommended for a recent diagnosis of invasive lobular carcinoma. Subtraction images from the contrast-enhanced MRI of this patient demonstrate left nipple retraction (circle) and non-mass enhancement in the central left breast (arrow), which represents invasive lobular carcinoma (ILC). The next best step would be MRI-guided biopsy to establish extent of disease. Of note, ILCs are difficult to detect mammographically due to their tendency to grow cell by cell in a single file without much mass effect or calcifications [3].

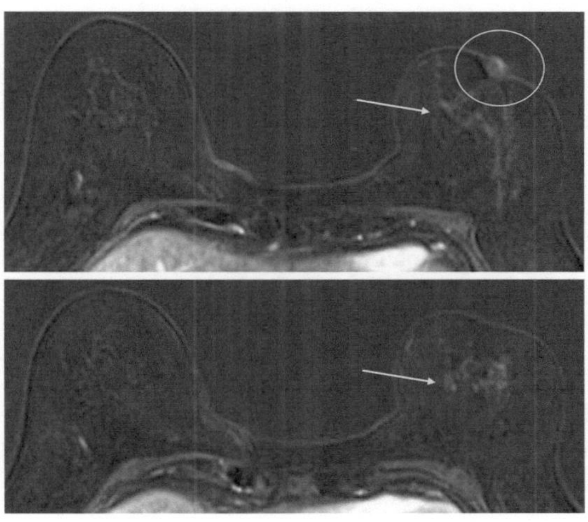

5a. d. Skin thickening and increased trabeculation.

Unilateral skin thickening and increased trabeculation are seen in the left breast. There is no architectural distortion, asymmetry, or discrete mass. Ultrasound findings confirm unilateral skin thickening and breast edema without a discrete mass. The patient also has left axillary lymphadenopathy seen on the MLO mammographic view.

5b. b. Inflammatory breast cancer.

Diffuse skin thickening and edema, trabecular changes without a discrete mass, and axillary lymphadenopathy are characteristic findings of inflammatory breast carcinoma [3, 8]. These findings can also be present in mastitis, however, less likely given the history of failed antibiotics. Risk factors for mastitis include breastfeeding and smoking (for infections outside of the puerperal period) [9]. Skin thickening and edema seen with systemic processes such as congestive heart failure is more likely bilateral. Post-radiation change can manifest as skin thickening and edema, sometimes persisting for years; however, no clinical history was provided to suggest this diagnosis. History of fever is also inconsistent with congestive heart failure or post-radiation change.

5c. a. Skin punch biopsy.

Tissue diagnosis is required to confirm inflammatory breast cancer; thus, skin punch biopsy is the next best step. Dermal lymphatic involvement is the pathologic hallmark of inflammatory breast cancer [8]. No intraparenchymal targets were identified on mammogram or ultrasound, thus choices b and c are not appropriate. In the absence of a biopsy target on conventional imaging, MRI can be obtained to help identify a biopsy target and document extent of disease [8]. This patient was ultimately diagnosed with inflammatory breast cancer via skin punch biopsy.

5d. c. Follow-up imaging.

Because the clinical and imaging manifestations of mastitis and inflammatory breast cancer are similar, follow-up with repeat ultrasound(s) after antibiotics (usually 7–14 days) is essential to rule out underlying inflammatory breast cancer. Serial ultrasound evaluations are recommended until complete resolution. For women presenting outside of the puerperal period or who are over 30 years old, such as this patient, mammography is also recommended to evaluate for underlying malignancy [9].

6a. c. Fine pleomorphic, regional.

Regional calcifications extend over more than one ductal distribution. They are defined as occupying a large proportion of the breast tissue that is >2 cm in greatest dimension [10].

6b. b. BI-RADS 4B.

Regional calcification distribution has a 26% likelihood of malignancy [10]. Fine pleomorphic calcification morphology is classified as suspicious, with a 29% likelihood of malignancy [10]. Thus, the most appropriate BI-RADS classification is 4B, moderately suspicious (>10% to ≤50% likelihood of malignancy) [10]. These calcifications were biopsied and resulted as ductal carcinoma in situ (DCIS). On mammography, DCIS usually presents as microcalcifications, while some may present as a mass or asymmetry, and least likely, as a palpable abnormality [11]. Calcification morphologies associated with DCIS include fine linear, fine-linear branching, amorphous, and fine pleomorphic [3, 11]. Table 4.1 lists the different types of suspicious calcification morphologies and their associated positive predictive value for breast cancer and BI-RADS assignments.

Table 4.1. Suspicious calcification morphologies and their positive predictive values for breast cancer [10, 11]

Calcification morphology	Positive predictive value for breast cancer	BI-RADS
Coarse heterogeneous	13%	4B
Amorphous	21%	4B
Fine pleomorphic	29%	4B
Fine linear or fine-linear branching	70%	4C

7a. c. Grouped coarse heterogeneous calcifications.

Coarse heterogeneous calcifications are defined as irregular, conspicuous calcifications that vary in size between 0.5 and 1 mm. The calcifications are too large to be punctate, and too irregular to be considered round. Grouped distribution is defined as relatively few calcifications occupying an area of breast tissue <2 cm, or at least 5 calcifications grouped within 1 cm of each other. Regional distribution describes calcifications spanning a larger area of >2 cm.

7b. c. BI-RADS 4B.

For assessment of calcifications, both the individual calcification morphology and distribution should be considered. Coarse heterogeneous calcifications are of moderate level of suspicion for malignancy. Differential diagnosis for coarse heterogeneous calcifications includes calcifying fibroadenomas or ductal carcinoma in situ. Thus, the distribution, including number of groups and laterality (e.g., bilateral versus unilateral), is essential for further risk stratification. Suspicious distributions include grouped, segmental, and linear, with grouped considered moderately suspicious and segmental or linear highly suspicious for malignancy. An isolated group of coarse heterogeneous calcifications in a grouped distribution together warrant a BI-RADS 4B.

8a. c. Spot compression.

A mixed density circumscribed mass is seen in the upper outer quadrant of the right breast (circles). Spot compression views are helpful for further evaluating masses. Magnification views are not needed for evaluations of masses unless there are associated calcifications [1].

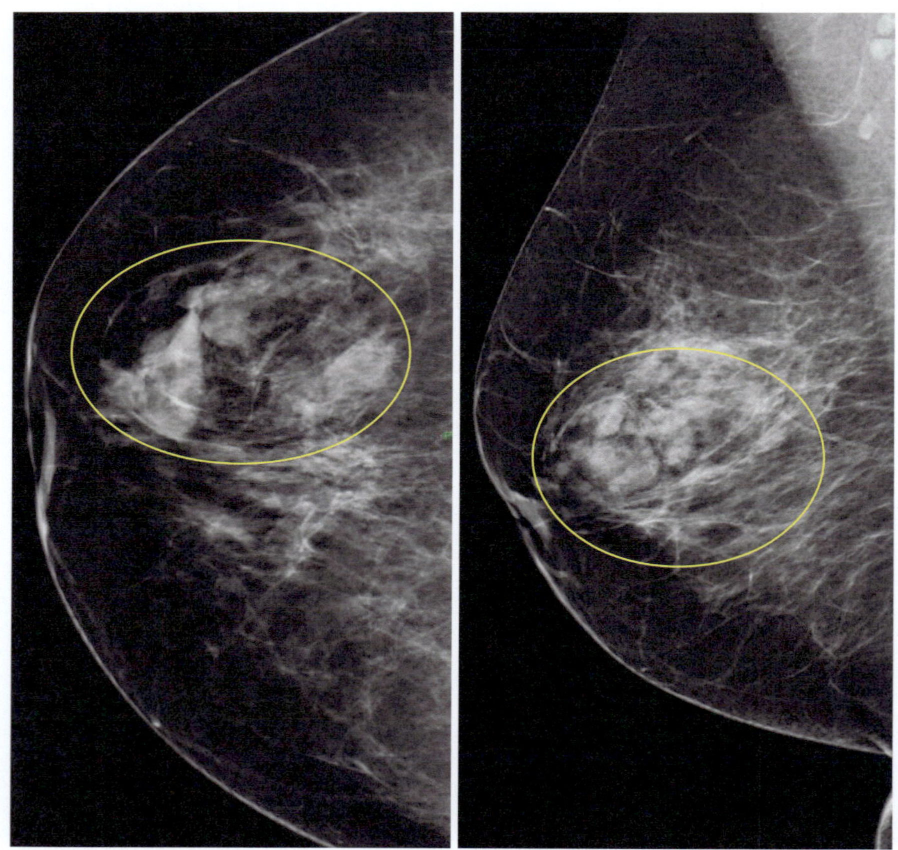

8b. a. BI-RADS 2.

Diagnostic mammogram demonstrates a hamartoma, also known as fibroadenolipoma, which is a benign mass containing fat and normal fibroglandular tissue. On mammogram, it appears classically as an oval mixed-density mass (depending on the ratio of fat to fibroglandular tissue) with a thin capsule or rim, and sometimes is described as a "breast within a breast" appearance. Hamartomas are benign and when classic-appearing should be left alone. If it contains suspicious calcifications or masses, then further imaging or biopsy may be warranted [3].

8c. b. Oval, circumscribed, parallel mass with mixed hypo- and hyperechoic echogenicity.

The below images demonstrate the common sonographic appearance of hamartomas, although the appearance can be variable depending on the composition [3]. Answer choice a describes the classic sonographic appearance of a fibroadenoma, which can be difficult to distinguish from hamartoma. Choice c incorrectly describes the margins and echogenicity. Choice d additionally incorrectly describes the shape and margins.

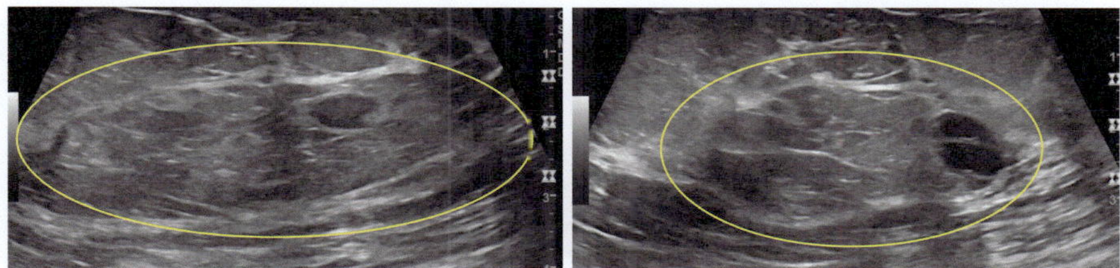

9. d. All of the above.

Given the history of anticoagulation, these findings most likely represent hematoma. However, without priors for comparison or more clinical context, all of the above should be on the differential for fluid-containing masses [3]. On mammography, hematomas most often present as a new mass, may be ill-defined or circumscribed, and blood may be seen tracking along connective tissue planes [12]. Ultrasound can show a hypoechoic fluid collection or a complex, heterogeneous cystic and solid mass as in this patient's imaging, depending on the amount of clotted versus free blood [12]. Aspiration of this patient's mass yielded bloody fluid, consistent with a hematoma (see below). Because of the overlap in imaging features of hematoma, abscess, and malignancy, imaging follow-up should be performed to confirm complete resolution [13].

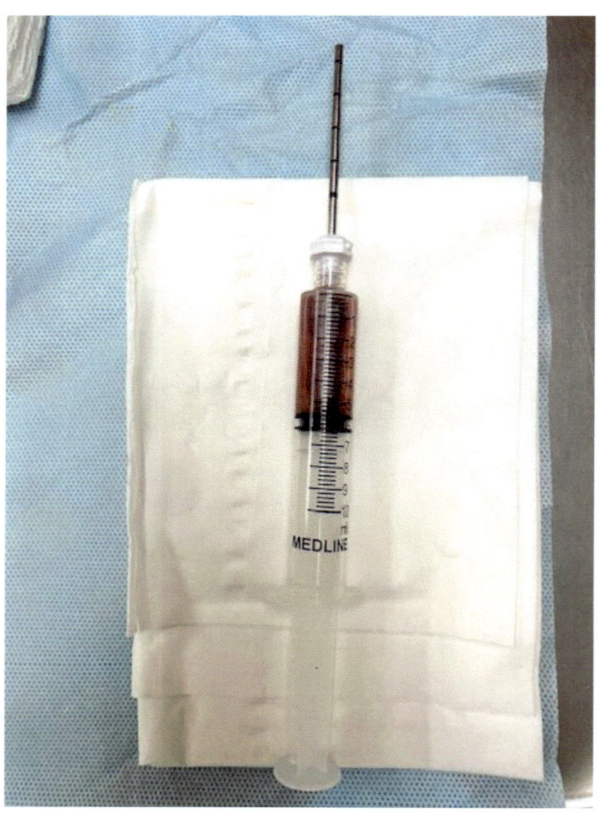

10a. a. Right upper outer quadrant.

On mammogram, there is an isodense mass in the right upper outer quadrant.

10b. a. BI-RADS 2.

Ultrasound confirms the classic appearance of a simple cyst, which is a circumscribed anechoic lesion with a thin posterior wall and posterior acoustic enhancement. Simple cysts are benign and no follow-up is necessary. Aspiration may be offered if the cyst is symptomatic, which yielded brown fluid in this case (image below) [3].

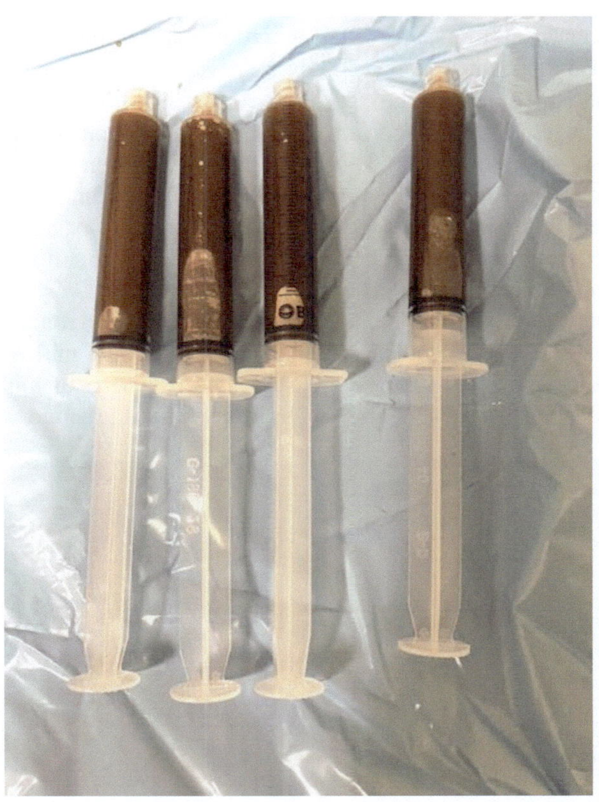

10c. a. BI-RADS 2.

BI-RADS assessment should be assigned based on imaging. Management, in this case, would be based on symptoms, but this does not change the suspicion for malignancy or malignant potential. Cysts are caused by fluid trapped within obstructed and dilated terminal ducts, and can enlarge and regress in response to hormones [3]. Thus, patients should be advised that even if aspirated, cysts can redevelop with fluid accumulation.

10d. c. Bloody.

Aspirated fluid should be sent for cytologic evaluation if it is bloody or if there is an associated intracystic solid mass. If there is an intracystic mass, core-needle biopsy of the solid component should be performed instead. For bloody cystic fluid, a marker can be placed in the cyst cavity at the time of aspiration to further guide future biopsy or surgical excision if cytology result is positive. All other types of cyst fluid can be discarded [3].

11a. b. Fat-fluid level.

Galactoceles are the most common benign breast lesions in lactating women and occur most frequently after cessation of breastfeeding when milk is retained and becomes stagnant. A cystic mass with a fat-fluid level is considered pathognomonic in the appropriate clinical setting. On ultrasound, the more echogenic superior portion of the lesion represents fat that has risen to the top, with the more anechoic inferior portion representing fluid. Mammographic appearance varies depending on the amount of fat and proteinaceous material, ranging from a pseudolipoma appearance (completely radiolucent mass due to high-fat content) to pseudohamartoma (due to variable proportions of milk and water) [14]. This patient's corresponding mammogram (see mammogram images below) presented as a round circumscribed mass. Aspiration is diagnostic and therapeutic, yielding milky fluid as in this patient's case (see image below). Note that aspiration of milk can also be obtained in a lactating adenoma or fibroadenoma with secretory changes [14].

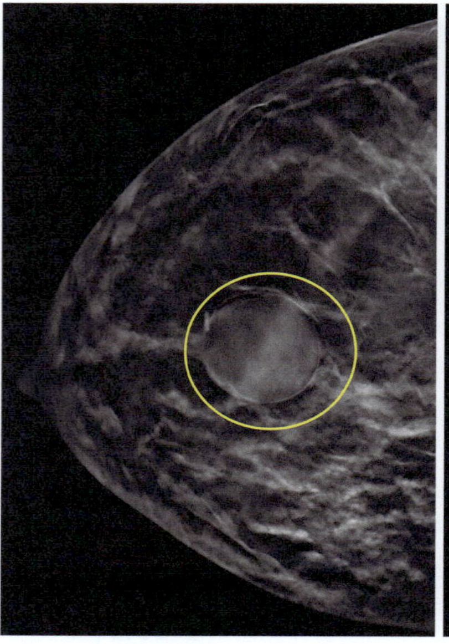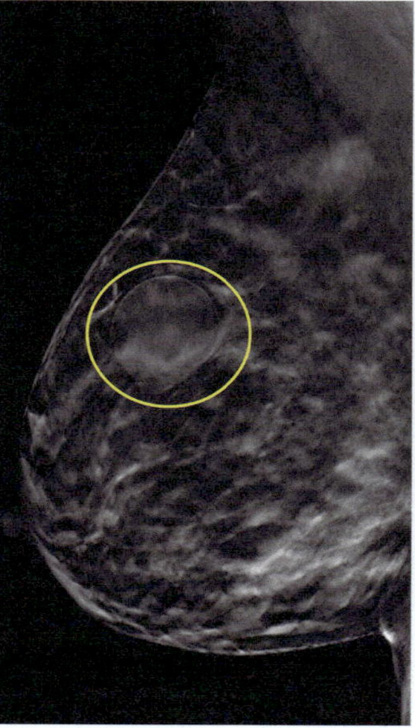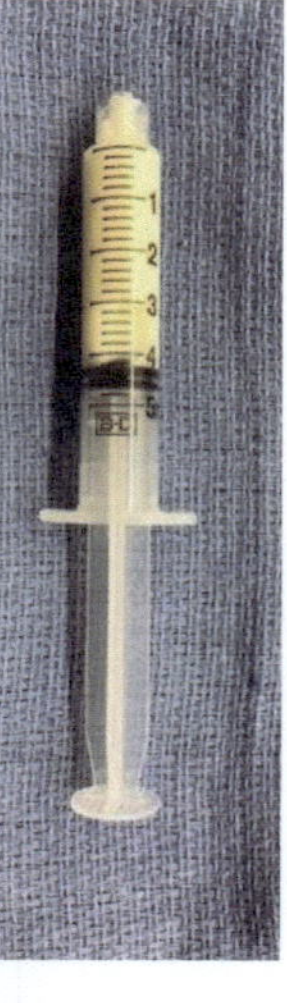

11b. b. Infection.

Infection is a common complication due to the rich nutrient content of galactoceles. Clinical suspicion can be confirmed with fine needle aspiration yielding mixed milky-purulent fluid [14].

12a. d. Right breast ultrasound.

Ultrasound is the most sensitive and appropriate diagnostic imaging modality for evaluating a palpable mass in pregnant or lactating women. Physiologic changes during pregnancy and lactation cause a diffuse, marked increase in parenchymal density which decreases the sensitivity of mammography. However, mammography should be performed if malignancy is suspected as it is more sensitive in detecting microcalcifications or subtle distortions [14].

12b. b. Ultrasound of the ipsilateral axilla.

Ultrasound demonstrates a large oval, circumscribed, heterogeneously isoechoic, vascular mass measuring 5.4 cm. While rare, pregnancy-associated breast cancer (PABC), defined as breast cancer diagnosed during pregnancy, lactation, or the first postpartum year, is the most common invasive cancer diagnosed during pregnancy and most commonly presents as a palpable mass [15]. Given its size, differential diagnosis including a malignant process warrants evaluation of the ipsilateral axilla.

12c. c. BI-RADS 4, ultrasound-guided core needle biopsy.

Although the axilla was negative for any findings and the mass has imaging features of a possible benign entity, such as a fibroadenoma or lactating adenoma, the mass remains suspicious given its large size and should be biopsied. Core biopsy is standard for further evaluation of breast masses during pregnancy and lactation [14]. Breast surgical consultation is premature at this stage.

12d. a. Milk fistula.

Milk fistula as a complication of biopsy in the lactating breast is rare but must be discussed with the patient. If desired and practical, the risk can be minimized by discontinuation of breastfeeding prior to biopsy. Risk of hematoma and infection are slightly increased during pregnancy or lactation due to increased vascularity, but not unique complications to the situation [14]. Vasovagal reaction can occur in any patient undergoing biopsy.

12e. d. Concordant, clinical follow-up to ensure resolution after cessation of breastfeeding.

Although PABC must be considered, the vast majority of palpable masses biopsied in pregnant or lactating women represent benign masses, including those unique to pregnancy and lactation such as lactating adenomas and galactoceles, or enlargement of pre-existing benign masses such as fibroadenomas and hamartomas [15].

Lactating adenomas may be indistinguishable from fibroadenomas on imaging. They can enlarge rapidly during pregnancy, and may be solitary, multiple, or bilateral. On ultrasound, they appear as oval, circumscribed masses with heterogeneous echogenicity due to cystic or necrotic spaces [3]. Lactating adenomas should regress following cessation of breastfeeding [3, 15]. If lactating adenomas persist, then surgical consultation is warranted.

13a. d. Focal asymmetry.

There is a right breast focal asymmetry (circles) corresponding to the area of the patient's palpable abnormality (note the adjacent BB marker).

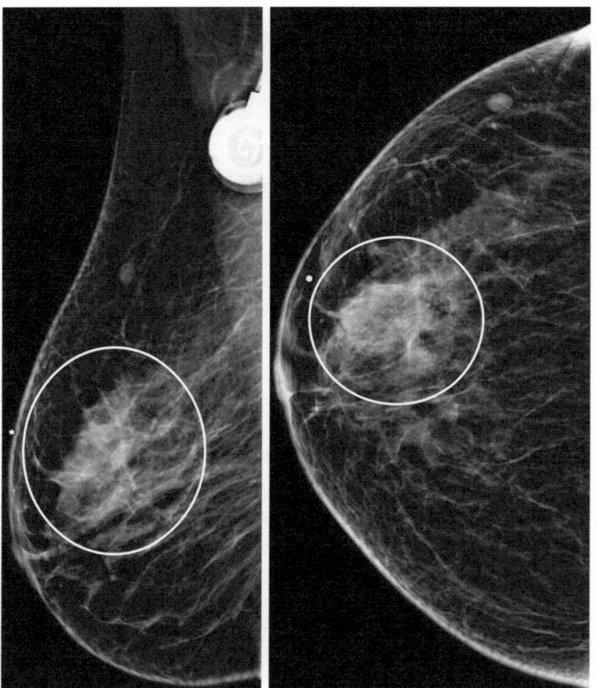

13b. a. Spot compression mammographic views and ultrasound.

Spot compression views are helpful for further evaluating masses and their margins. If the mass persists and remains suspicious, further evaluation with ultrasound is warranted. Rolled views are obtained by moving hemispheres of the breast in opposite directions. For example, rolled views in CC would involve moving the superior and inferior breast in opposite directions and would help localize lesions seen in CC view only. Exaggerated cranio-caudal views pull either the lateral breast tissue (XCCL) or the medial breast tissue

(XCCM) into the detector, which are not needed since the full extent of the lesion is seen. Magnification views are not needed for evaluations of masses unless there are associated calcifications [1].

13c. b. Ultrasound-guided core needle biopsy.

The finding persists with spot compression mammographic views, confirming a true and suspicious lesion in a patient with a history of malignancy. Ultrasound reveals a corresponding hypoechoic mass with microlobulated margins. These findings are suspicious for malignancy and warrant ultrasound-guided core needle biopsy. For this patient, pathology yielded carcinoma with signet ring cells, consistent with gastric origin and therefore metastatic gastric carcinoma to the breast. Gastric cancer with breast metastasis is rare and most commonly presents as a palpable abnormality [16].

While the ultrasound findings could represent an abscess, the clinical history does not support answer choice a. Choices c and d are incorrect because there is a sonographic correlate, so ultrasound-guided biopsy should be performed.

13d. b. The most common location for extramammary metastases to the breast is the upper-outer quadrant.

Choice b is a true statement; the upper-outer quadrant is the most common location for both extramammary metastases and primary breast cancer, thought to be due to the increased blood supply in this region. Choice a is incorrect as breast metastases from extramammary cancers are rare, with prevalence ranging from 0.5 to 6.6% of all malignant tumors in the breast. Choice c is incorrect; the extramammary malignancies that most commonly metastasize to the breast are melanoma, lymphomas, ovarian, lung, neuroendocrine tumors, and sarcomas. Choice d is incorrect; common imaging findings depend on hematogenous disseminated versus lymphatic spread, and are outlined in Table 4.2 [17].

Table 4.2. Common imaging findings on mammography and ultrasound of breast metastases from extramammary cancers [17]

Common findings	Imaging differentiators from primary breast cancer
Hematogenous spread • Round masses with circumscribed margins (on mammography, masses are high density) • ± microlobulated or indistinct margins • Rare calcifications (more likely seen with ovarian cancer metastases) Lymphatic spread • Skin thickening • Trabecular thickening • Axillary lymphadenopathy	Generally, metastatic lesions are not associated with spiculated margins, or skin or nipple retraction due to absence of desmoplastic reaction

14a. c. Ultrasound-guided core needle biopsy.

While the most likely palpable breast mass in a patient of this age is a fibroadenoma, this patient's presentation demonstrates some atypical imaging features in addition to rapid growth over the last three months. Differential diagnoses for fibroadenomas with atypical imaging features include juvenile fibroadenoma (rapidly growing mass primarily seen in adolescents), complex fibroadenoma (which have slightly increased risk of invasive breast cancer in both breasts), phyllodes tumor, lactational adenoma (common during pregnancy), or malignant masses (including BRCA-associated breast cancers which can mimic fibroadenoma). Because these etiologies often cannot be differentiated on imaging, biopsy is warranted for probable fibroadenomas with atypical features or clinical concern for malignancy or phyllodes, rendering answer choice c the most appropriate.

Answer choice a is inappropriate because even classic appearing features of fibroadenomas typically warrant short-term imaging follow-up for 2 years to confirm stability. Because classic features of fibroadenoma are not present, short-term interval follow-up by imaging alone is inappropriate. Answer choice d, direct surgical consultation, may be appropriate following biopsy.

14b. c. Microlobulated margins.

Fibroadenomas classically appear on ultrasound as oval, parallel, circumscribed, homogeneously hypoechoic masses with echogenic, thin fibrous internal septations. While fibroadenomas can have gentle undulations, microlobulated margins are atypical. This patient's ultrasound demonstrates atypical features, including mildly indistinct and microlobulated margins. Up to 80% of fibroadenomas exhibit internal vascularity on Doppler imaging. Posterior features vary depending on the fibroadenoma's composition, with epithelial-dominant lesions demonstrating posterior enhancement and hyalinized-dominant lesions demonstrating posterior acoustic shadowing.

14c. b. >20%.

Probably benign lesions with interval growth >20% should undergo biopsy.

15a. b. BI-RADS 0, left breast spot compression views and ultrasound recommended.

BI-RADS 0 is appropriate because additional views are warranted to further evaluate findings seen in the left breast.

15b. b. 2.

There are two abnormalities in the left breast: an irregular, spiculated hyperdense mass in the left axilla and an area of architectural distortion in the left
breast at 12 o'clock. Spot compression and targeted ultrasound should be
obtained for focal asymmetries and apparent masses to distinguish between
true lesions and summation artifacts such as from overlapping fibroglandular
tissue [18]. Magnification views are useful for evaluating calcifications, which
are not present in these two areas of concern [18].

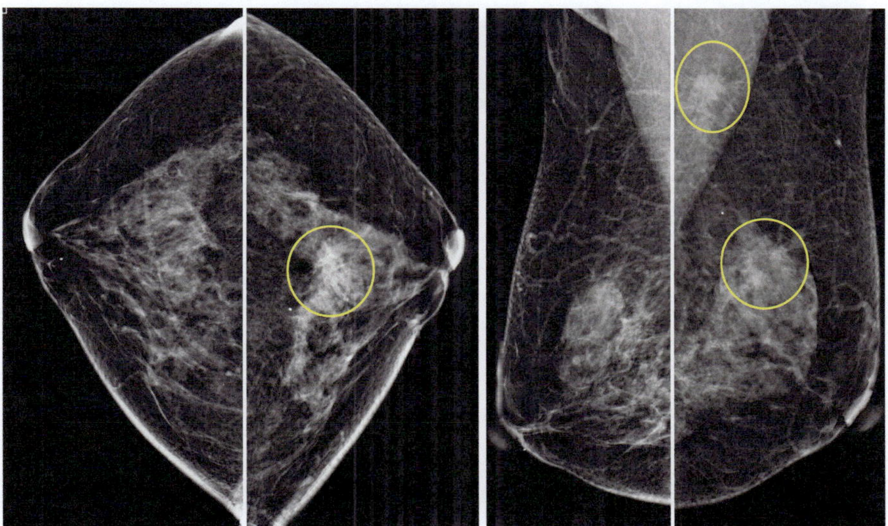

15c. d. BI-RADS 4.

Both lesions persisted with spot compression views with sonographic correlates, confirming true lesions. Suspicious features on mammogram (spiculated margins, architectural distortion), and on ultrasound (spiculated and
angular margins, not parallel orientation, posterior shadowing, and markedly
hypoechoic echotexture) are concerning for malignancy and warrant tissue
diagnosis, and thus should be categorized as BI-RADS 4 [10]. This case
resulted as biopsy-proven multicentric invasive lobular carcinoma.

16a. a. Architectural distortion.

A subtle architectural distortion is seen in the right lower inner quadrant, at 5:00, 3 cm from the nipple. An architectural distortion describes distorted breast parenchyma which appears as linear spiculations radiating from a focal point without a discernible central mass.

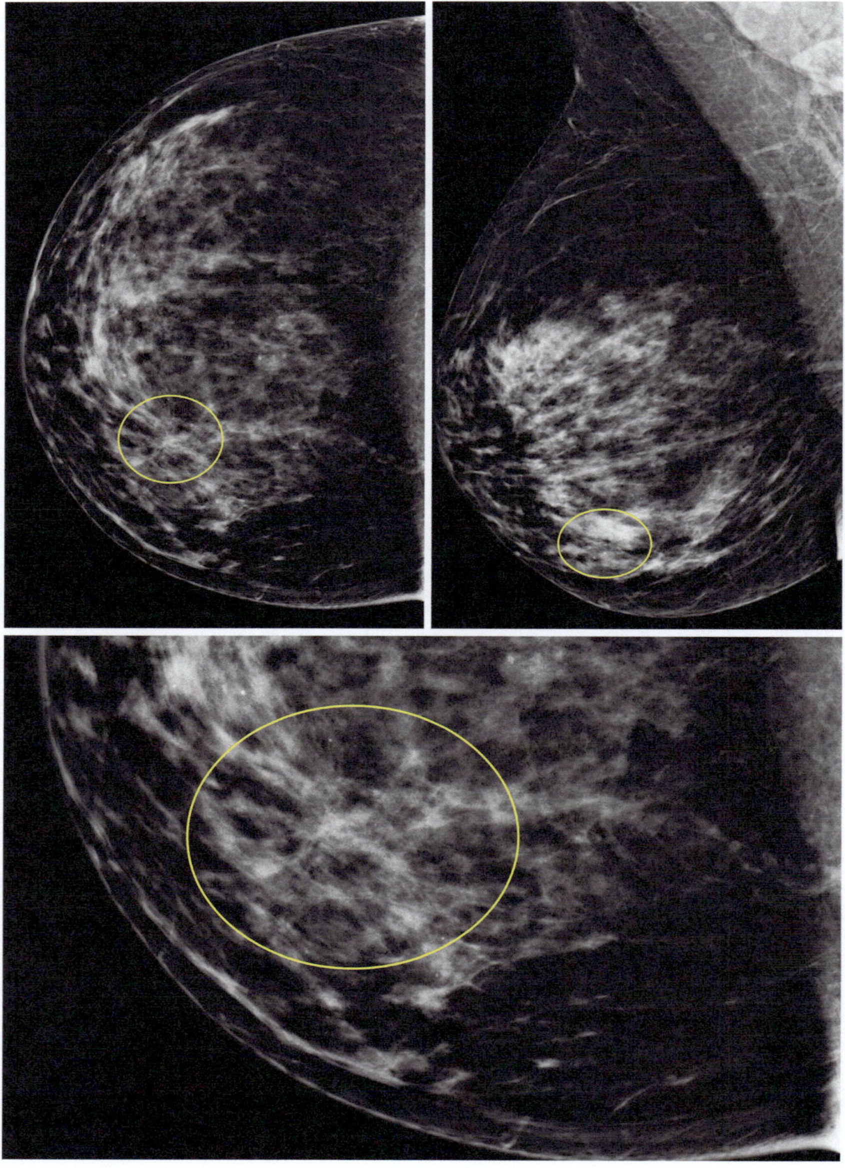

Table 4.3 lists the benign, high-risk, and malignant etiologies that can manifest as architectural distortion in the breast.

Table 4.3. Differential diagnosis for architectural distortion [19]

Risk category	Etiology
Benign	Postsurgical scar
	Fat necrosis
	Sclerosing adenosis
	Focal fibrosis
	Diabetic mastopathy
	Normal overlapping tissue
High-risk	Radial scar or complex sclerosing lesion
Malignant	Invasive ductal carcinoma
	Tubular carcinoma
	Invasive lobular carcinoma
	Ductal carcinoma in situ (uncommon)

16b. e. BI-RADS 4, stereotactic core needle biopsy.

Stereotactic core needle biopsy is the most appropriate next step. Choice a is inappropriate because BI-RADS 1 is reserved for a completely negative exam. Choices b and c are incorrect because there is a new finding that could represent a malignancy and warrants further management, specifically biopsy. Choice d is incorrect because there is no sonographic correlate.

16c. a. Malignant concordant.

Tubular carcinoma (TC) is a rare, slow-growing, low-grade type of invasive ductal carcinoma which represents 1–2% of all breast cancers and has generally favorable prognosis. The most common mammographic appearance is a subtle developing asymmetry, distortion, or spiculated mass, which may be visible as a one-view-only finding. Up to 50% of TCs have associated amorphous or pleomorphic microcalcifications. TC can be slow growing for years, emphasizing the importance of continuous evaluation of mammographically stable lesions. Standard treatment is breast-conserving surgery with or without radiation therapy [20].

17a. c. Bilateral axillary lymphadenopathy.

The current screening mammogram demonstrates new bilateral axillary lymphadenopathy, with increased size and opacity of multiple lymph nodes compared to one year prior. No new breast masses are seen. The breast density does appear less dense, but this is normal with aging.

17b. c. Diagnostic ultrasound.

Axillary lymph nodes with abnormal mammographic features or substantial interval enlargement warrant further evaluation with diagnostic ultrasound if there is no underlying clinical explanation [21]. Diagnostic MRI is not appropriate before an ultrasound is obtained. Clinical follow-up only is inappropriate as there is interval change seen on screening mammogram that requires further work-up.

17c.	a. Cortical thickness greater than 3 mm.

For axillary lymphadenopathy, the threshold for cortical thickness is 3 mm. While size is important, morphology is the most important factor in evaluation of abnormal lymph nodes [22].

17d.	c. Question the patient about her medical history, including underlying systemic diseases and concurrent illnesses.

Axillary lymphadenopathy seen on breast imaging can be a sign of systemic benign and malignant processes [21, 22]. Thus, more information should be obtained regarding the patient's history.

17e.	d. BI-RADS 4, recommends ultrasound-guided core needle biopsy of the largest axillary lymph node.

In the absence of any known systemic causes, bilateral abnormal axillary lymphadenopathy should be assigned a BI-RADS 4. Ultrasound-guided core needle biopsy of either the largest, the most suspicious appearing, or most accessible lymph node should be performed to rule out malignant processes such as lymphoma or leukemia, which can present as bilateral axillary lymphadenopathy. If lymphoma or leukemia are suspected, samples should be sent in formalin for pathology and saline for flow cytometry, which requires fresh cells for fluorescence-activated cell sorting [22]. This patient's biopsy resulted as lymphoma.

The most common cause of axillary lymphadenopathy is nonspecific reactive hyperplasia, followed by metastatic breast cancer. Leukemia and lymphoma are the most common extramammary malignant causes of bilateral axillary lymphadenopathy, followed by metastatic melanoma and ovarian cancer [22].

Typical Benign and Malignant Causes of Unilateral and Bilateral Axillary Lymphadenopathy [22].

Laterality	Benign causes	Malignant causes
Unilateral	*Infectious:* Mastitis Upper extremity infection Cat-scratch disease *Other:* Recent vaccination	Metastatic primary breast cancer
Bilateral	*Infectious:* Tuberculosis Human immunodeficiency virus Mononucleosis *Inflammatory:* Rheumatoid arthritis Psoriatic arthritis Systemic lupus erythematosus Systemic sclerosis Dermatomyositis/polymyositis Granulomatosis with polyangiitis Sarcoidosis	Lymphoma Leukemia Metastatic extramammary malignancy (melanoma, ovarian cancer)

18a. b. Ultrasound.

For a patient under 30 years old, the most appropriate initial study for evaluation of a palpable breast mass is an ultrasound [23].

18b. b. Abscess.

Ultrasound images show a subareolar heterogeneous slightly irregular collection with peripheral vascularity, which most likely represents an abscess in the setting of a nipple piercing and clinical symptoms of fever and erythema. A helpful way to classify breast abscess for purposes of treatment management is by puerperal (within the breastfeeding period) or nonpuerperal (outside of the breastfeeding period) clinical presentation. Puerperal abscess is most common in primiparous mothers and improves with antibiotics and drainage. Risk factors for nonpuerperal abscess include nipple piercings, Black race, obesity, tobacco smoking, recent breast intervention, and steroids. Nonpuerperal abscesses tend to be central (periareolar) but can also be peripheral. While nonpuerperal abscesses are also treated with percutaneous drainage and antibiotics, additional management includes cessation of controllable risk factors (e.g., smoking) [9]. This patient underwent percutaneous drainage (image a), which yielded a mixture of purulent and bloody fluid (image b). Immediate post-drainage ultrasound showed near resolution of the collection (image c). Cultures were positive for *Staphylococcus aureus*.

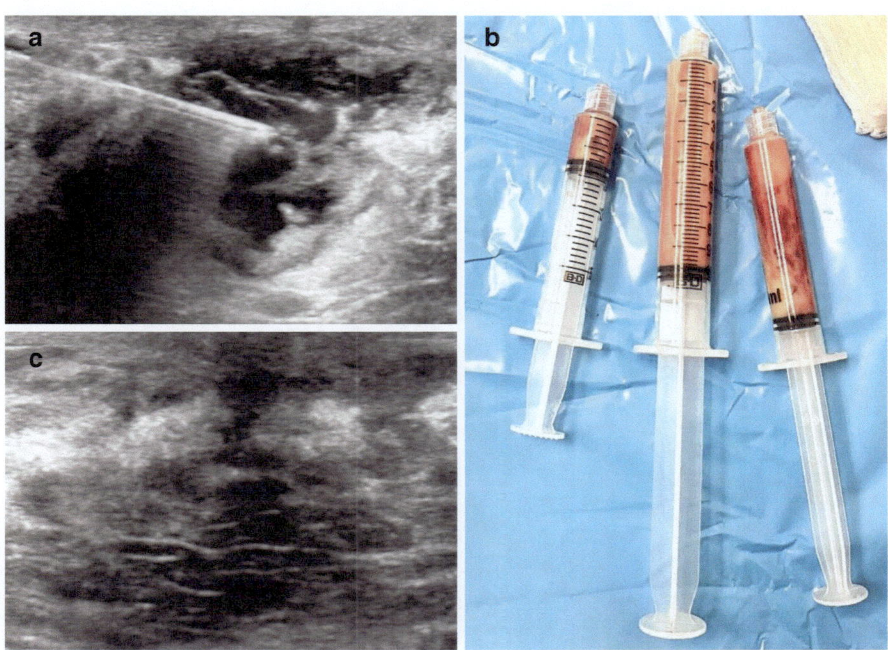

19a. a. Mammogram.

In a female patient 40 years of age or older, diagnostic mammogram is the most appropriate initial imaging study for a palpable abnormality. If mammogram findings are suspicious, then diagnostic ultrasound should be performed next. If the patient had a recent mammogram (i.e., within the past 6 months), then ultrasound may be appropriate, but this information was not provided in this scenario [23].

19b. a. Margins.

A large, hyperdense spiculated mass in the left upper outer quadrant corresponds to the patient's palpable abnormality. The most suspicious feature of this mass is the spiculated margins, which is a common feature of breast cancer [3]. Additional findings on this mammogram include unilateral axillary lymphadenopathy and focal skin thickening, which increase suspicion for malignancy. There is no obvious nipple retraction or extensive calcifications. The size of the mass is also not as relevant as small lesions can be malignant and very large masses can be benign.

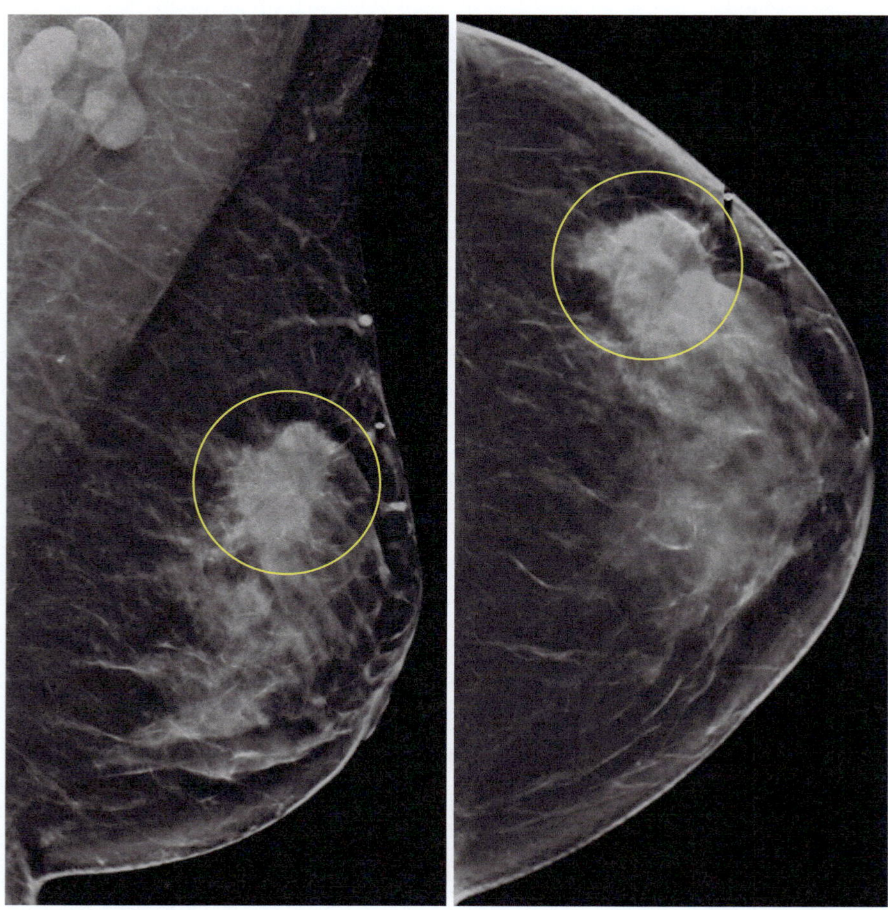

19c. b. Invasive ductal carcinoma.

Based on the mammographic findings, diagnostic ultrasound was performed in this patient demonstrating a large, irregular, hypoechoic, and vascular mass with indistinct and angular margins corresponding to the patient's palpable abnormality. Ultrasound-guided core needle biopsy of the mass revealed IDC.

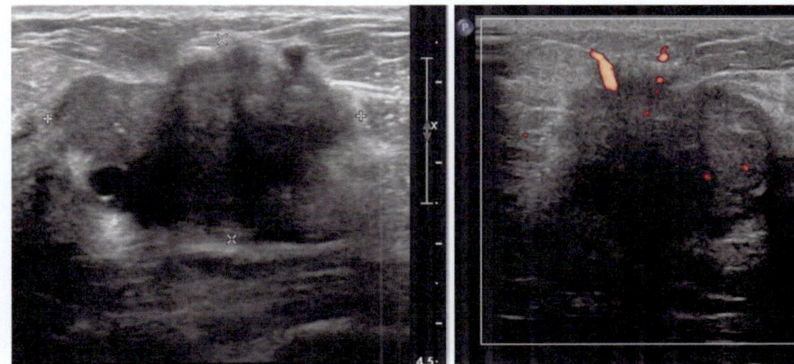

Invasive ductal carcinoma (IDC), is the most common breast cancer, accounting for almost 90% of all breast cancers, and classically presents as a hard palpable breast mass that appears as a high-density irregular spiculated mass on mammography. On occasion, adjacent pleomorphic calcifications are present which represent ductal carcinoma in situ (DCIS) [3]. DCIS presents most commonly as microcalcifications, and less frequently as a mass or palpable abnormality [11]. Metastatic extramammary malignancy that occurs in the breast tends to lack spiculation due to lack of desmoplastic reaction [17]. Post-biopsy scar can appear as a spiculated mass, but this information was not provided in the clinical scenario. While suspicious, the differential diagnosis for spiculated masses may include benign etiologies (see Table 4.4).

Table 4.4. Differential diagnosis of spiculated breast masses [3]

Risk category	Etiology
Malignant	Invasive ductal carcinoma
	Invasive lobular carcinoma
	Tubular carcinoma
High-Risk	Radial scar
Benign	Post biopsy scar
	Fat necrosis (atypical)
	Sclerosing adenosis
	Proliferative fibrocystic change (rare)

20a. c. Ultrasound-guided core needle biopsy.

This patient's ultrasound demonstrated a predominantly hypoechoic, parallel, avascular mass corresponding to her palpable abnormality. The mass demonstrates circumscribed margins with some areas of microlobulated and indistinct margins. While this finding could represent a fibroadenoma, especially in a patient of this age, the mass has some atypical features including microlobulated and indistinct margins. Core needle biopsy was performed and resulted in triple-negative IDC.

Triple-negative breast cancer is cancer that tests negative for estrogen receptors, progesterone receptors, and excess HER2 protein. Triple-negative breast cancers may grow so rapidly that they do not produce spiculated margins, and instead have smooth or "pushing" borders [3]. They are commonly reported to appear on imaging as masses with benign features, such as round shape and circumscribed margins [3, 24]. On mammogram, spot compression views may be required to reveal irregular shape or suspicious microlobulated or indistinct margins [3]. Common ultrasound appearance includes hypoechoic irregular mass with circumscribed margins [24].

Diagnostic mammogram was recommended for this patient to complete preoperative/pre-treatment evaluation, which demonstrates a round mass in the left breast lower inner quadrant corresponding to the biopsy and BB markers.

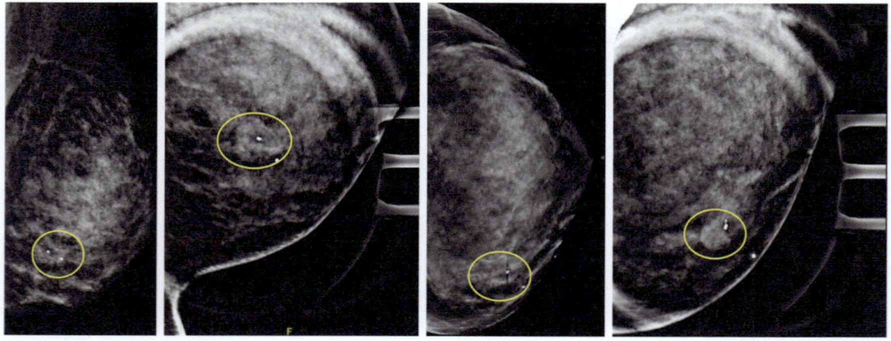

20b. a. Triple-negative IDC tends to affect younger women.

Triple-negative IDC is more likely to be diagnosed in people younger than age 50 years, Black and Hispanic women, and people with a BRCA1 mutation. Triple-negative breast cancer is considered to be more aggressive and has a poorer prognosis than other types of breast cancer as it does not respond to traditional hormone-responsive therapies [24]. It tends to be higher grade than other types of breast cancer and usually is of a cell type called "basal-like." About 10–20% of breast cancers are triple-negative breast cancers.

21a. d. All of the above.

A homogeneous mass with circumscribed borders is the most common mammographic appearance of PASH, as identified in the example image below. The mass (yellow circle) demonstrates a microclip and was biopsy-proven PASH.

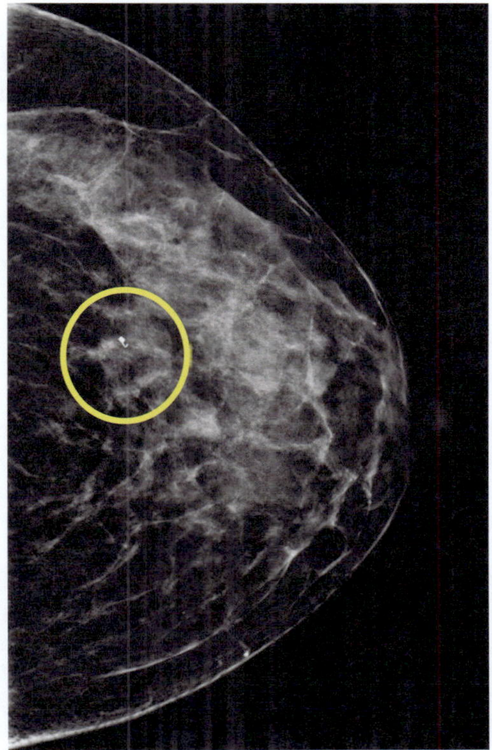

Focal asymmetry is the second most common finding, followed by mammo-graphically occult. PASH rarely presents as an architectural distortion or an irregular mass [25].

On ultrasound, this patient's lesion demonstrates the characteristic appearance of PASH as a circumscribed, round or oval hypoechoic mass with anechoic foci (yellow arrows). The anechoic foci are helpful features for differentiating PASH from fibroadenomas [25].

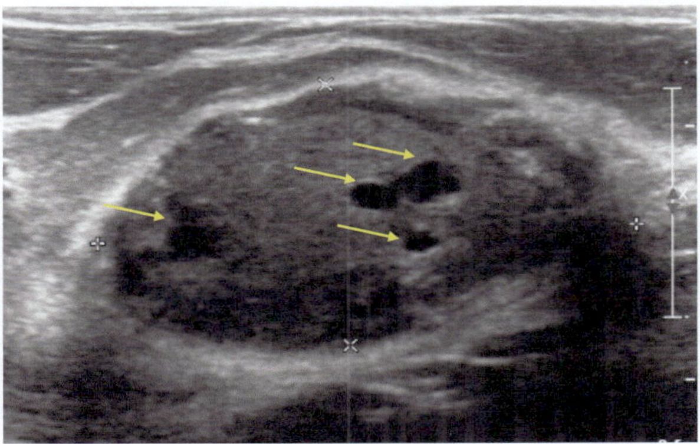

21b. c. PASH is a high-risk lesion with malignant potential.

PASH is a benign disease of the breast, characterized by the statement in answer choice a. It is thought to be a hormonal proliferative response of myofibroblasts, and thus more commonly seen in premenopausal women. The slit-like spaces seen in PASH can be mistaken for a low-grade angiosarcoma, but the entities can be differentiated on the basis of malignant cytologic features and immunohistochemical staining markers [25]. While there are no treatment guidelines for PASH, it is an important entity to recognize given its benign and malignant imaging and histopathologic mimics.

22a. a. Increased trabeculation and skin thickening involving the entire right upper outer breast and enlarged right axillary lymph node.

CC and MLO mammographic views demonstrate increased trabeculation and skin thickening involving the entire right upper outer breast, extending from anterior to posterior depth (circle). Additionally, at least three enlarged right axillary lymph nodes are seen, the largest measuring up to 24 mm (arrow).

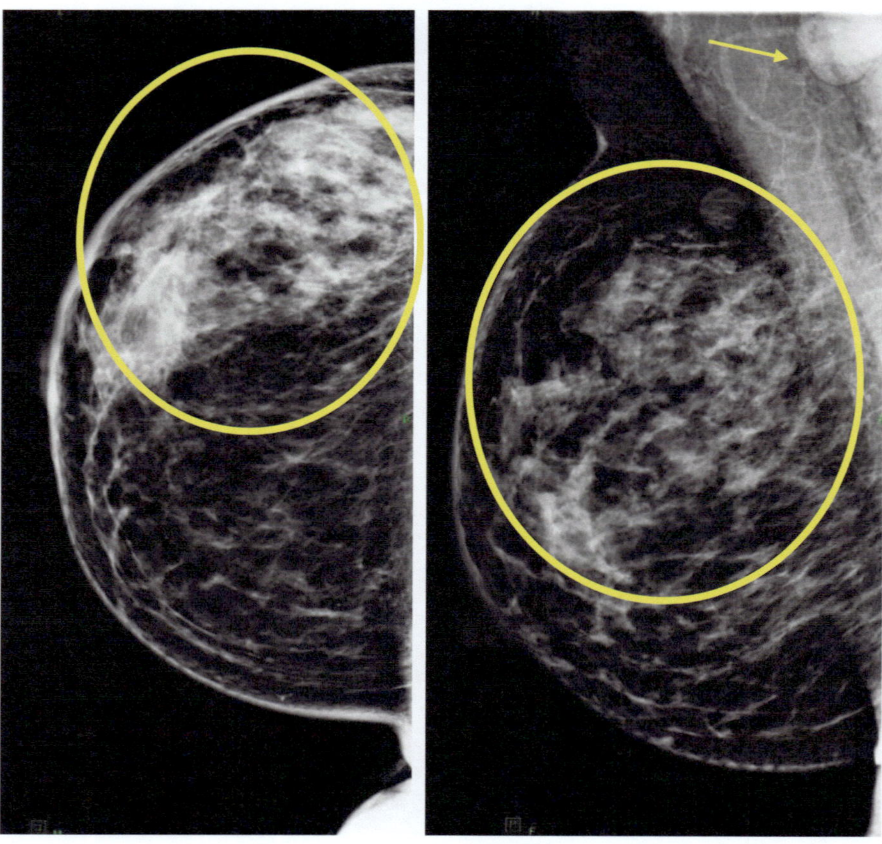

22b. d. BI-RADS 4, recommends ultrasound-guided core needle biopsy of the largest hypoechoic area.

Ultrasound shows multiple similar appearing hypoechoic areas throughout the right upper outer quadrant (images a–d). Three enlarged right axillary lymph nodes are also seen (image e).

This patient has failed antibiotic treatment. Given the ultrasound findings, ultrasound-guided core needle biopsy should be performed to rule out cancer. The differential diagnosis for these findings includes cancer (particularly inflammatory breast cancer), infection, and granulomatous mastitis.

22c. e. Benign and Concordant, surgical consultation for further management.

This patient should be referred for surgical consultation for further management. Idiopathic granulomatous mastitis (IGM) is a rare benign inflammatory breast condition characterized by lobulocentric granulomas. Table 4.5 lists the various risk factors, clinical presentation, and imaging findings for diagnosis of IGM. Treatment for IGM includes oral steroids (first-line), immunosuppressive and prolactin-lowering medications (second-line), and surgical excision for those in whom medication therapy is unsuccessful [26].

23a. c. Focal breast pain.

Clinically significant breast pain is considered focal and noncyclical breast pain [27].

23b. a. No imaging needed.

Non-focal (greater than one quadrant), diffuse, or cyclical pain without other suspicious clinical findings is generally considered clinically insignificant, and imaging is usually not appropriate. For clinically significant breast pain, appropriate imaging for evaluation is subsequently determined by age. Ultrasound is usually appropriate for patients aged under 30 years, and mammography with ultrasound for patients aged 30 years and older [27].

Table 4.5. Characteristics, imaging findings, and diagnosis of idiopathic granulomatous mastitis

Risk factors	Affects parous premenopausal women with a history of lactation
Clinical presentation and course	Unilateral palpable tender mass
	Persistent or recurrent disease
Mammographic findings[a]	Focal or global asymmetry
	Irregular focal mass
	Skin thickening with edema or trabecular thickening
	Axillary lymphadenopathy
Ultrasound findings[a]	Irregular hypoechoic masses
	Skin thickening and edema
	Axillary lymphadenopathy
	Abscess with draining cutaneous sinus tract (may cause misdiagnosis of IGM as chronic, relapsing abscesses and thus do not get biopsied [1])
Diagnosis	Requires biopsy

[a] Imaging findings are nonspecific

23c. d. Clinical follow-up.

Breast pain is a common complaint and reason for breast imaging. However, there is limited literature evaluating the role of imaging in breast pain and the association of breast pain with cancer [28]. ACR provides guidelines for the initial screening of breast pain only [27]. A review of available literature found that reported rates of malignancy associated with breast pain were low (0-2.3%), and that mammography combined with ultrasound has a nearly 100% negative predictive value in women with isolated breast pain [28]. Breast MRI and PET-CT have no role in imaging for breast pain. Biopsy is inappropriate in the absence of suspicious imaging findings.

24a. c. BI-RADS 4.

Suspicious calcification distributions include regional, grouped, linear, or segmental, with segmental distribution giving the highest positive predictive value for breast cancer (see Table 4.6) [3]. Fine pleomorphic calcification morphology is classified as suspicious, with a 29% likelihood of malignancy [3]. Thus, the most appropriate BI-RADS classification is 4, suspicious for malignancy. The morphology and distribution is concerning for ductal carcinoma in situ (DCIS) [11].

24b. c. Biopsy the posterior aspect of the region of calcifications.

Breast cancer spanning greater than 5 cm is usually treated with mastectomy, whereas breast cancer spanning less than 5 cm can be managed with lumpectomy [29]. Thus, stereotactic biopsy approach aids in diagnosis and determining extent of disease. However, approach to stereotactic biopsy of morphologically similar segmental calcifications may differ by institution. Some prefer a single biopsy within the area of abnormality, whereas others prefer biopsy of the anterior and posterior aspects of the abnormality to confirm disease extent [29]. One single institution retrospective 5-year review of 32 cases demonstrated 100% pathological concordance between anterior and posterior paired biopsy sites, suggesting that a single biopsy site may be adequate in these cases [29].

Table 4.6. Calcification distributions and their positive predictive values for breast cancer [1]

Suspicious calcification distribution	Positive predictive value for breast cancer
Diffuse	0%
Regional	26%
Grouped	31%
Linear	60%
Segmental	62%

25a. d. Smudgy on CC view and layering on ML view.

The calcifications are typical of milk of calcium, which are dependent calcium layering within breast cyst and typically appears as "tea cup" or "crescent shaped" on a true lateral view or occasionally on the MLO view. The calcifications appear smudged on the CC view due to being viewed en face [3].

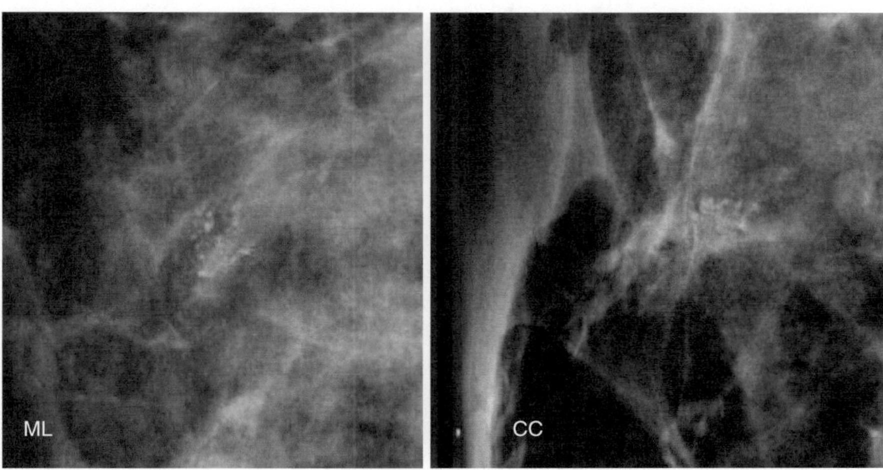

25b. a. BI-RADS 2: Recommend routine annual mammography.

Milk of calcium represents sedimented calcifications that form in benign cysts, enlarged fluid-filled acini, or ductules. Their unique appearance on mammogram is caused by calcifications floating within these fluid-filled cysts or cystic structures. When the patient is upright (i.e., mediolateral view), the calcifications layer dependently and appear dense, linear, or curvilinear and always parallel to the floor. On CC view, the en face calcifications appear smudgy, amorphous, or fuzzy. They are considered benign calcifications [3].

26. c. Focal asymmetry.

Per BI-RADS lexicon, the four types of asymmetries are asymmetry, global asymmetry, focal asymmetry, and developing asymmetry [10]. A focal asymmetry is a less than one quadrant sized, fibroglandular-like density seen in one breast on two orthogonal mammographic views, and lacks convex, mass-like borders [3]. If there is no sonographic correlate, this finding can be assigned a BI-RADS 3 (probably benign) since it has been shown to have a 0.5–1% probability of cancer if the finding is stable over 2–3 years [3]. Developing asymmetries are focal asymmetries that increase in size or are more conspicuous compared to prior studies, and thus more suspicious with a greater than 2% chance of malignancy and should be biopsied [3]. Unilateral and suspicious asymmetries are not part of the BI-RADS lexicon.

27. a. Return to screening.

This patient has an enlarging palpable mass which should be further evaluated despite negative mammographic and sonographic findings as some malignancies may be occult on mammography or ultrasound. Targeted ultrasound re-evaluation of the lump can be performed in a clinical setting with high suspicion. Breast MRI has high sensitivity and can improve detection of cancers that may be clinically, mammographically, or sonographically occult [30]. If MRI cannot be obtained, the patient should at least be referred for surgical consultation. Return to screening is the least appropriate answer in this situation.

28a. b. Air.

Neurofibromatosis 1 (NF1), also known as Von Recklinghausen disease, is a systemic neurocutaneous disorder that can affect the breast. In the breast, these skin lesions can mimic intraparenchymal breast masses. On mammography, skin lesions may be surrounded by air that gets trapped during mammographic compression, which helps differentiate these findings from intraparenchymal breast masses [3].

28b. a. Autosomal dominant.

29. d. Poland syndrome.

The patient has a unilateral absence of the left pectoralis muscle, which is seen in Poland syndrome [3].

30. a. Duct ectasia.

Ultrasound images show subareolar simple fluid-filled tubular structures converging toward the nipple, consistent with duct ectasia. Duct ectasia can be unilateral or bilateral, and is common and benign. It can occasionally be associated with nipple discharge and contain proteinaceous contents. However, solitary duct ectasia or the presence of an intraductal mass may necessitates a biopsy [3].

31. b. Supportive care.

Diagnostic mammogram right MLO image shows BB markers next to a tubular density overlying the breast. Corresponding ultrasound images show a hypoechoic tubular structure without color Doppler flow. This patient presents with typical physical exam and imaging findings of Mondor disease, an acute thrombophlebitis of the superficial veins of the breast. Mondor disease is self-limited and resolves over 2–12 weeks, thus supportive care is the most appropriate answer [3].

Table 4.7. Benign and malignant causes of axillary lymph node hyperdensities [31]

Malignant	Benign
Causes of calcifications: • Metastatic disease from occult breast primary • Metastatic disease from other primaries (e.g., ovarian carcinoma)	Causes of calcifications: • Fat necrosis • Tuberculosis • Prior granulomatous disease Causes of hyperdensities: • Gold therapy (e.g., for rheumatoid arthritis) • Silicone injection or extracapsular implant rupture • Tattoo pigment

32. b. It almost always coexists with breast ductal carcinoma.

Paget disease of the nipple is a distinct clinical entity characterized by infiltration of the nipple epidermis by malignant cells. More than 90% of Paget disease cases are associated with underlying ductal carcinoma in situ or invasive carcinoma of the breast. Typical symptoms are similar to dermatitis, including nipple erythema and eczematous changes, but sometimes progress to ulceration and nipple destruction if untreated. While some women have symptoms, the nipple itself and mammogram are normal in 50% of cases [3].

33. d. Obtain more history from the patient.

There are several benign and malignant causes of calcifications in axillary lymph nodes seen on mammography. On ultrasound, there are several benign causes of hyperdensity that can mimic calcifications (see Table 4.7) [31]. Thus, more history should be obtained from the patient first. The mammogram magnification view shows a few hyperdense foci within the left axillary lymph node. However, the lymph node otherwise retains a normal morphologic appearance on mammography and ultrasound (thin cortex with fatty hilum), suggesting a possible benign etiology. This patient had received several new tattoos on her left arm within the last year; thus, these hyperdensities were due to tattoo pigment mimicking calcifications.

References

1. Mandell J. Core Radiology: A Visual Approach to Diagnostic Imaging. 1st ed. Cambridge, Massachusetts: Cambridge University Press; 2013.
2. Horvat JV, Keating DM, Rodrigues-Duarte H, Morris EA, Mango VL. Calcifications at Digital Breast Tomosynthesis: Imaging Features and Biopsy Techniques. RadioGraphics. 2019;39:307–18.
3. Ikeda DM, Miyake KK. The Requisites: Breast Imaging. 3rd ed. St. Louis, Missouri: Elsevier; 2017.
4. Tayyab SJ, Adrada BE, Rauch GM, Yang WT. A pictorial review: multimodality imaging of benign and suspicious features of fat necrosis in the breast. Br J Radiol. 2018;91:20180213.

5. Giess CS, Raza S, Birdwell RL. Distinguishing Breast Skin Lesions from Superficial Breast Parenchymal Lesions: Diagnostic Criteria, Imaging Characteristics, and Pitfalls. RadioGraphics. 2011;31:1959–72.

6. Strachowski L, Mercado CL. Papilloma, Benign. In: StatDx. Elsevier. 2020. https://app.statdx.com/document/papilloma-benign/967bd637-b8ee-4ddf-8482-b03e4060b4b0?searchTerm=intraductal%20papilloma. Accessed 27 Dec 2020.

7. Nicholson BT, Harvey JA. Cohen MA. Nipple-Areolar Complex: Normal Anatomy and Benign and Malignant Processes. RadioGraphics; 2009. p. 509–23.

8. Yeh ED, Jacene HA, Bellon JR. What Radiologists Need to Know about Diagnosis and Treatment of Inflammatory Breast Cancer: A Multidisciplinary Approach. RadioGraphics. 2013;33:2003–17.

9. Trop I, Dugas A, David J, et al. Breast Abscesses: Evidence-based Algorithms for Diagnosis, Management, and Follow-up. RadioGraphics. 2011;31:1683–99.

10. D'Orsi CJ, Sickles EA, Mendelson EB, Morris EA, et al. ACR BI-RADS® Atlas. VA, American College of Radiology: Breast Imaging Reporting and Data System. Reston; 2013.

11. Parikh U, Chhor CM, Mercado CL. Ductal Carcinoma In Situ: The Whole Truth. AJR. 2018;210:246–55.

12. Mahoney MC, Ingram AD. Breast Emergencies: Types, Imaging Features, and Management. American Journal of Roentgenology. 2014;202:W390–9.

13. Lehman CD, Lee AY, Lee CI. Imaging Management of Palpable Breast Abnormalities. American Journal of Roentgenology. 2014;203:1142–53.

14. Sabate JM, Clotet M, Torrubia S, et al. Radiologic Evaluation of Breast Disorders Related to Pregnancy and Lactation. RadioGraphics. 2007;27:S101–24.

15. Breast Imaging of Pregnant and Lactating Women. In: ACR Appropriateness Criteria. American College of Radiology. 2018. https://acsearch.acr.org/docs/3102382/Narrative/. Accessed 22 Dec 2020.

16. Ma Y, Liu W, Li J, Xu Y, Wang H. Gastric cancer with breast metastasis: Clinical features and prognostic factors. Oncol Lett. 2018;16(5):5565–74.

17. Bitencourt AG, Gama RR, Graziano L, et al. Breast metastases from extramammary malignancies: multimodality imaging aspects. Br J Radiol. 2017;90:20170197.

18. Giess CS, Frost EP, Birdwell RL. Interpreting One-View Mammographic Findings: Minimizing Callbacks While Maximizing Cancer Detection. RadioGraphics. 2014;34:928–40.

19. Durand M, Berg W. Architectural Distortion. In: StatDx. Elsevier. 2020; https://app.statdx.com/document/architectural-distortion/15726ab4-2cbb-4f15-ab47-d4cf97f748bb. Accessed 27 Dec 2020

20. Berg WA, Oligane H, Yang WT. Tubular and Tubulolobular Carcinoma. In: StatDx. Elsevier. 2020; https://app.statdx.com/document/tubular-and-tubulolobular-carcinoma/df0c87f7-1c8e-41dc-98ce-e73d7ea97577. Accessed 27 Dec 2020

21. Cao MM, Hoyt AC, Bassett LW. Mammographic Signs of Systemic Disease. RadioGraphics. 2011;31:1085–100.

22. Net JM, Mirpuri TM, Plaza MJ, et al. Resident and Fellow Education Feature: US Evaluation of Axillary Lymph Nodes. RadioGraphics. 2014;34:1817–8.

23. Palpable Breast Masses. In: ACR Appropriateness Criteria. American College of Radiology. 2016. https://acsearch.acr.org/docs/69495/Narrative/. Accessed 15 Feb 2021.

24. Krizmanich-Conniff KM, Paramagul C, Patterson SK, et al. Triple Receptor-Negative Breast Cancer: Imaging and Clinical Characteristics. AJR. 2012;198:458–64.

25. Jones KN, Glazebrook KN, Reynolds C. Pseudoangiomatous Stromal Hyperplasia: Imaging Findings With Pathologic and Clinical Correlation. AJR. 2010;195:1036–42.

26. Pluguez-Turull CW, Nanyes JE, Quintero CJ, et al. Idiopathic Granulomatous Mastitis: Manifestations at Multimodality Imaging and Pitfalls. RadioGraphics. 2018;38:330–56.

27. Pain B. In: ACR Appropriateness Criteria. American College of Radiology. 2018; https://acsearch.acr.org/docs/3091546/Narrative/. Accessed 16 Feb 2021

28. Holbrook A. Breast Pain, A Common Grievance: Guidance to Radiologists. AJR. 2020;214:259–64.

29. Raj SD, Sedgwich EL, Severs FJ, Hilsenbeck SG, Want T, Sepulveda KA. Stereotactic Biopsy of Segmental Breast Calcifications: Is Sampling of Anterior and Posterior Components Necessary? Acad Radiol. 2016;23:682–6.
30. ACR Practice Parameter for the Performance of Contrast-Enhanced Magnetic Resonance Imaging (MRI) of the Breast. 2018. https://www.acr.org/-/media/ACR/Files/Practice-Parameters/MR-Contrast-Breast.pdf?la=en. Accessed 12 Jul 2021.
31. Honegger M, Hesseltine S, Gross J, Singer C, Cohen J. Case Report: Tattoo Pigment Mimicking Axillary Lymph Node Calcifications on Mammography. AJR. 2004;183:831–2.

Breast MRI

Melissa M. Joines, Iram Dubin, and Shabnam Mortazavi

M. M. Joines (✉) · S. Mortazavi
Department of Radiology, David Geffen School of Medicine at UCLA,
Los Angeles, CA, USA
e-mail: MJoines@mednet.ucla.edu; SMortazavi@mednet.ucla.edu

I. Dubin
Department of Radiology, Olive View-UCLA Medical Center, Sylmar, CA, USA

Department of Radiology, David Geffen School of Medicine at UCLA,
Los Angeles, CA, USA

© The Author(s), under exclusive license to Springer Nature
Switzerland AG 2022
L. Chow, B. Li (eds.), *Absolute Breast Imaging Review*,
https://doi.org/10.1007/978-3-031-08274-0_5

1a. Based on the MR images, what is the most likely diagnosis?

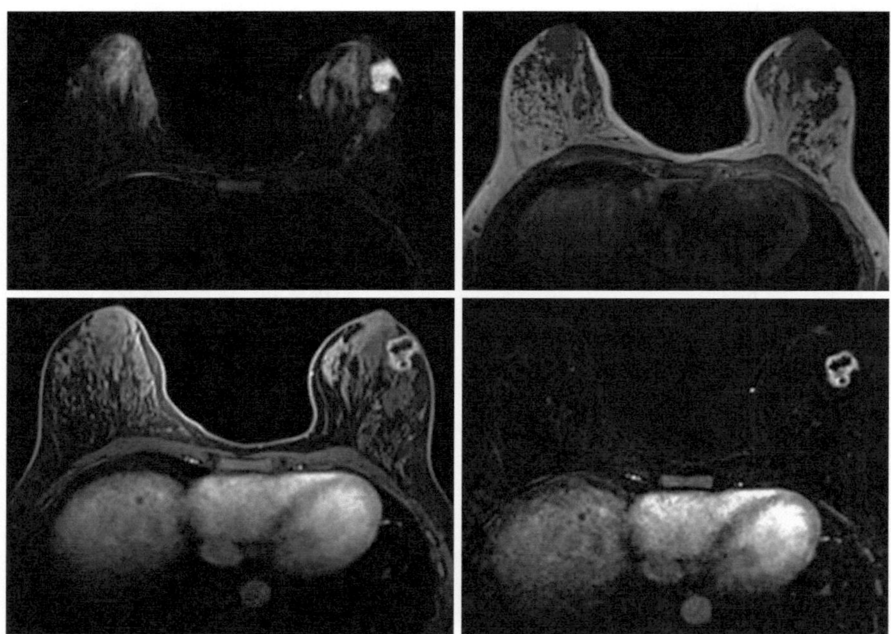

    (a) Fibroadenoma.
    (b) Mucinous Carcinoma.
    (c) Lipoma.
    (d) Fat necrosis.

1b. Where is the finding located within the breast in the image above?
    (a) Medial breast at anterior depth.
    (b) Medial breast at posterior depth.
    (c) Lateral breast at anterior depth.
    (d) Lateral breast at posterior depth.

2. What is usually associated with mucinous carcinoma?
    (a) Seen more frequently in women older than 65 years of age.
    (b) Hypointense on STIR imaging.
    (c) Strongly associated with BRCA2 mutation.
    (d) Worse prognosis than the "not otherwise specified" subtype.

3. Based on the MR images, what is the most likely diagnosis?

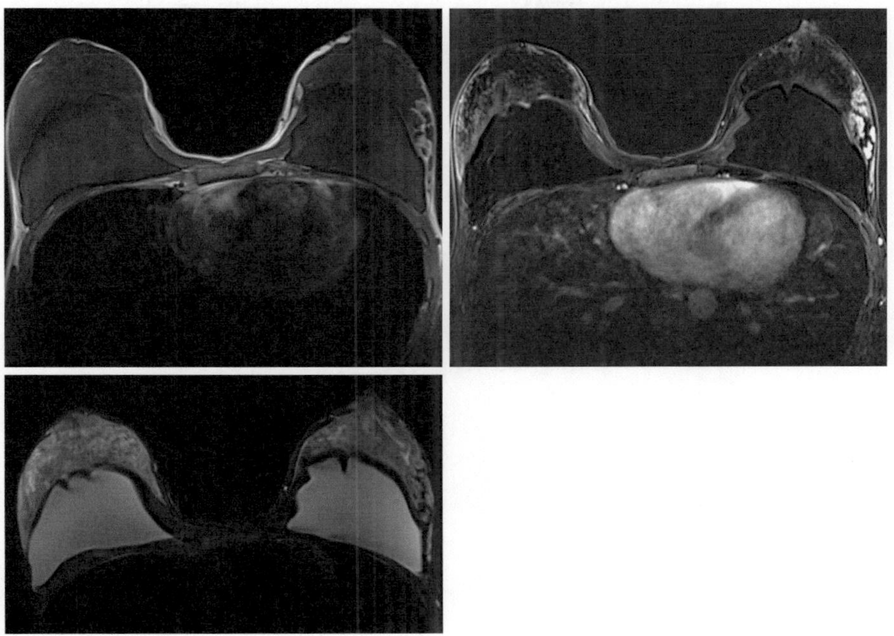

   (a) Invasive ductal carcinoma.
   (b) Complicated cyst.
   (c) Hamartoma.
   (d) Implant rupture.

4. What is the most likely diagnosis in this subtracted enhanced axial image in an asymptomatic patient without history of prior surgery in the right breast?

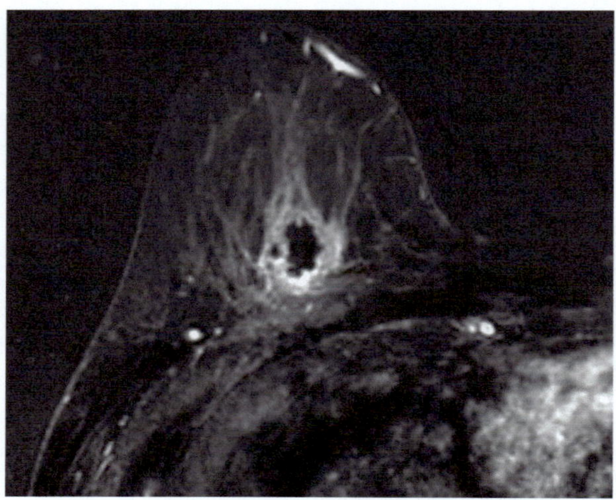

    (a) Abscess.
    (b) Seroma.
    (c) Necrotic breast cancer.
    (d) Calcified fibroadenoma.

5. The left internal mammary lymph node located at the level of the arrow is in what space?

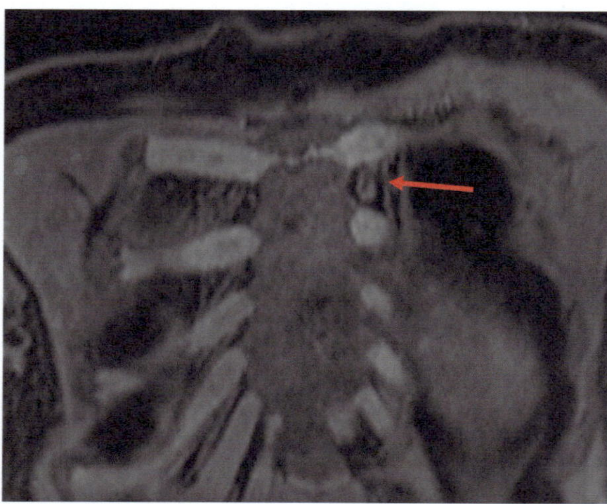

    (a) First intercostal space.
    (b) Supraclavicular space.
    (c) Prevascular space.
    (d) Second intercostal space.

6. A 52-year-old woman with biopsy-proven DCIS in the right breast undergoes MRI to evaluate for extent of disease. What does the MRI show?

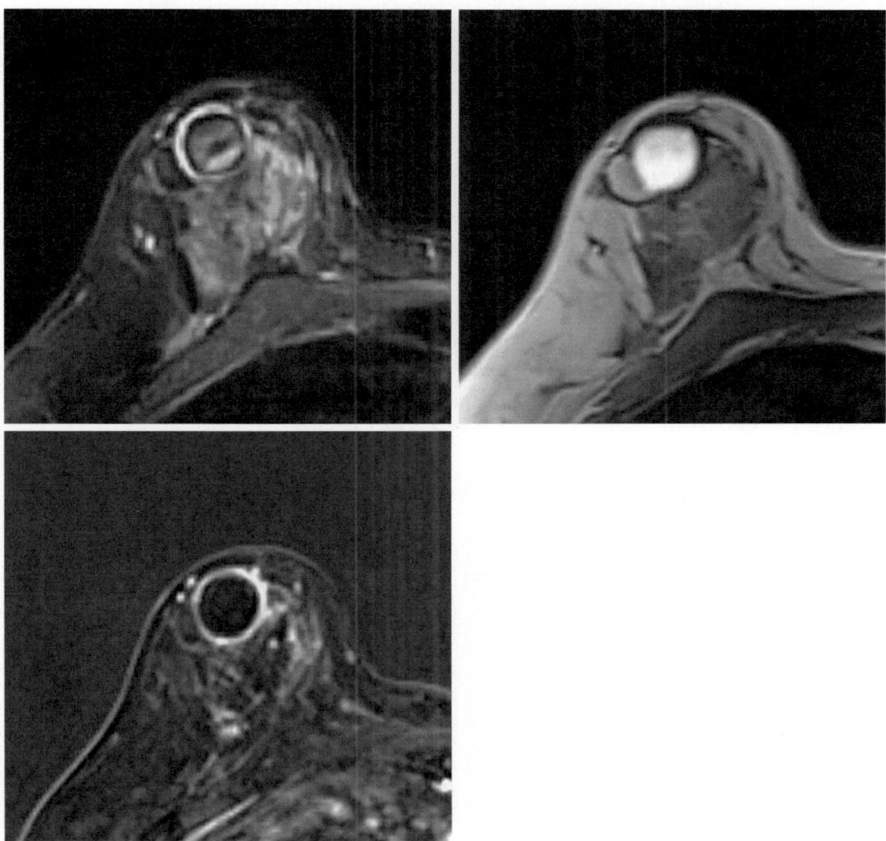

    (a) Cyst.
    (b) Lipoma.
    (c) Hematoma.
    (d) Fibroadenoma.

7. Which entity is least associated with the imaging appearance below?

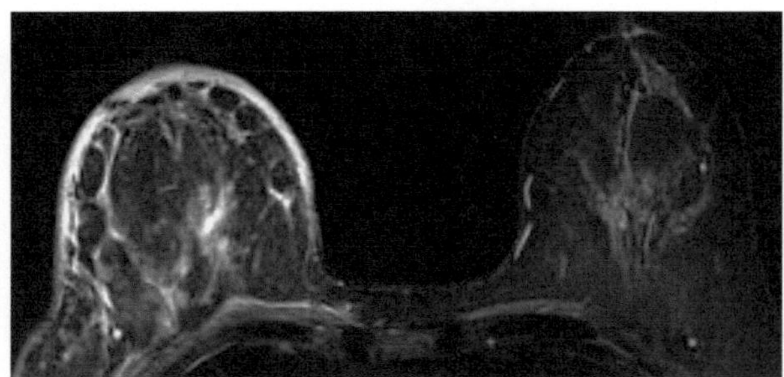

    (a) Post-radiation change.
    (b) Congestive heart failure.
    (c) Mastitis.
    (d) Inflammatory breast carcinoma.

8. Given the two images of the right breast from the same patient with known malignancy, what is the accurate description of disease distribution?

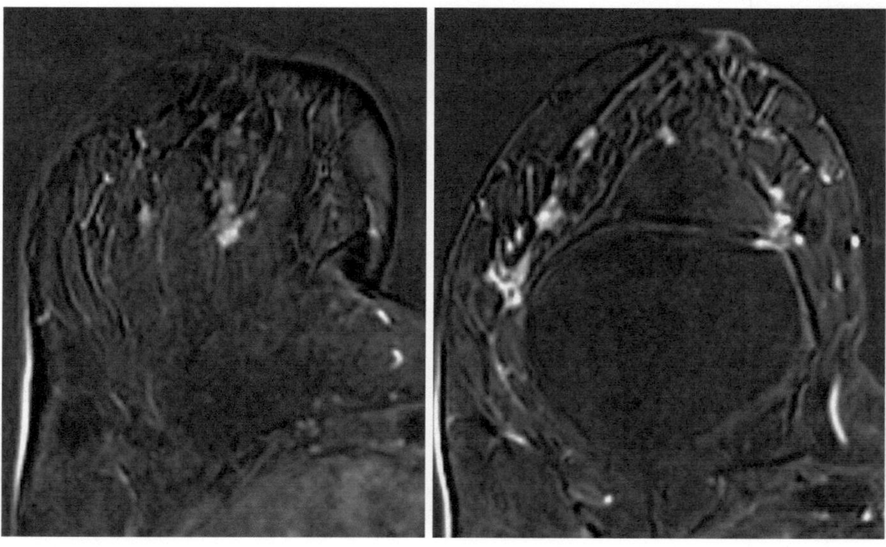

    (a) Multicentric.
    (b) Multifocal.
    (c) Multisegmental.
    (d) Focal.

9a. Which of the following MR artifacts is circled in yellow?

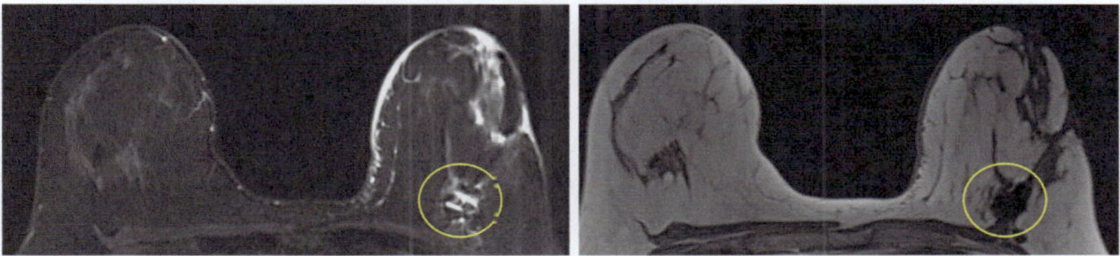

    (a) Chemical shift.
    (b) Aliasing.
    (c) Susceptibility.
    (d) Zipper.

9b. What imaging parameters would minimize the artifact in the above image?
    (a) Narrow bandwidth.
    (b) Increased field strength.
    (c) Short TE.
    (d) Long TR.

10a. 55 year old woman with history of IDC status post mastectomy over 5 years ago. Based on the MR images, what type of reconstruction did this patient have?

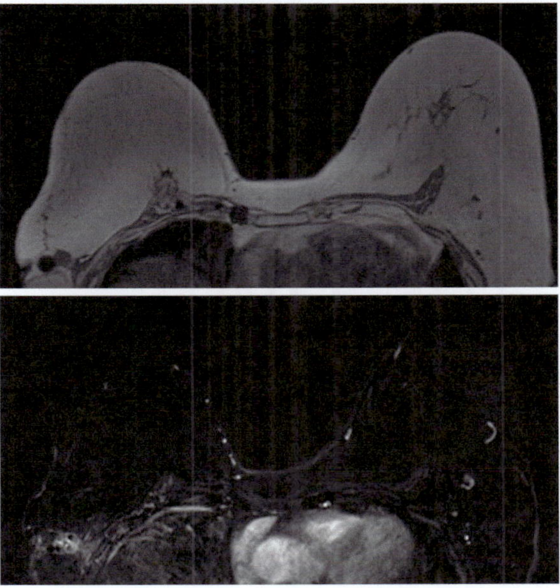

    (a) Deep Inferior Epigastric Perforator (DIEP) flap.
    (b) Implant.
    (c) Transverse Rectus Abdominus Myocutaneous (TRAM) flap.
    (d) Superior Inferior Epigastric Artery (SIEA) flap.

10b. The below finding (arrow) is compatible with:

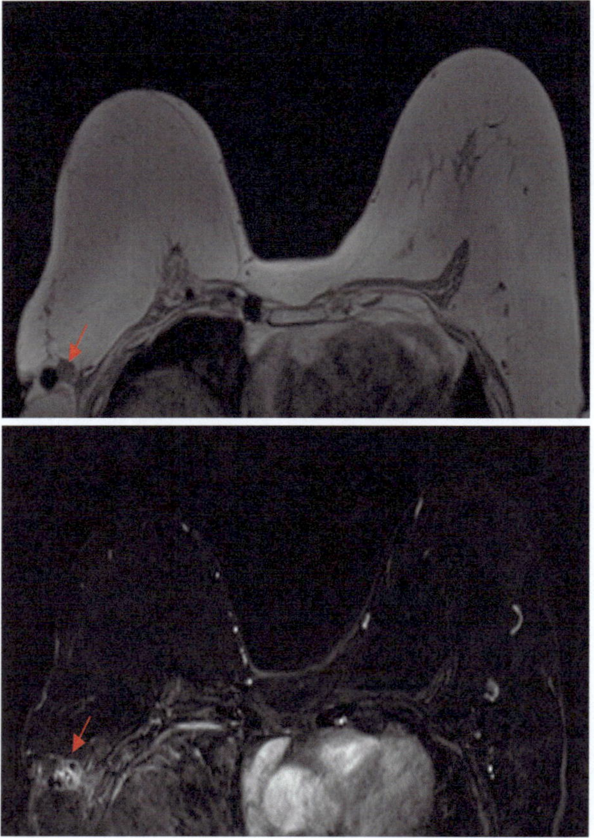

(a) Seroma.
(b) Fat necrosis.
(c) Recurrence.
(d) Hematoma.

11. A 65-year-old woman with a history of IDC status post-mastectomy. Based on the MR images what type of reconstruction did this patient have?

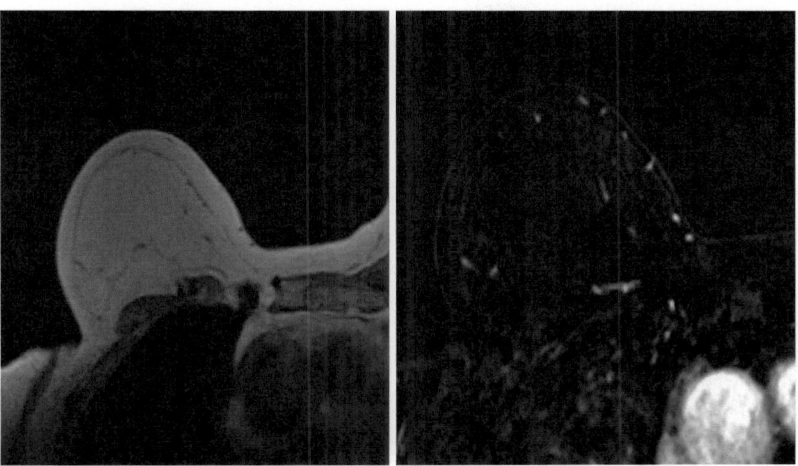

    (a) DIEP flap.
    (b) Implant.
    (c) TRAM flap.
    (d) No reconstruction was performed.

12. A 60-year-old woman with a history of silicone implants. The below findings suggest a prior history of:

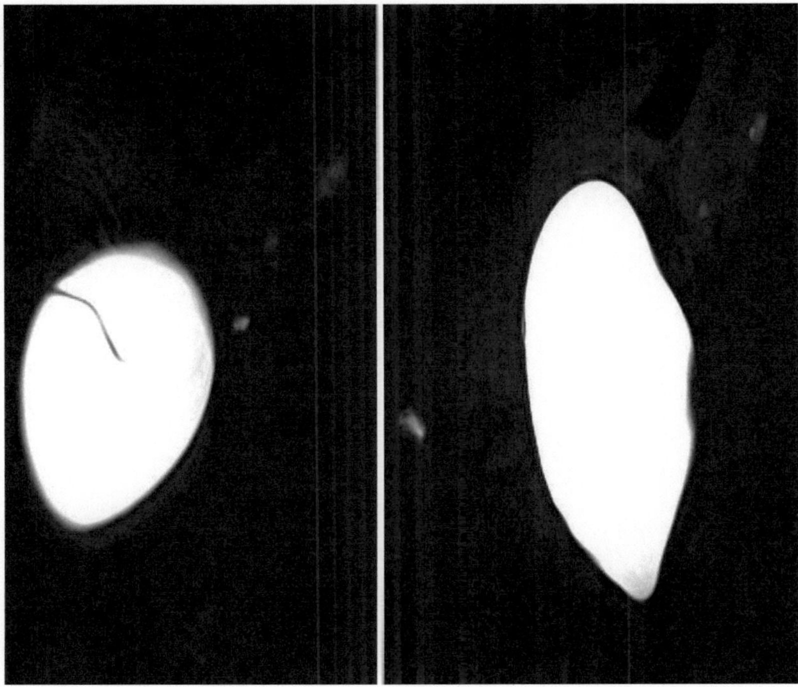

(a) Subcutaneous fat injections.
(b) Intracapsular rupture.
(c) Gold therapy.
(d) Extracapsular rupture.

13. A 42-year-old woman who is 8 weeks post-partum. The below findings are consistent with:

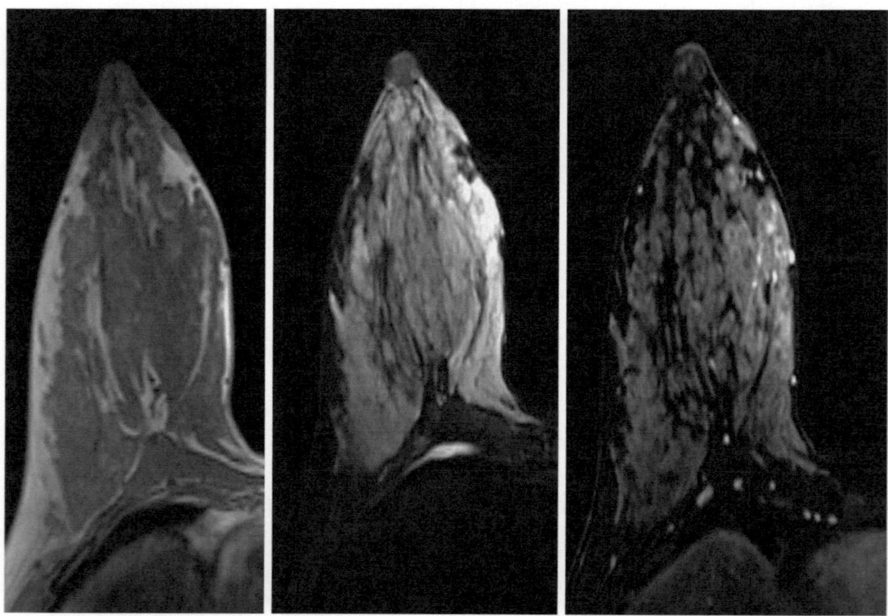

(a) Mastitis.
(b) Lactation changes.
(c) Inflammatory breast cancer.
(d) Multicentric IDC.

14. Identify the level of the axillary lymph node circled in red:

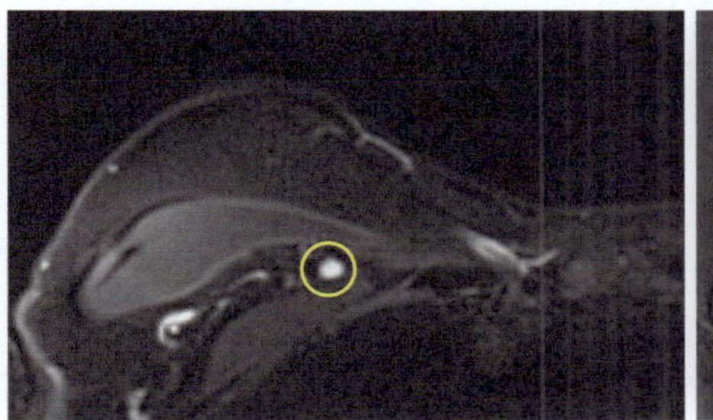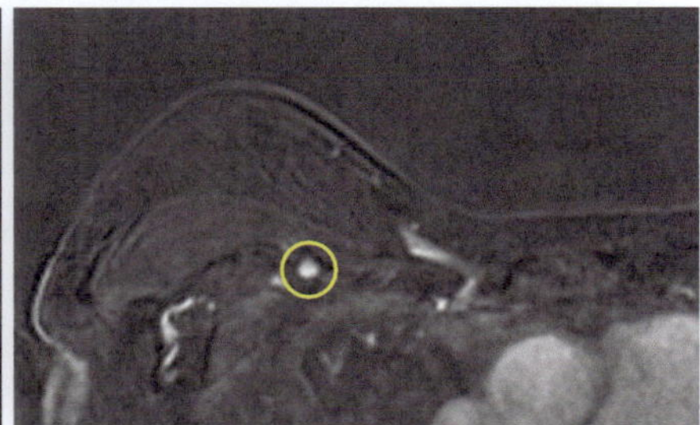

   (a) Level I.
   (b) Level II.
   (c) Level III.
   (d) Level IV.

15. Post-contrast MR images are obtained on a 65-year-old woman. Which of the following BI-RADS distribution descriptor for the non-mass enhancement in the right breast is most accurate?

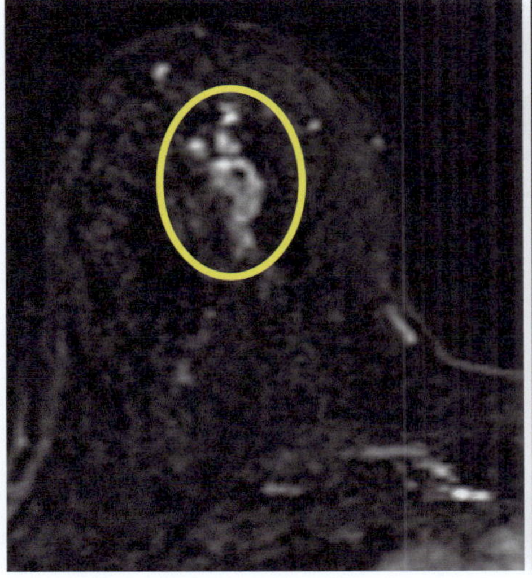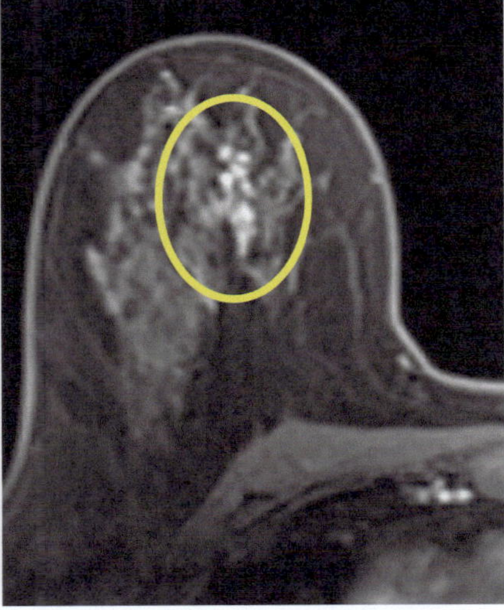

   (a) Regional.
   (b) Focal.
   (c) Linear.
   (d) Segmental.
   (e) Diffuse.

16. Which of the following is NOT a descriptor used when describing background parenchymal enhancement on breast MRI?

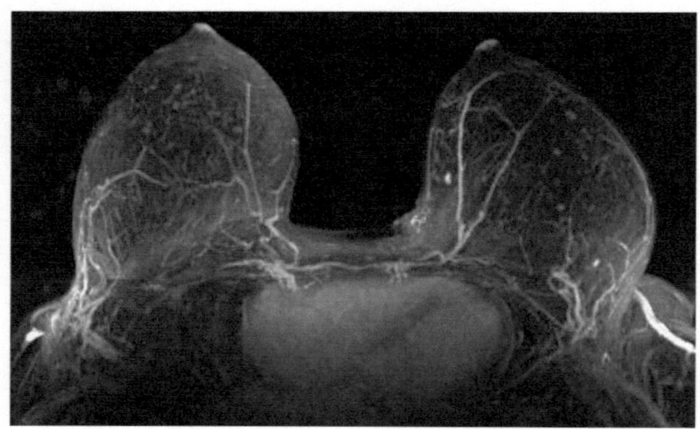

   (a) Moderate.
   (b) Extreme.
   (c) Minimal.
   (d) Mild.
   (e) Marked.

17. Which of the following MR artifacts is shown below?

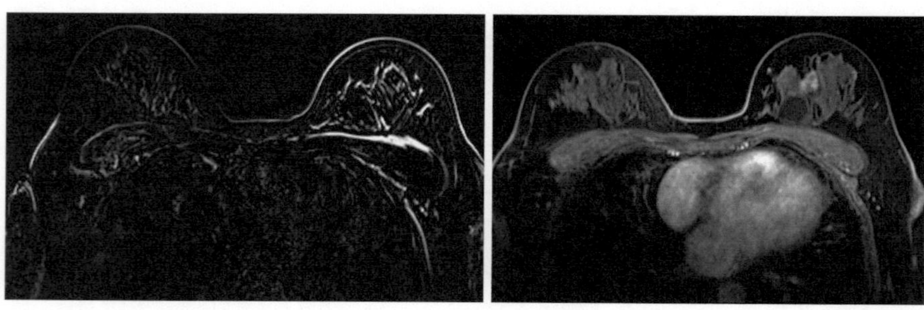

   (a) Misregistration.
   (b) Incomplete fat saturation.
   (c) Ghosting.
   (d) Radiofrequency.

18. A 45-year-old female presents for screening breast MRI. What is the best next step?

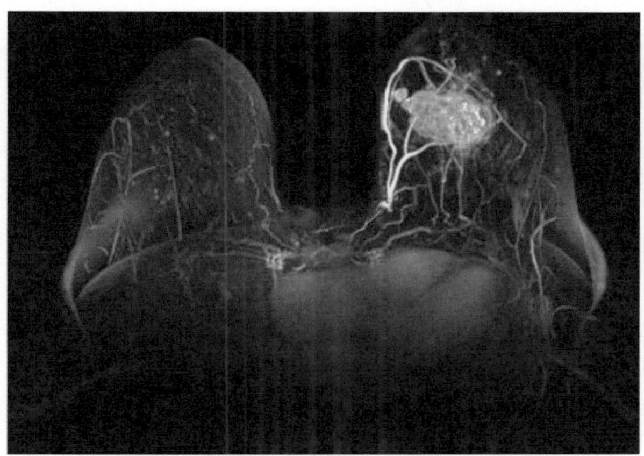

 (a) Second look breast ultrasound.
 (b) Surgical excision.
 (c) Neoadjuvant chemotherapy.
 (d) MRI guided biopsy.

19. Review the breast MR sequences below. Which of the following sequences (not shown) is also performed as part of a diagnostic breast MRI exam?

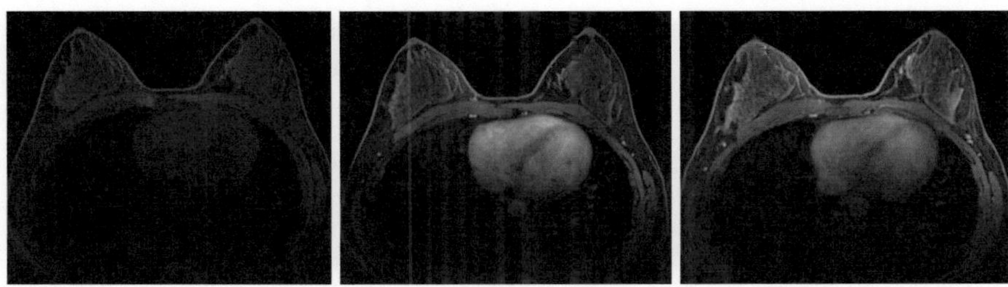

 (a) T2-weighted/Bright fluid sequence.
 (b) Pre-Contrast T1.
 (c) Early phase post-contrast T1.
 (d) Late phase post-contrast T1.

20a. A 45-year-old woman presents for high-risk screening breast MRI. What is
the most appropriate BI-RADS internal enhancement descriptor for the
mass shown?

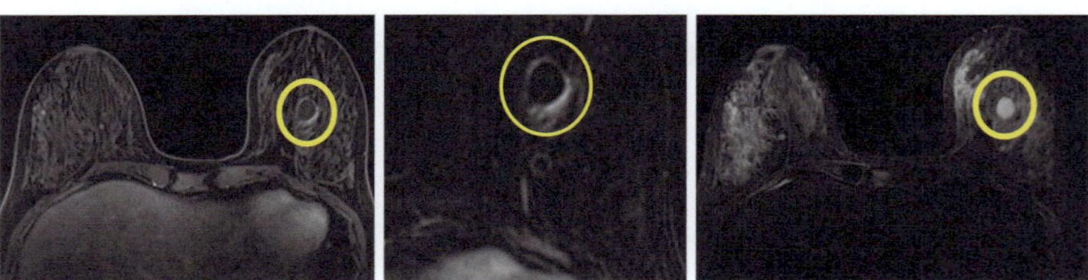

(a) Dark internal septations.
(b) Heterogeneous internal enhancement.
(c) Rim enhancement.
(d) Stippled, punctate.
(e) Homogeneous internal enhancement.

20b. What is the most likely diagnosis for the finding in the prior question?
(a) Fibroadenoma.
(b) Inflamed cyst.
(c) Mucinous carcinoma.
(d) Invasive ductal carcinoma.
(e) Intramammary lymph node.

21a. A 30-year-old woman presents for high-risk screening breast MRI. What is
the most appropriate BI-RADS non-mass enhancement pattern in the left
breast shown below?

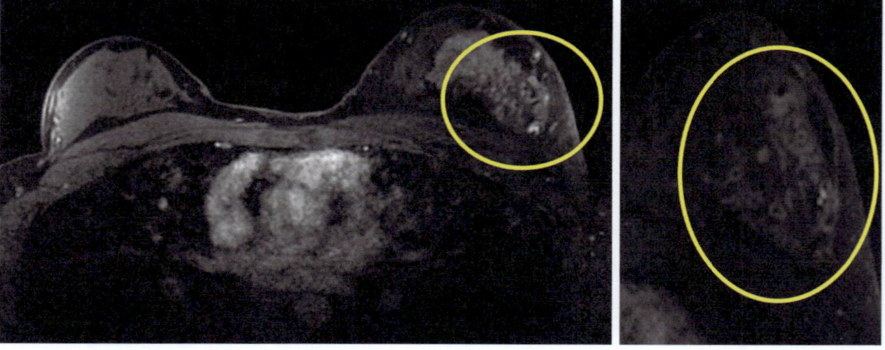

(a) Heterogeneous internal enhancement.
(b) Clustered ring.
(c) Stippled, punctate.
(d) Homogeneous internal enhancement.
(e) Clumped.

21b. What is the most appropriate BI-RADS assessment for the case presented in the prior question?
   (a) BI-RADS Category 1: Negative.
   (b) BI-RADS Category 2: Benign.
   (c) BI-RADS Category 3: Probably Benign.
   (d) BI-RADS Category 4: Suspicious.
   (e) BI-RADS Category 0: Incomplete.

21c. What is the most likely diagnosis?
   (a) Fibrocystic change.
   (b) DCIS.
   (c) Pseudoangiomatous stromal hyperplasia.
   (d) Atypical lobular hyperplasia.

22. Review the kinetic curve graph below. Which kinetic curve enhancement pattern on breast MRI is most suggestive of a malignancy?

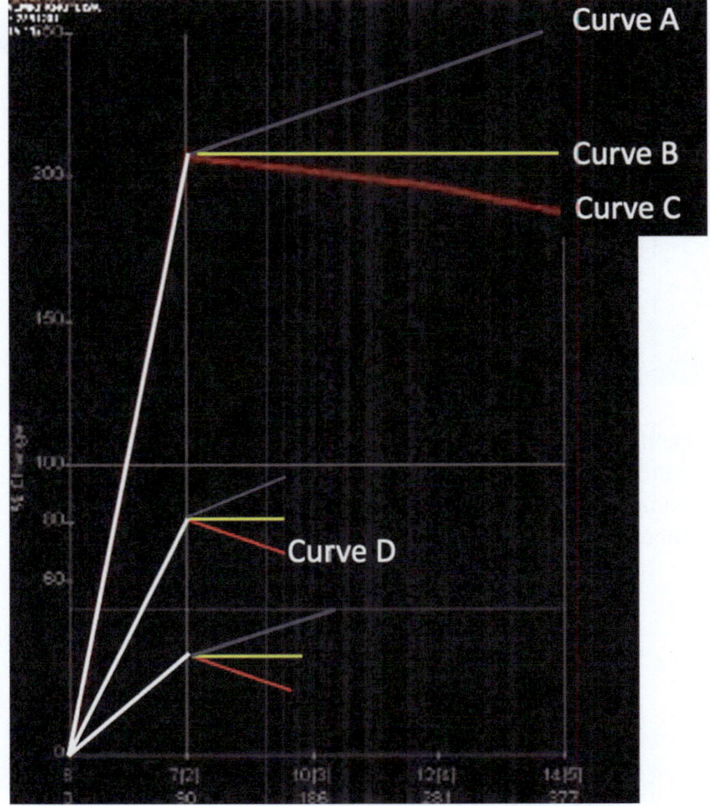

   (a) Curve A.
   (b) Curve B.
   (c) Curve C.
   (d) Curve D.

23. For the delayed phase, washout is less than or equal to ___% of the initial enhancement.
    (a) 5%.
    (b) 10%.
    (c) 15%.
    (d) 20%.

24. Based on the MR images, what is the most likely diagnosis in this 45-year-old patient?

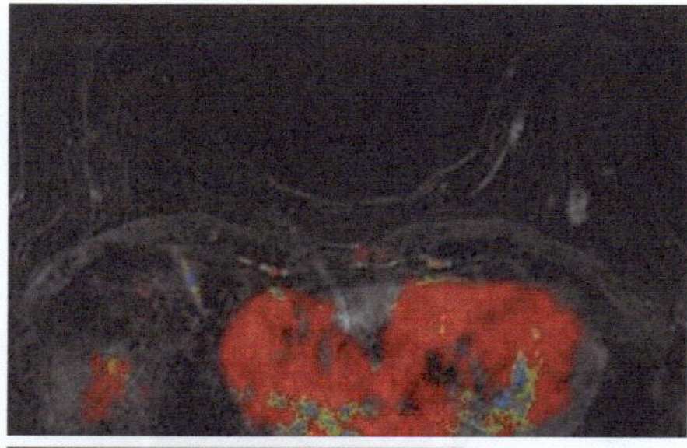
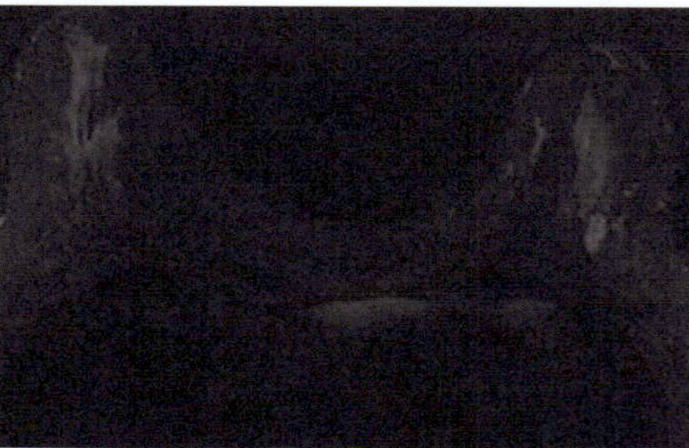
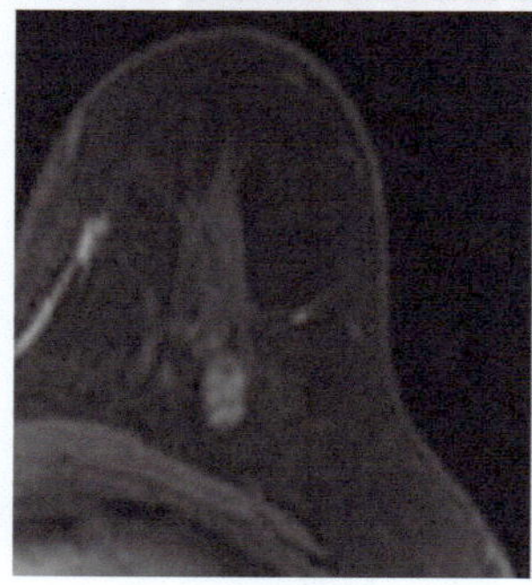

    (a) Papillary Carcinoma.
    (b) Fibroadenoma.
    (c) Complicated cyst.
    (d) Tubular carcinoma.

25. Based on the MR images below, what is the most likely diagnosis?

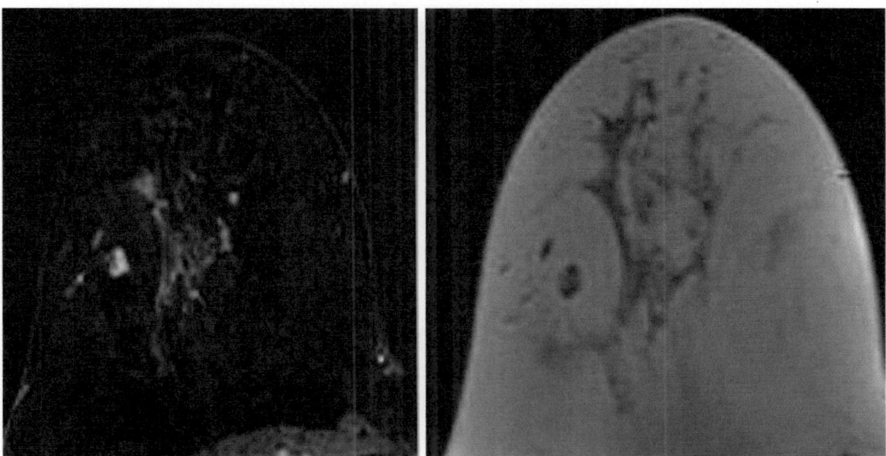

   (a) Fibroadenoma.
   (b) Complicated cyst.
   (c) Intramammary lymph node.
   (d) DCIS.

26. A 40-year-old patient underwent screening breast MRI shown below. Which of the following indications does not qualify for high-risk screening breast MRI, per the American Cancer Society Guidelines?

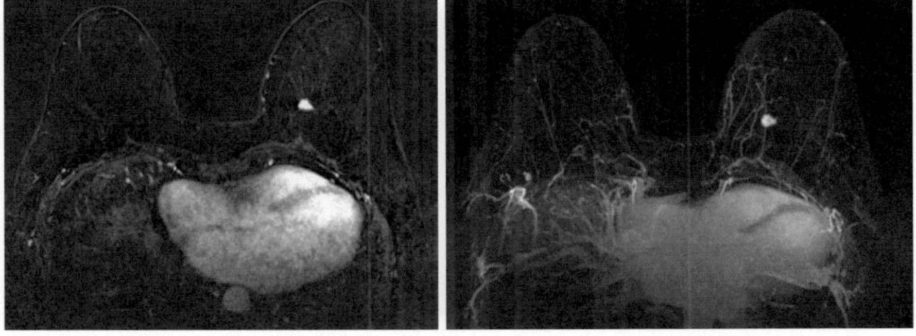

   (a) Known BRCA 1 or 2 mutation.
   (b) First-degree relative with a known BRCA mutation, but untested.
   (c) Personal history of LCIS.
   (d) History of mantle field radiation between the ages 10 and 30 years.
   (e) History of Cowden syndrome.

27. A patient is status post mantle field radiation for Hodgkin's Lymphoma at age 16. When should she begin screening for breast MRI?
    (a) Eight years after radiation therapy but not before the age of 25 years.
    (b) Screening breast MRI is not indicated in this patient population.
    (c) Screening breast MRI should begin at the age of 30 years.
    (d) Screening breast MRI should begin at the age of 40 years once mammography screening starts.

28. A patient presented with metastatic axillary lymphadenopathy consistent with breast primary. Breast MRI will identify the breast primary lesion in what percentage of cases?

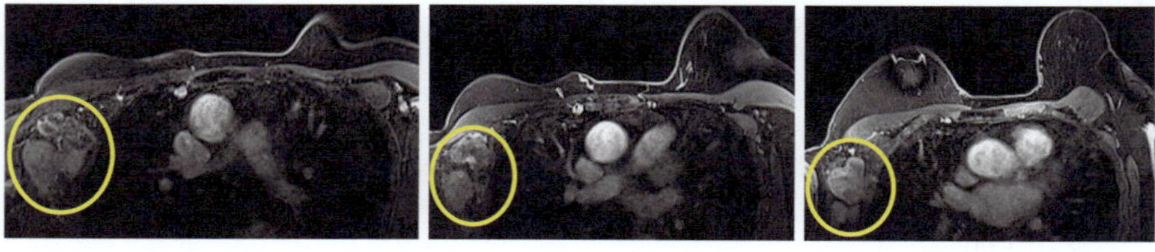

    (a) 10–20%.
    (b) 20–30%.
    (c) 40–50%.
    (d) 70–80%.

29. A high-risk patient presents for screening. The right breast shows a small enhancing focus. The kinetic curve for this focus is also shown. Which is the most appropriate BI-RADS?

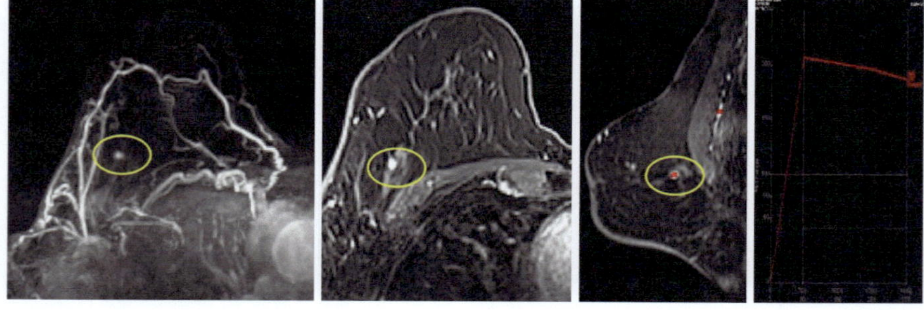

    (a) BI-RADS Category 2. Benign, focus is too small to characterize.
    (b) BI-RADS Category 3. Probably Benign. Recommend 6-month follow-up MRI.
    (c) BI-RADS Category 0. Assessment Incomplete. Recommend second-look ultrasound.
    (d) BI-RADS Category 4. Suspicious. Recommend second-look ultrasound. If no sonographic correlate, MRI biopsy should be performed.

30. Which of the following is NOT an indication for breast MRI?
    (a) A 45-year-old woman with dense breasts and average lifetime risk.
    (b) A 32-year-old woman status post neoadjuvant chemotherapy for breast cancer.
    (c) A 55-year-old woman with newly diagnosed breast cancer and suspected chest wall involvement.
    (d) Evaluation of silicone implant integrity in a 65-year-old woman with a new breast contour deformity and inconclusive breast ultrasound.
    (e) Screening of the contralateral breast in a 40-year-old woman with newly diagnosed breast cancer.

31. Which of the following is a correct statement regarding breast MRI in pregnancy and lactation?
    (a) Contrast-enhanced breast MRI is an absolute contraindication in lactation.
    (b) No special consideration for a lactating patient to receive a non-contrast MRI.
    (c) Gadolinium-based contrast media have been classified by the Food and Drug Administration as pregnancy class B drugs.
    (d) Gadolinium-based contrast agents pass through the placental barrier but do not enter fetal circulation.

32. What is the feature that makes a focus more suspicious?
    (a) Washout kinetics.
    (b) Fatty hilum.
    (c) Hyperintense signal on fluid-sensitive sequences.
    (d) Persistent kinetics.

33. What is the most appropriate description of the finding indicated by the arrow?

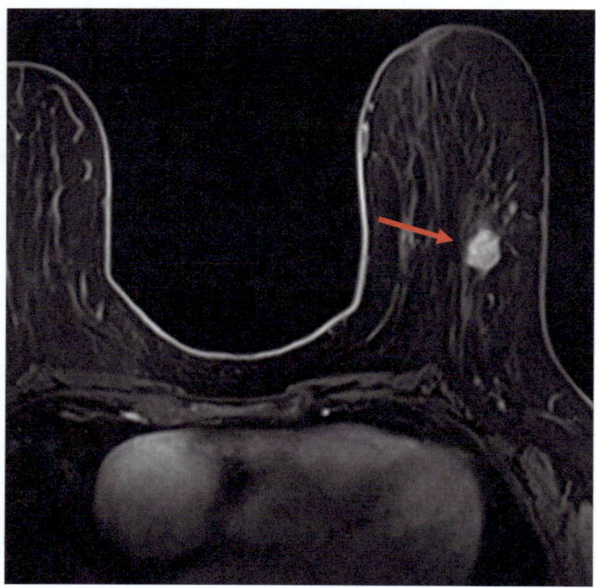

   (a) Homogenously enhancing round mass with irregular margins.
   (b) Homogenously enhancing round mass with indistinct margins.
   (c) Homogenously enhancing focus with indistinct margins.
   (d) T2 hyperintense oval mass with irregular margins.

34. What is the shape description and most appropriate BI-RADS category for the finding in the right breast?

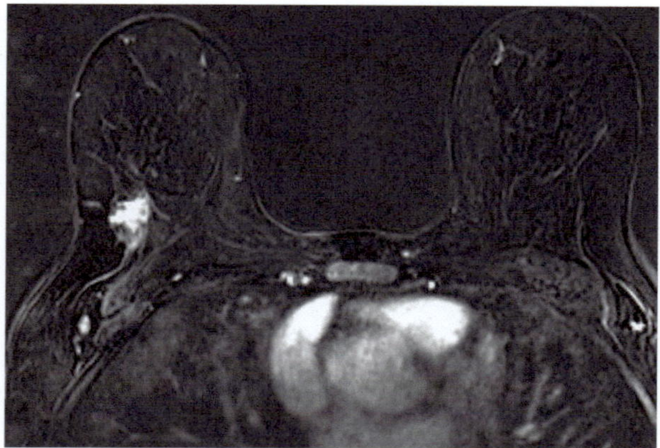

   (a) Irregular mass; BI-RADS Category 3.
   (b) Irregular mass; BI-RADS Category 4.
   (c) Oval mass; BI-RADS Category 3.
   (d) Oval mass; BI-RADS Category 4.

35. The MRI shows a biopsy-proven malignancy in the right breast which measures 3 cm in maximum dimension without other suspicious findings in either breast. Based on the 8th edition of TNM staging, what is the appropriate T stage for this mass?

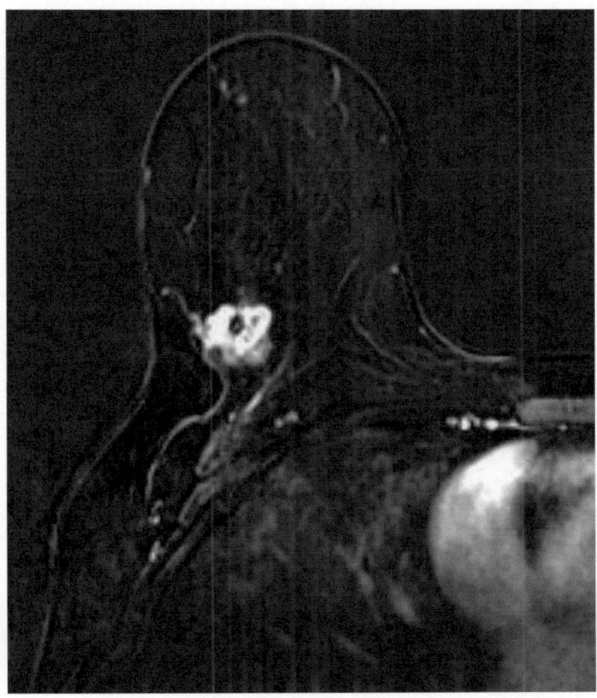

   (a) T1.
   (b) T2.
   (c) T3.
   (d) More information is needed to assign the T staging.

36. What is the sequence shown and what is the appropriate description of amount of fibroglandular tissue?

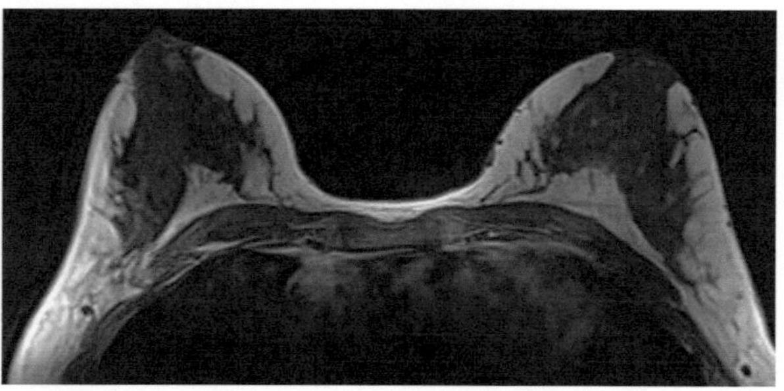

(a) Precontrast T1 non-fat saturated; Extreme fibroglandular tissue.
(b) Precontrast T1 non-fat saturated; Almost entirely fat.
(c) Contrast-enhanced T1 non-fat saturated; Extreme fibroglandular tissue.
(d) Precontrast T1 non-fat saturated; Assessment of the amount of fibroglandular tissue is not part of the MRI lexicon and should be assessed only in mammogram.

37. The mass in the left breast is a biopsy-proven malignancy. What other suspicious finding is in the below image?

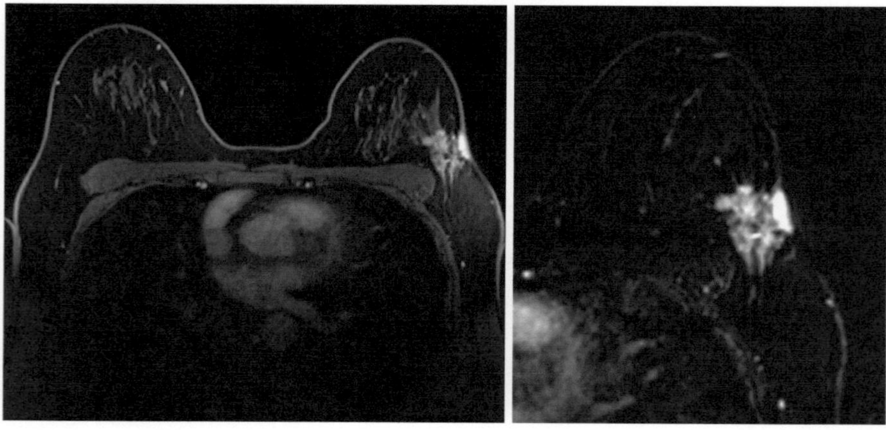

(a) Skin retraction and enhancement.
(b) Nipple retraction.
(c) Left axillary lymphadenopathy.
(d) Chest wall invasion.

38. Which of the following is not depicted in the below image?

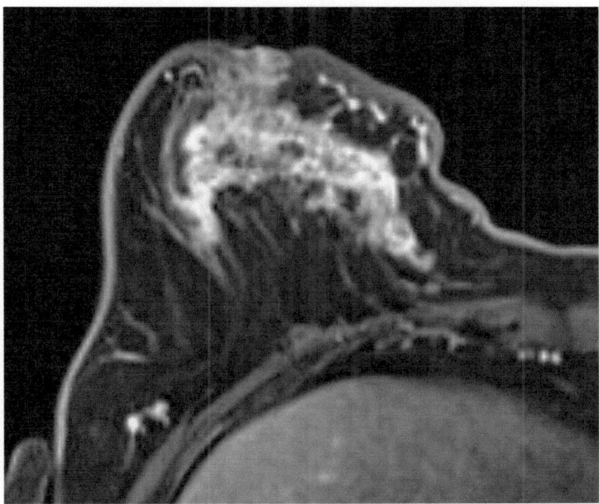

    (a) Nipple inversion.
    (b) Nipple invasion.
    (c) Skin thickening.
    (d) Chest wall invasion.

39. What is the most appropriate assessment and recommendation of the finding in the left breast in this asymptomatic patient with a recent history of lumpectomy?

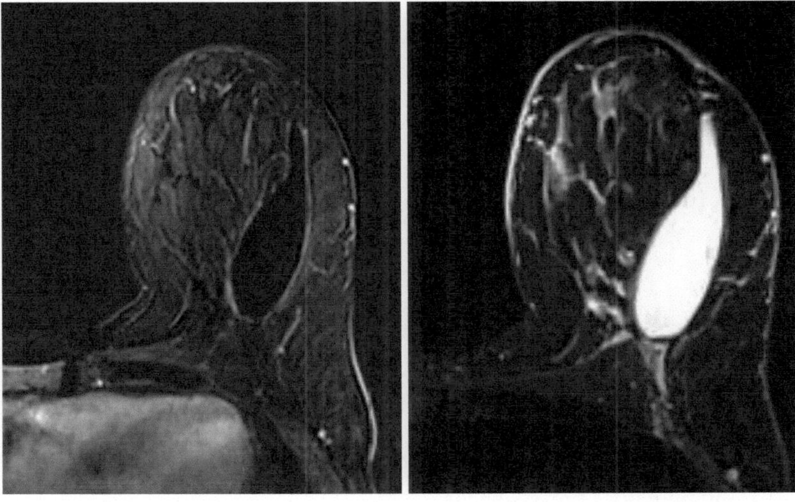

    (a) Cyst; recommend cyst aspiration.
    (b) Cyst; recommend short term follow-up breast MRI to ensure resolution.
    (c) Suspicious mass; recommend targeted second-look ultrasound and core needle biopsy.
    (d) Benign seroma; no action is needed.

40. What is an appropriate description of the margin of the mass shown in the MRI?

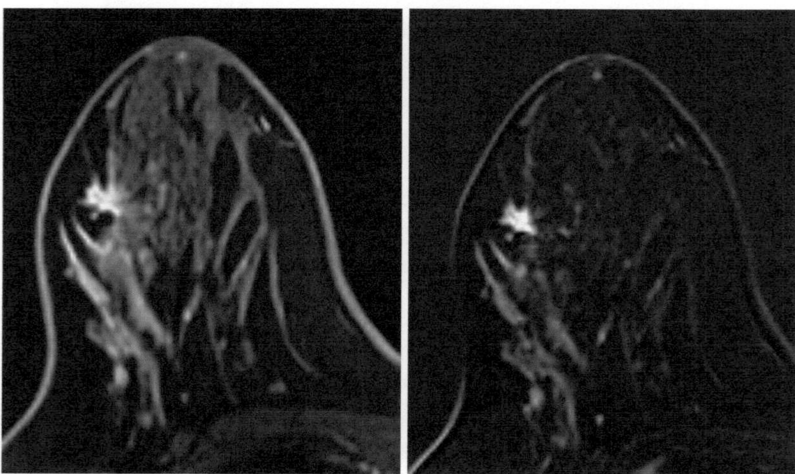

(a) Microlobulated.
(b) Spiculated.
(c) Circumscribed.
(d) Angular.

41. Based on the ultrasound and corresponding MRI finding in the right breast, what is the most likely diagnosis?

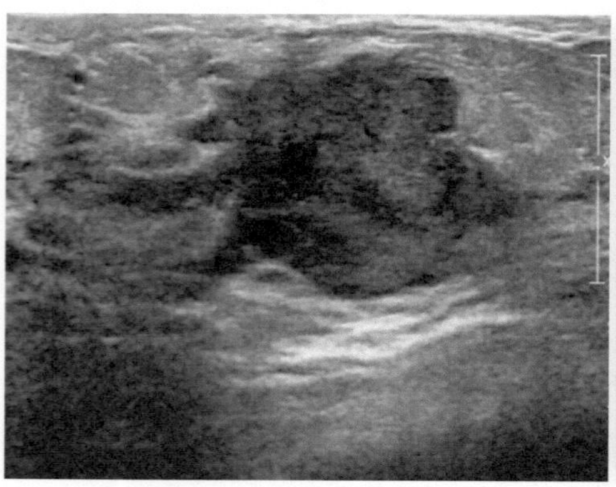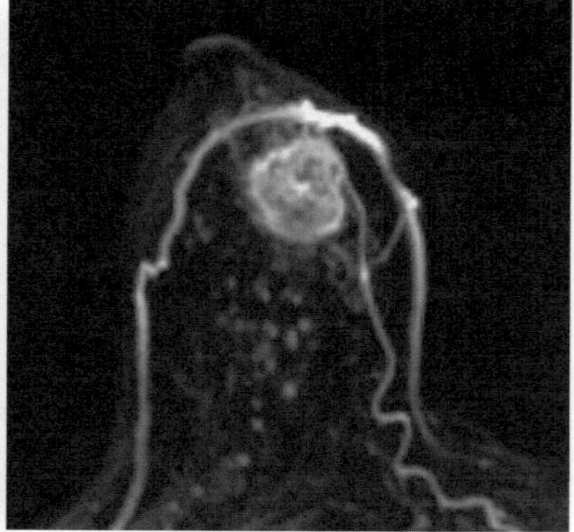

(a) Invasive ductal carcinoma.
(b) Inflammatory breast cancer.
(c) Breast abscess.
(d) Fibroadenoma.

42. Which of the following is NOT correct regarding screening breast MR in high-risk women?
    (a) Screening breast MRI is indicated in a patient with a 25% lifetime risk of breast cancer due to strong family history.
    (b) Li-Fraumeni syndrome, Cowden and Bannayan-Riley-Ruvalcaba syndromes are associated with an increased risk of developing breast cancer.
    (c) 30% of all breast cancer occurs in women with a family history of breast cancer (familial breast cancer).
    (d) Increased risk of breast cancer is only associated in patients with BRCA1 mutation, and not in patients with BRCA2 mutation.

43. Which of the following is NOT a contraindication for contrast-enhanced breast MRI?
    (a) Pregnancy.
    (b) Port-A-Cath.
    (c) Metallic foreign body in the eye.
    (d) Non-MRI-conditional implanted device.

44. What artery is denoted by the arrow in the axial enhanced T1 image and corresponding MIP image?

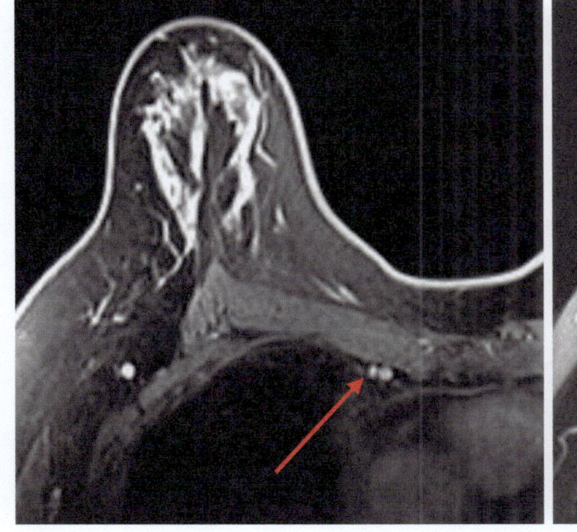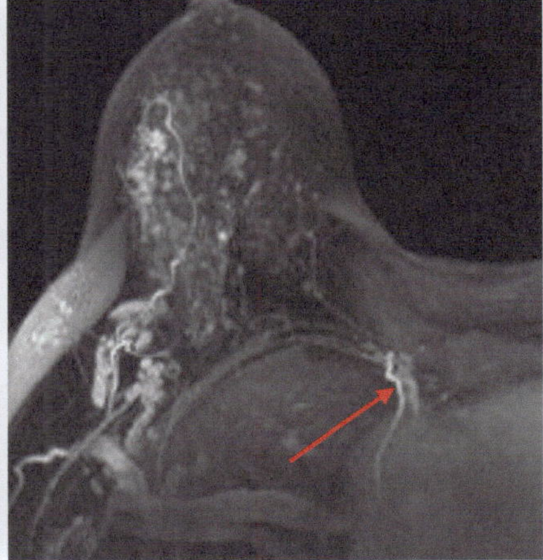

    (a) Lateral thoracic artery.
    (b) Intercostal artery.
    (c) Internal mammary (thoracic) artery.
    (d) Epigastric artery.

Answers

1a. b. Mucinous carcinoma.

1b. c. Lateral breast at anterior depth.

2. a. Seen more frequently in women older than 65 years.

Mucinous carcinoma of the breast, also known as colloid carcinoma, is a subtype of invasive ductal carcinoma. It tends to occur in women older than 65 years. Malignant cells in mucinous carcinoma secrete large quantities of extracellular mucin-producing high-signal intensity on T2-weighted images on MRI. The masses can be lobulated, oval, or round with circumscribed or irregular margins. They may also present with a thickened, enhancing, or irregular rim [1].

3. c. Hamartoma.

Breast hamartomas are benign lesions composed of fibrous, glandular, and fatty tissue surrounded by a thin capsule. Their appearance is frequently described as a "breast within a breast." Breast hamartomas are commonly asymptomatic or they may present as a painful mass. The MRI demonstrates a fat-containing mass with intermixed areas of fat and heterogeneous enhancement in the left lateral breast. The fat-containing components follow fat signal intensity on all MR sequences. Mammogram demonstrates a circumscribed mass (circled) with areas of internal lucency reflective of the inherent fat component. Ultrasound demonstrates a heterogeneous mass (arrows) with mixed hypoechoic and hyperechoic areas reflective of the fat and fibroglandular tissue.

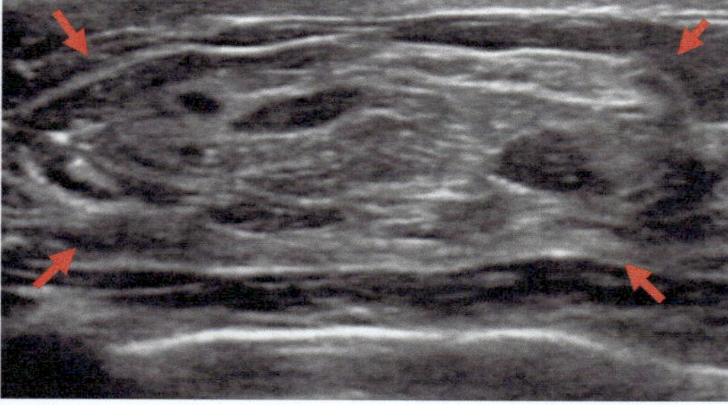

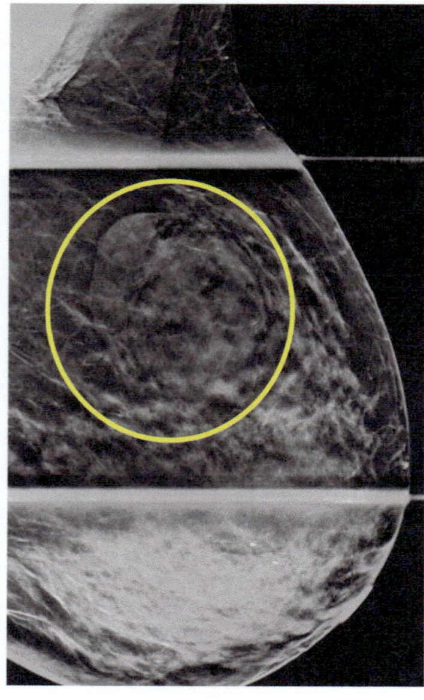

4. c. Necrotic breast cancer.

Irregular thick rim enhancement with central necrosis is suspicious for necrotic breast cancer.

Choice a is incorrect because the patient is asymptomatic.

Choice b is incorrect because there is no history of surgery in the right breast. A breast seroma does not present with thick irregular rim enhancement and usually has a smooth wall with thin peripheral enhancement.

Choice d is incorrect. A calcified fibroadenoma does not demonstrate enhancement.

5. d. Second intercostal space.

The "sternal angle of Louis" also known as the sternal angle is located at the sternomanubrial junction. It demarcates where the costal cartilages of the second rib articulates with the sternum. Internal mammary lymph nodes located at this level are therefore located in the second intercostal space.

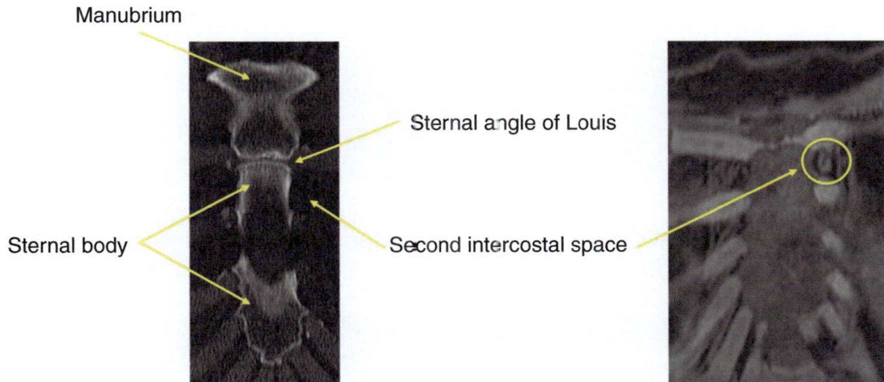

6. c. Hematoma.

The images demonstrate a round, intrinsically T1 hyperintense lesion with associated STIR hyperintensity and fluid–fluid layer in the right breast. In the context of recent stereotactic biopsy, this lesion represents a post-biopsy hematoma. Mild uniform thin rim enhancement seen on the post-contrast subtraction sequence is likely reflective of post-biopsy changes.

7. b. Congestive heart failure.

The image demonstrates diffuse parenchymal edema with associated skin thickening in the right breast. These findings are nonspecific and may be seen in the setting of post-radiation change, mastitis, lymphedema, and inflammatory breast cancer. This may also occur with SVC syndrome or upper extremity DVT. Although congestive heart failure may produce similar imaging findings, it would be expected to occur bilaterally.

8. a. Multicentric.

Multicentric breast cancer is defined as two or more foci of cancer in different quadrants of the breast.

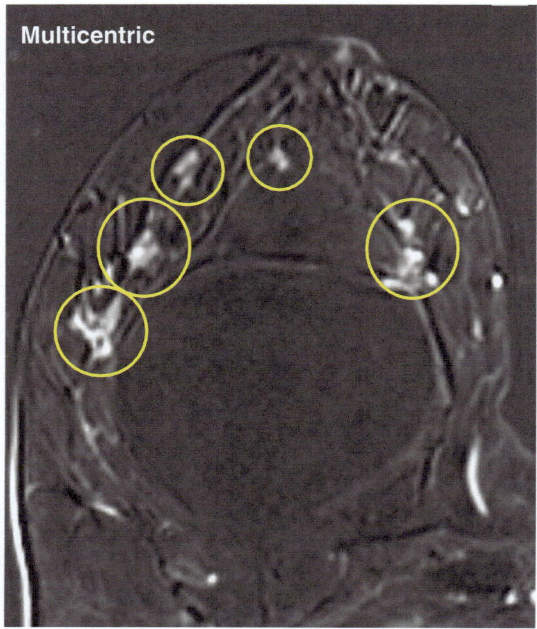

Multifocal breast cancer refers to two or more foci of cancer within the same breast quadrant [2].

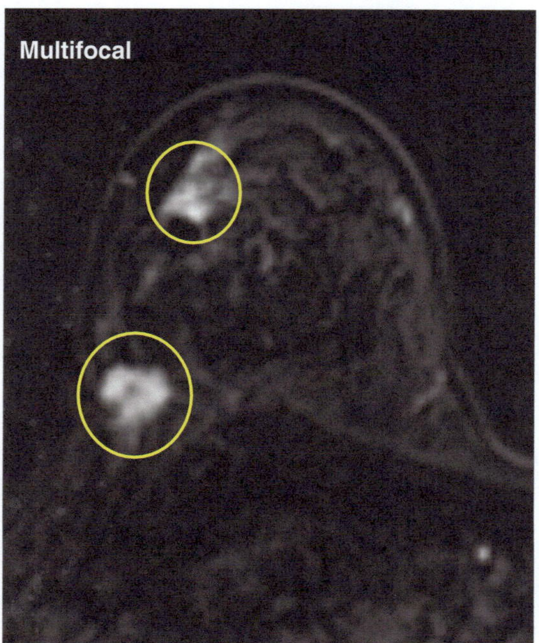

9a. c. Susceptibility.

MR images demonstrate magnetic susceptibility artifact from a BioZorb implantable marker embedded with titanium clips. This artifact is the result of signal change due to local magnetic field inhomogeneities introduced by the metallic object into the otherwise homogenous external magnetic field. This artifact is useful for localization of metal within the breast.

9b. c. Short TE.

Susceptibility artifact may be reduced by decreasing the field strength, decreasing the TE, increasing the receiver bandwidth, and employing spin echo and fast spin echo rather than gradient echo imaging.

10a. c. Transverse Rectus Abdominus Myocutaneous (TRAM) flap.

MR images demonstrate a transverse rectus abdominis mycocutaneous (TRAM) flap reconstruction status post-mastectomy. The rectus abdominis muscle has a dual blood supply provided by the superior and inferior epigastric vessels. MRI demonstrates replacement of the native breast glandular tissue by adipose tissue and the presence of a line of intermediate signal intensity that separates the native tissue from the flap reconstruction. A key feature that distinguishes the TRAM flap from other reconstructive surgeries (i.e., muscle sparing-free TRAM flap, DIEP flap) is the presence of an atrophied rectus abdominal muscle along the anterior chest wall. The T1-weighted image below of the TRAM flap shows the atrophied rectus abdominus muscle anterior to the chest wall (arrow).

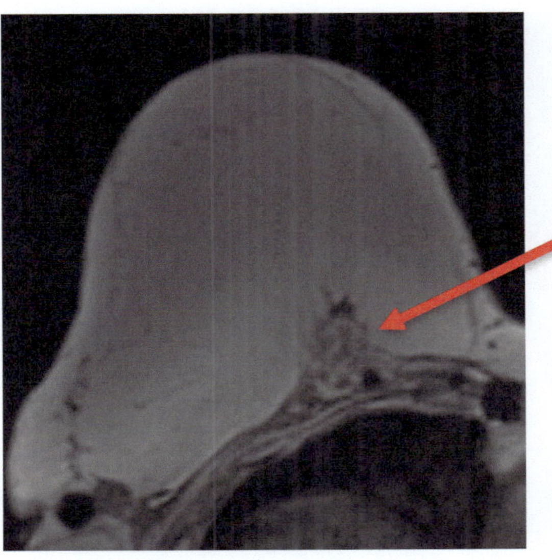

10b. c. Recurrence.

Axial T1 non-fat saturated images show a T1 isotense irregular mass. There is suspicious enhancement of the mass on post-contrast images. There is no fat signal in the mass. Therefore, this finding is most likely a recurrence out of the choices. Fat necrosis is unlikely given the lack of fat signal within the mass [3, 4].

11. a. DIEP flap.

MR images demonstrate deep inferior epigastric perforator (DIEP) flap reconstruction, which involves removal and transfer of a portion of the patient's lower abdominal skin and subcutaneous soft tissue along with perforating vessels originating from the inferior epigastric artery. DIEP flap can be differentiated from a TRAM flap by the absence of the atrophied rectus abdominis muscle and its vascular pedicle in the reconstructed breast and the characteristic removal of a segment of costal cartilage of the ipsilateral third or fourth rib, which is performed to expose the internal mammary vessels required for anastomosis [5].

12. d. Extracapsular rupture.

Sagittal silicone-selective MR images of the breast are presented. Silicone-selective sequences result in the purposeful suppression of water and fat so that only hyperintense silicone-containing structures remain visible. This case demonstrates hyperintense, silicone-laden lymph nodes, which may be seen in the context of extracapsular implant rupture or gel bleed. This patient had a prior history of extracapsular rupture. The current implant is intact. Circled are silicone laden axillary lymph nodes.

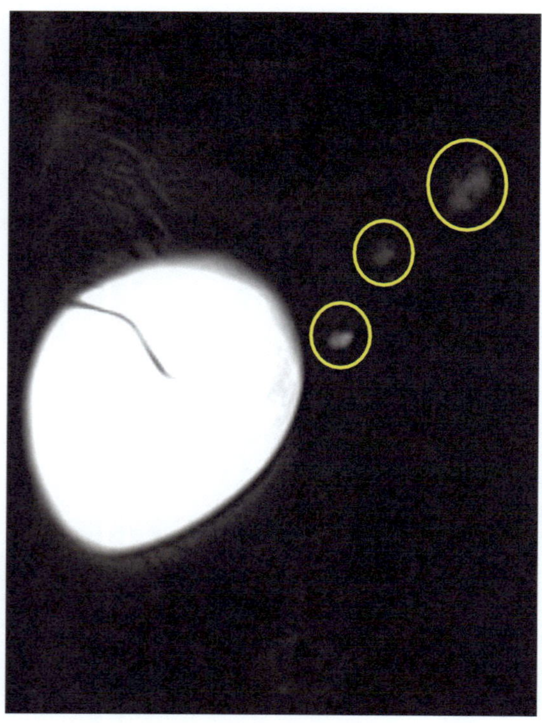

13. b. Lactational changes.

MR images demonstrate increased glandular density, increased T2-weighted signal, duct ectasia, and rapid glandular contrast enhancement in the bilateral breasts consistent with lactation changes. Increased enhancement from hypervascularity in the bilateral breasts may limit evaluation for breast cancer in lactating patients. Women undergoing MRI should be instructed to nurse or pump immediately before imaging or imaging may be postponed until after cessation of lactation, depending upon the patient's underlying risk for breast cancer.

14. b. Level II.

The pectoralis minor muscle serves as a landmark separating the axilla into three levels. Level I is located inferolateral to the pectoralis minor. Level II is located posterior to the pectoralis minor. Level III is located superomedial to the pectoralis minor. MR images demonstrate a Rotter node, otherwise known as an interpectoral lymph node, which is located in the level II axillary space [6].

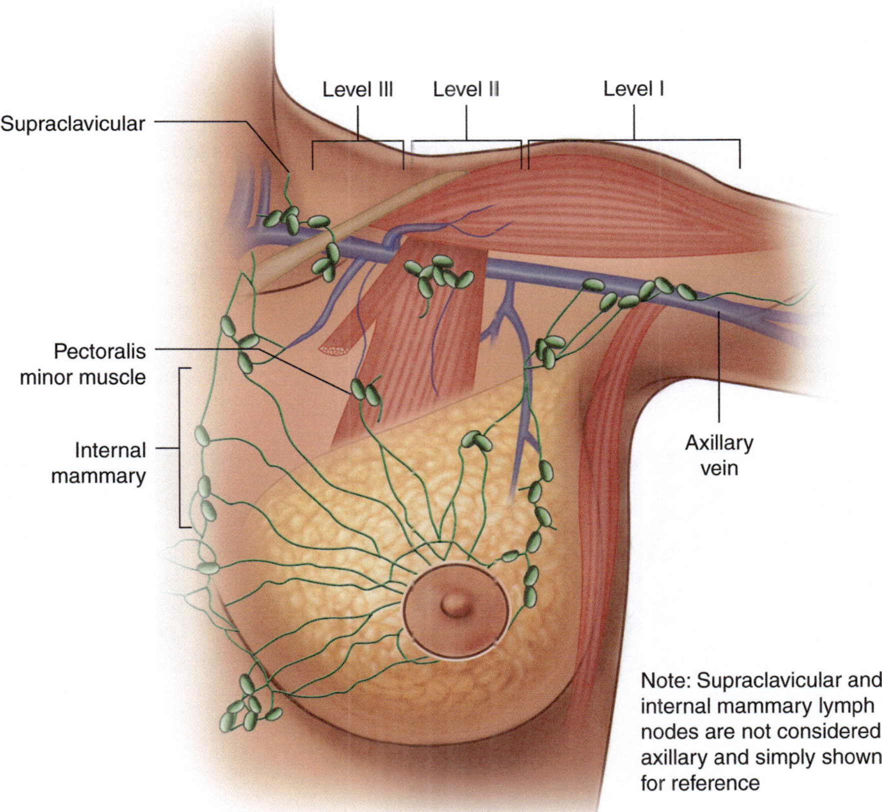

15. c. Linear.

Non-mass enhancement is defined in the BI-RADS lexicon as an area of enhancement that does not meet criteria for a mass. Non-mass enhancement lacks convex borders and has intervening fat or fibroglandular tissue between the enhancing areas. This case features non-mass enhancement in the right breast in a linear distribution. Linear non-mass enhancement is described as along a line in a ductal or non-ductal distribution. The linear enhancement may branch, as in this case. The distribution of non-mass enhancement may be described as diffuse, regional, multiple regions, segmental, linear, or focal. The positive predictive value (PPV) for malignancy with linear enhancement is 30%. The linear non-mass enhancement in this case was biopsied as ductal carcinoma in situ (DCIS) [7].

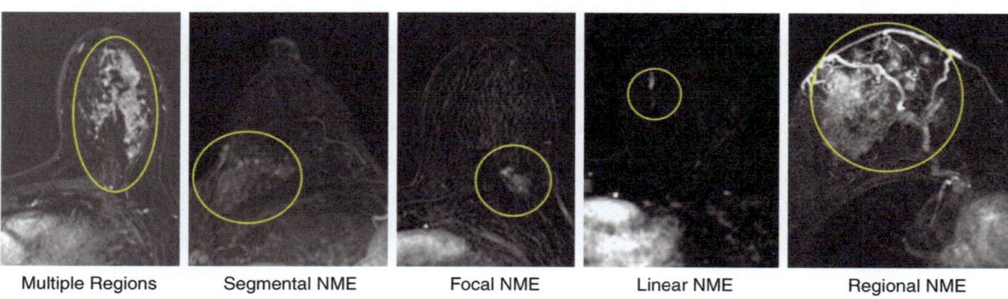

16. b. Extreme.

Normal parenchymal enhancement at breast MR imaging is termed background parenchymal enhancement (BPE). The BI-RADS lexicon contains 4 categories of BPE: minimal, mild, moderate, and marked. BPE is based on both the amount and degree of normal parenchymal tissue enhancement. BPE is assessed on the first postcontrast MIP image at approximately 90 seconds. It can also be symmetric or asymmetric. BPE can occur regardless of the menstrual cycle or menopausal status of the patient. Hormonal influences, breast vascular supply, and the permeability of the contrast agent into the breast tissue can all affect BPE. Examples of BPE on breast MRI are shown below [8].

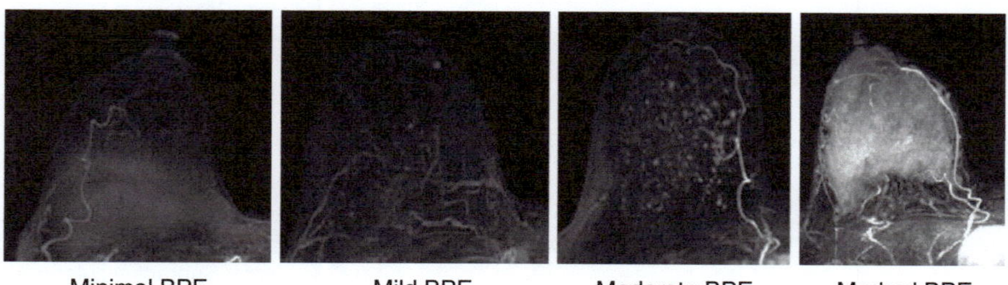

17. a. Misregistration.

Misregistration artifact is the result of motion artifact between the unenhanced and contrast-enhanced images, resulting in an area that mimics enhancement on subtraction images. In this case, there is apparent enhancement along the left pectoralis musculature on the subtraction image. However, the post-contrast non-subtracted images do not show this enhancement, in keeping with artifact. Often this apparent enhancement on the subtraction image is due to pectoralis muscle relaxation between the pre- and post-contrast series [9].

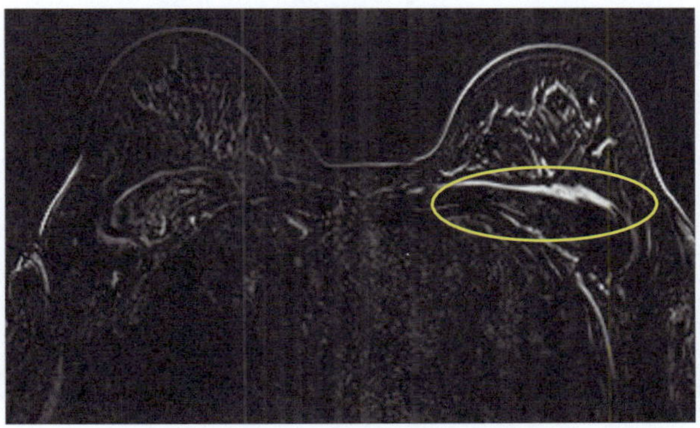

18. a. Second look breast ultrasound.

Masses identified on MRI should be evaluated with a breast ultrasound. Ultrasound is a useful tool that enables ultrasound biopsy of suspicious lesions detected on breast MRI. Ultrasound biopsy is preferred over MRI biopsy as it is less expensive, more comfortable, and less time consuming.

19. a. T2-weighted/Bright fluid sequence.

In order to receive ACR accreditation for breast MRI, the following sequences should be performed: T2-weighted or bright fluid series (can be a STIR sequence), multi-phase T1-weighted series (pre-contrast T1 with fat suppression and dynamic post-contrast series at 90 seconds for a total of four post-contrast sequences).

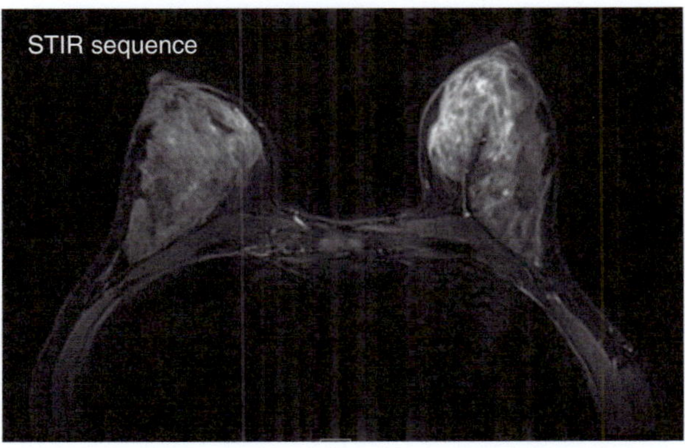

20a. c. Rim enhancement.

20b. Inflamed cyst.

The internal enhancement patterns used to describe masses include homogeneous, heterogeneous, rim enhancement, and dark internal septations. Rim enhancement, as shown in this case, is an enhancement that is more pronounced at the periphery of the mass. Rim enhancement of a solid mass is a suspicious finding. Cysts can enhance peripherally, as in this case, and are bright on fluid-sensitive sequences. Smooth inner and irregular outer rim enhancement is classic for an inflamed cyst, also known as the "solar eclipse sign." Irregular inner and outer rim enhancement is an enhancement pattern seen in breast malignancies [7].

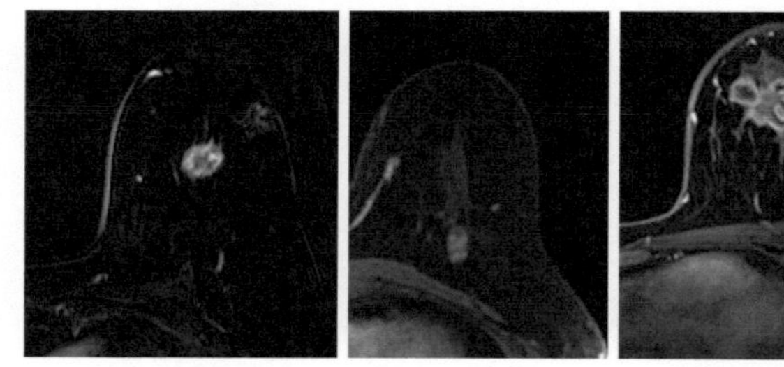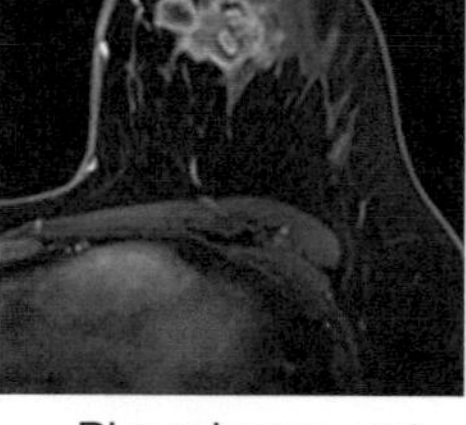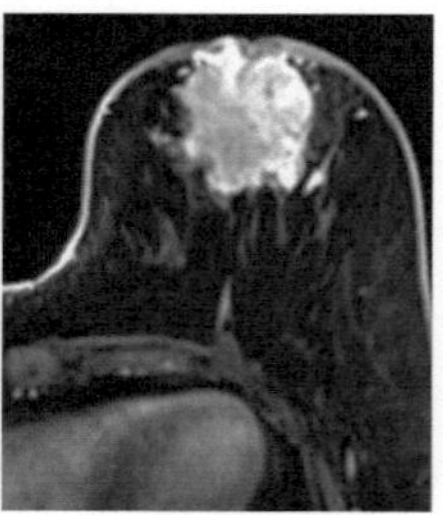

Heterogeneous   Non enhancing internal septations   Rim enhancement   Homogeneous

21a. b. Clustered ring.

21b. d. BI-RADS Category 4: Suspicious.

21c. b. DCIS.

Non-mass enhancement (NME) is the enhancement of an area that is not a mass or focus. NME is an enhancement that is discrete from the surrounding breast tissue. The internal enhancement characteristics of NME can be described as homogeneous, heterogeneous, clumped, or clustered ring. Of note, stippled, punctate is no longer a BI-RADS term used to describe NME.

NME showing a clustered ring pattern of enhancement is suggestive of malignancy. Clustered ring enhancement looks like "punched out holes." This non-mass enhancement pattern is thought to reflect periductal enhancement and is the result of contrast pooling in the periductal stroma or ductal walls. This has a high PPV value for malignancy, and thus DCIS (answer D) is the most appropriate answer choice. The most appropriate BI-RADS assessment is BI-RADS Category 4, suspicious. Given that clustered ring enhancement is strongly suggestive of malignancy, biopsy is the most appropriate next step [7].

22. c. Curve C.

23. b. 10%.

Kinetic techniques are dynamic measurements in which the uptake and washout of contrast material is assessed for a period of time after contrast injection. Lesion enhancement depends on perfusion, capillary permeability, blood volume, contrast distribution volume, and local vascular anatomy and physiology.

The kinetic information is expressed as a time intensity curve (TIC). TICs can be divided into three main shapes reflecting the initial enhancement phase and the delayed enhancement phase. The initial phase enhancement pattern reflects enhancement within the first 2 mins after contrast injection and the delayed phase pattern occurs after 2 mins.

The initial phase of enhancement is determined by comparing the differences in signal intensity between the pre- and post-contrast sequences. An intensity increase of <50% is classified as "slow," 50–100% is classified as "medium," and >100% enhancement is classified as "fast."

Delayed phase enhancement is classified as persistent, plateau, and washout. Persistent curves show continued increases in enhancement throughout the delayed phase. Plateau curves remain constant in signal intensity after the upstroke of enhancement. Washout curves show decreasing signal intensity after peak enhancement.

In general, for the delayed phase, persistent is greater than or equal to 10% of the initial enhancement, plateau is equal to the initial enhancement, and washout is less than or equal to 10% of the initial enhancement. Malignant masses tend to have fast washout enhancement and benign lesions show more persistent kinetics. However, there is overlap in enhancement kinetics of benign and malignant masses and lesion morphology should also be taken into consideration when evaluating masses [7].

24. b. Fibroadenoma.

The MR features of fibroadenomas are variable.They typically appear as oval masses with circumscribed margins and are hypointense to isointense on T1-weighted images. The T2 or STIR signal intensity varies and depends on the amount of myxoid (bright) and fibrous (dark) tissue within the mass. They also show variable enhancement and may have dark internal septations [10].

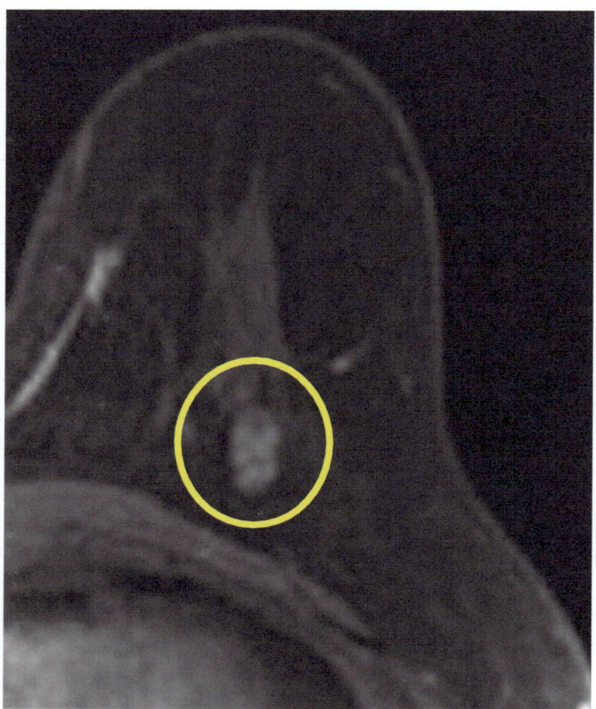

25. c. Intramammary lymph node.

The MR images include a post-contrast subtracted image and a T1-weighted image. The mass in question is consistent with an intramammary lymph node. Imaging characteristics of an intramammary lymph node on MR include a reniform shape, a fatty hilum, and a feeding vessel. The fatty hilum is best seen on the T1-weighted image without fat suppression. Intramammary lymph nodes can show avid enhancement and may show rapid washout kinetics. However, recognition of the lymph node morphology is important in making the diagnosis. Lymph nodes are also hyperintense on fluid-sensitive sequences.

A complicated cyst may show rim enhancement or no enhancement. It may show hyperintense signal on both fluid-sensitive and T1-weighted sequences.

A fibroadenoma is oval and may or may not enhance. It should not contain fat centrally. DCIS generally shows non-mass enhancement [11].

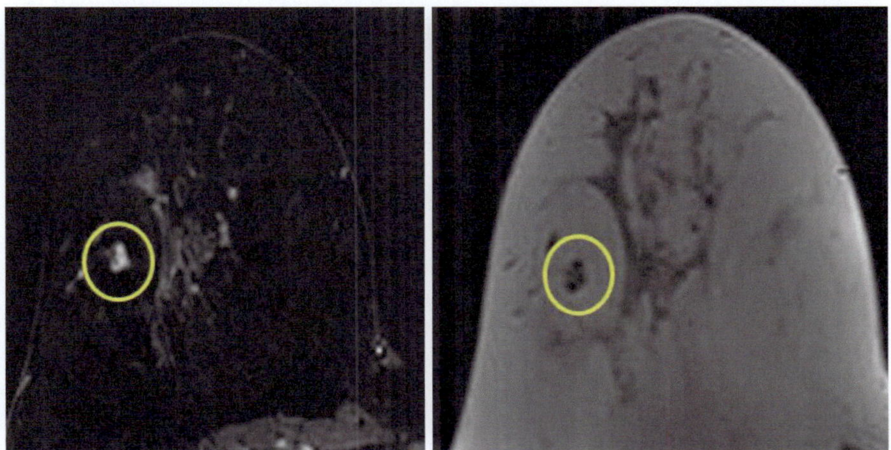

26. c. Personal history of LCIS.

The American Cancer Society Guidelines for Screening Breast MRI recommend annual screening breast MRI in the following high-risk groups:

- Known BRCA mutation
- First-degree relative of BRCA carrier, but untested
- Lifetime risk of 20–25% or greater, as defined by BRCAPRO or other models that are largely dependent on family history
- Radiation to the chest between the ages 10 and 30 years
- Li-Fraumeni syndrome and first-degree relatives
- Cowden and Bannayan-Riley-Ruvalcaba syndromes and first-degree relatives

Insufficient Evidence to Recommend for or Against MRI Screening:

- Lifetime risk 15–20%, as defined by BRCAPRO or other models that are largely dependent on family history
- Lobular carcinoma in situ (LCIS) or atypical lobular hyperplasia (ALH)
- Atypical ductal hyperplasia (ADH)
- Heterogeneously or extremely dense breasts on mammography
- Women with a personal history of breast cancer, including DCIS

Recommend Against MRI Screening:

- Women at <15% lifetime risk [12]

27. a. Eight years after radiation therapy but not before the age of 25 years.

Increased breast cancer risk has been consistently shown in those women with a history of Hodgkin's disease who underwent mantle field radiation. The risk seems to be greatest in women who received radiation between the ages 10 and 30 years. Therefore, screening breast MRI should be performed in this high-risk subgroup 8 years after radiation therapy or beginning at the age of 25 years, whichever occurs first [12].

28. d. 70–80%.

This case shows bulky right axillary lymph nodes in keeping with nodal metastasis. Less than 1% of all breast cancers present with metastatic LAD without a primary breast lesion detected clinically or with mammography. Breast MRI may identify the site of primary breast carcinoma and affect patient management. Breast MRI detects mammographically occult breast cancer in 62–86% of patients, thus answer choice d is most correct. Most occult tumors identified on breast MRI are less than 2 cm. Breast MRI is indicated for the evaluation of unilateral metastatic axillary lymphadenopathy with an unknown primary malignancy [13, 14].

29. d. BI-RADS Category 4. Suspicious. Recommend second-look ultrasound. If no sonographic correlate, MRI biopsy should be performed.

The post-contrast MR images show an isolated enhancing focus in the right breast. The kinetic enhancement pattern is suspicious, showing rapid washout. The most appropriate BI-RADS, in this case, is a BI-RADS 4, suspicious. A second-look ultrasound should be performed to identify a sonographic correlate. If a sonographic correlate is not identified, an MRI biopsy should be performed.

There are no formal guidelines to assign a breast MRI a BI-RADS 3, probably benign assessment; therefore, this should be avoided.

When a suspicious finding is seen on breast MRI, it should NOT be given a BI-RADS 0 assessment. An incomplete assessment (BI-RADS 0) should not be given when recommending targeted US in order to determine the feasibility of performing a biopsy using sonographic guidance. These cases should be given a Category 4 or 5 assessment (suspicious or highly suggestive of malignancy). If a suspicious abnormality is detected, the report should indicate that a biopsy should be performed (either with ultrasound or MR guidance) [7].

30. a. A 45-year-old woman with dense breasts and average lifetime risk.

The indications for breast MRI include the following:

- High-risk screening.
- Extent of ipsilateral disease and screening of the contralateral breast.
- Evaluate involvement of adjacent structures, including pectoralis muscle, chest wall, skin, and nipple.

- Evaluate treatment response following neoadjuvant chemotherapy.
- Metastatic adenopathy of unknown primary (suspect breast origin).
- Evaluation of positive margins following lumpectomy.
- Implant evaluation (silicone implants; can be non-contrast).
- Evaluation of equivocal mammographic and/or sonographic findings. (Problem-solving breast MRI should not be used in place of a complete diagnostic mammographic and sonographic work-up and should not be used as an alternative to biopsy suspicious findings.)
  - *Breast MRI should not be used for screening average-risk women with dense breasts [15].

31. b. No special consideration for a lactating patient to receive a non-contrast MRI.

There are no contraindications for a lactating patient to receive a non-contrast or a contrast-enhanced MRI.

Gadolinium-based contrast agents have been classified by the Food and Drug Administration as pregnancy class C drugs (no adequate and well-controlled studies in humans have been performed, although animal reproduction studies have shown an adverse effect on the fetus) and not class B.

Gadolinium-based contrast agents pass through the placental barrier and enter the fetal circulation. They are then filtered by the fetal kidneys and excreted into the amniotic fluid, where they may remain for a prolonged period [16, 17].

32. a. Washout kinetics.

A focus is a unique punctate enhancing dot usually <5 mm, which is nonspecific, is too small to be characterized morphologically, and has no corresponding finding on the precontrast sequence.

A focus may be benign or malignant. The following features make a focus more likely to be benign: hyperintense signal on fluid sensitive sequences (e.g., STIR or T2-weighted imaging), fatty hilum, persistent enhancement kinetics, and stability compared to prior exams.

The following features make a focus more suspicious: hypointense signal on T2-weighted imaging, washout kinetics, and an increase in size compared to prior studies [18].

33. a. Homogenously enhancing round mass with irregular margins.

This MRI is an axial contrast-enhanced image with fat suppression. The clue for contrast-enhanced image is the cardiac enhancement. Therefore, choice d is incorrect.

A mass is a 3-D, space-occupying structure with convex outward contour. A focus is a unique punctate enhancing dot usually <5 mm, which is nonspecific, is too small to be characterized morphologically, and has no corresponding finding on the precontrast sequence.

BI-RADS descriptors of a mass on MRI include shape, margin, and internal enhancement characteristics.

MRI BI-RADS shape descriptors are oval, round, and irregular.

MRI BI-RADS margin descriptors are circumscribed and not circumscribed. Not circumscribed is further classified as irregular or spiculated. An indistinct margin is not part of the MRI lexicon for mass. Therefore, choices b and c are incorrect.

Internal enhancement characteristics are homogenous (confluent and uniform), heterogeneous (nonuniform, with areas of variable signal intensity), rim enhancement, and dark internal septations. Homogeneous enhancement is confluent and uniform [18].

34. b. Irregular mass; BI-RADS Category 4.

The lesion's shape is neither round nor oval. For MRI, use of this descriptor usually implies a suspicious finding. Given the heterogeneous enhancement with irregular shape and margin, this finding is suspicious for malignancy. Thus, BI-RADS Category 4 assessment is most appropriate [18].

35. b. T2.

Based on the 8th edition of AJCC for breast cancer, T category is based primarily on the size of the invasive component of cancer. The largest contiguous dimension of a tumor focus is used, and small satellite foci of noncontiguous tumor are not added to the size. Please refer to Chap. 10, question 25b explanation for full table of Tumor Staging.

- T1: tumor 20 mm or less in greatest dimension.
- T2: tumor more than 20 mm but not more than 50 mm in greatest dimension.
- T3: tumor more than 50 mm in greatest dimension.
- T4: tumor of any size with direct extension to chest wall and/or to the skin (ulceration or skin nodules) [19].

36. a. Precontrast T1 non-fat saturated; Extreme fibroglandular tissue.

The presented sequence is precontrast T1 non-fat saturated. Note, that there is no contrast in the heart. Assessment of the amount of fibroglandular tissue is part of the MRI lexicon. The four categories of breast composition are defined by the visually estimated content of fibroglandular tissue (FGT) within the breasts. If the breasts are not of apparently equal amounts of FGT, the breast with the most FGT should be used to categorize breast composition.

Examples of 4 categories of breast composition in the MRI (non-fat saturated pre-contrast T1 axial image):

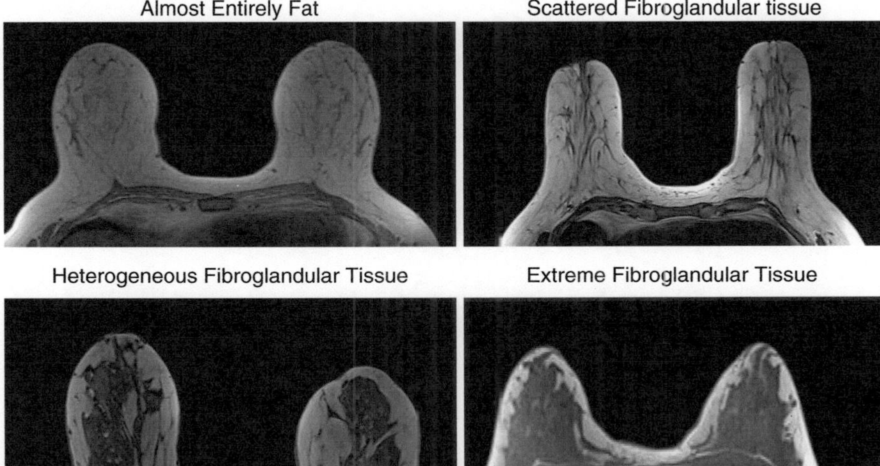

37. a. Skin retraction and enhancement.

The arrow demonstrates enhancement of the skin. The presence of localized skin involvement increases the T staging to T4b.

There is normal nipple enhancement and morphology. There is no evidence of axillary lymphadenopathy or chest wall invasion.

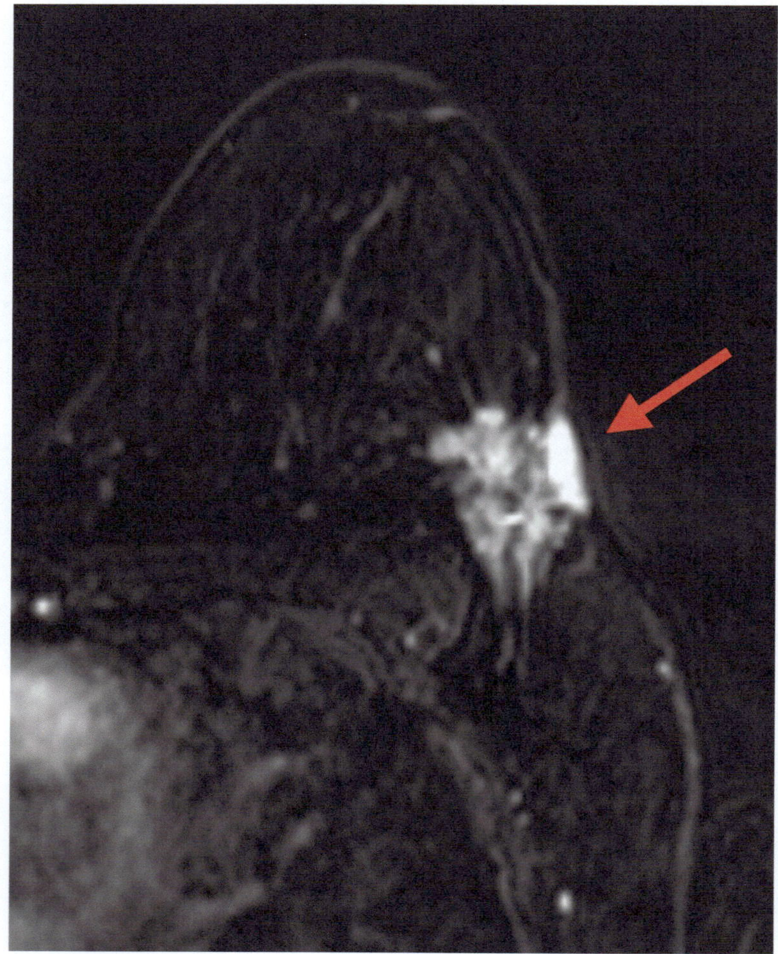

38. d. Chest wall invasion.

The circle demonstrates nipple retraction and invasion. The nipple is retracted with subareolar abnormal enhancement. The arrow shows skin thickening.

There is preserved fat plane between the malignancy and the chest wall posteriorly.

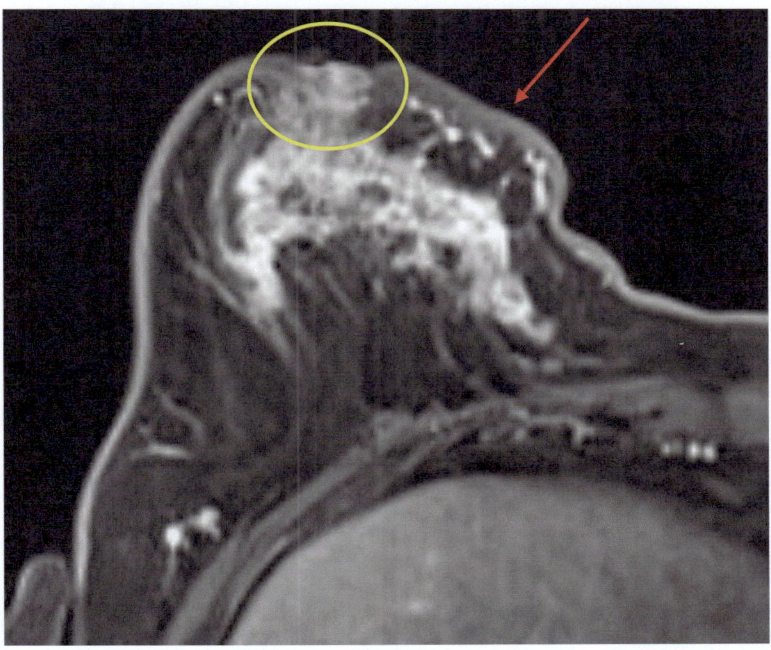

39. d. Benign seroma; no action is needed.

There is an oval circumscribed mass showing fluid signal without enhancement which is consistent with a benign postsurgical seroma given recent lumpectomy. Note that there is no peripheral thickening or enhancing solid component. Therefore, targeted second look ultrasound or short-term follow-up is not an appropriate recommendation. Patient is asymptomatic and no aspiration is indicated. Most seromas will resolve over time.

40. b. Spiculated.

The BIRADS descriptor of margin for mass in MRI are:

- Circumscribed
- Not circumscribed
  - irregular
  - spiculated

Angular and microlobulated margins are sonographic descriptors and are not included in the MRI lexicon for margin description.

The circle demonstrates a spiculated enhancing mass in the right breast. Note that there is a susceptibility artifact in the posterior border of the mass representing a biopsy clip (arrow) [18].

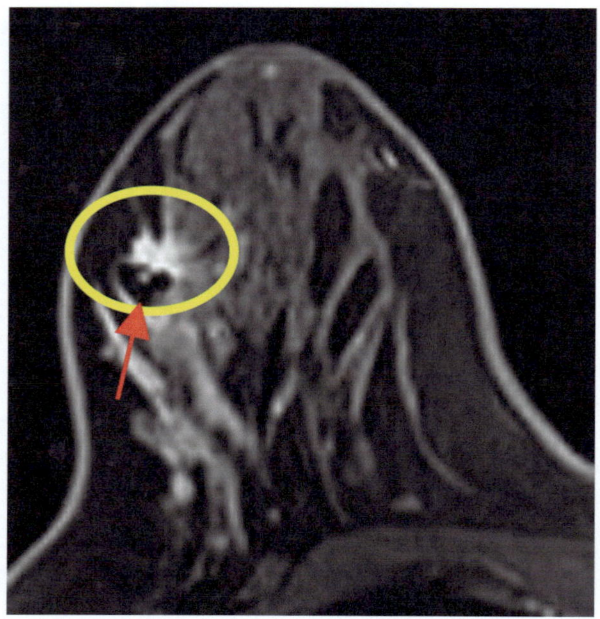

41. a. Invasive ductal carcinoma.

The most common primary breast cancer is invasive ductal carcinoma (about 75% of all primary breast cancers). Inflammatory breast cancer (IBC) is a rare subtype of breast cancer that accounts for 2%–5% of all breast cancers and presents with breast skin edema and thickening as well as skin enhancement. There is no skin thickening or skin enhancement on this MRI.

A breast abscess demonstrates a rim-enhancing mass on MRI without internal enhancement. There is often overlying skin thickening without skin enhancement.

Fibroadenomas usually present as an oval circumscribed mass with or without enhancement on MRI. The margins of the mass shown are irregular; thus, answer choice d would not be appropriate.

42. d. Increased risk of breast cancer is only associated in patients with BRCA1 mutation, and not in patients with BRCA2 mutation.

Both BRCA1 and BRCA2 mutations are associated with an increased risk of breast cancer. For women with a history of mantle or chest radiation therapy who received a cumulative dose of 10 Gy or more before the age of 30 years, contrast-enhanced breast MRI should be performed annually beginning at age 25 or 8 years after radiation therapy, whichever is later. Known genetic predisposition for breast cancer is BRCA1 or BRCA2 mutation. Other less common gene mutations include TP53 and CHEK2 (Li-Fraumeni syndrome), PTEN

(Cowden and Bannayan-Riley-Ruvalcaba syndromes), CDH1 (hereditary diffuse gastric cancer), STK11 (Peutz-Jeghers syndrome), PALB2 (interacts with BRCA2), and ATM (ataxia-telangiectasia) genes.

Thirty percent of all breast cancer occurs in women with a family history of breast cancer (familial breast cancer). According to the American College of Radiology (ACR), breast MRI is indicated in women with greater than or equal to 20% lifetime risk of breast cancer [20].

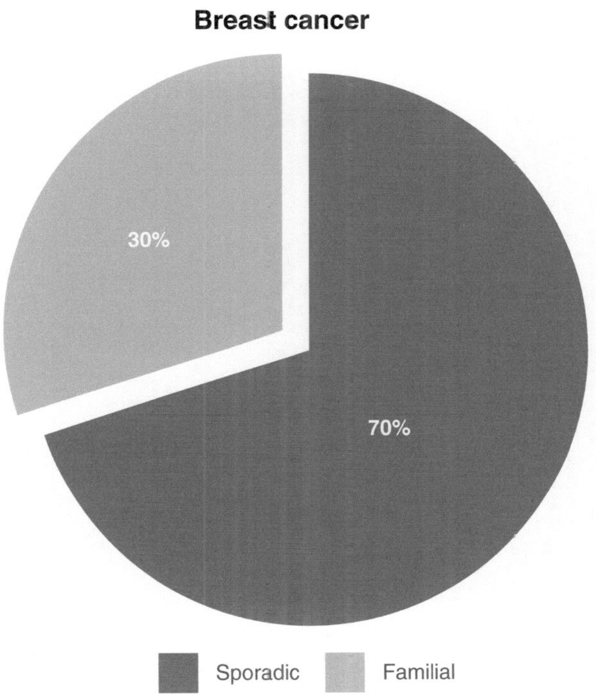

43. b. Port-a-cath.

Port-a-Cath is not a contraindication for breast MRI.

In pregnancy, gadolinium-based contrast agents (GBCAs) cross the placental barrier, enter the fetal circulation, and pass via the kidneys into the amniotic fluid. Although no definite adverse effects of GBCA administration on the human fetus have been documented, the potential bioeffects of fetal GBCA exposure are not well understood. GBCA administration should therefore be avoided during pregnancy unless no suitable alternative imaging is possible and the benefits of contrast administration outweigh the potential risk to the fetus.

Only a tiny fraction of a GBCA administered to a lactating woman is excreted into the breast milk, and only a similarly small portion of the excreted milk is absorbed by the infant's gut. Moreover, intravenous administration of a GBCA to neonates and infants is considered safe and performed routinely in clinical practice. ACR contrast manual suggests that it is safe for the mother and infant to continue breast-feeding after receiving contrast. Ultimately, an informed decision to temporarily stop breast-feeding should be up to the mother after these facts are communicated. If the mother remains concerned about any potential effects to the infant, she may abstain from breast-feeding from the time of contrast administration for a period of 12–24 h. There is no value to stop breast-feeding beyond 24 h [21, 22].

44. c. Internal mammary (thoracic) artery.

The vessel shown by thin arrow is the right internal mammary vein that runs parallel to the internal mammary artery shown by thick arrow.

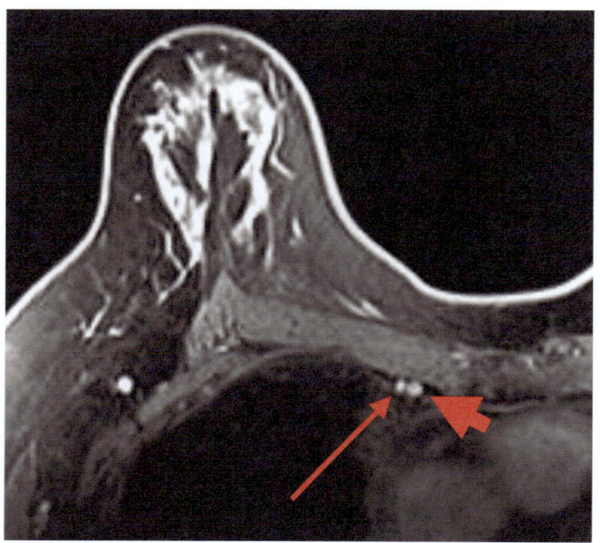

References

1. Bitencourt AG, Graziano L, Osorio CA, Guatelli CS, Souza JA, Mendonca MH, et al. MRI features of mucinous cancer of the breast: correlation with pathologic findings and other imaging methods. AJR Am J Roentgenol. 2016;206(2):238–46.
2. Bozzini A, Renne G, Meneghetti L, Bandi G, Santos G, Vento AR, et al. Sensitivity of imaging for multifocal-multicentric breast carcinoma. BMC Cancer. 2008;8:275.
3. Adrada BE, Whitman GJ, Crosby MA, Carkaci S, Dryden MJ, Dogan BE. Multimodality imaging of the reconstructed breast. Curr Probl Diagn Radiol. 2015;44(6):487–95.
4. Peng C, Chang CB, Tso HH, Flowers CI, Hylton NM, Joe BN. MRI appearance of tumor recurrence in myocutaneous flap reconstruction after mastectomy. AJR Am J Roentgenol. 2011;196(4):W471–5.
5. Hedegard W, Niell B, Specht M, Winograd J, Rafferty E. Breast reconstruction with a deep inferior epigastric perforator flap: imaging appearances of the normal flap and common complications. AJR Am J Roentgenol. 2013;200(1):W75–84.
6. Ecanow JS, Abe H, Newstead GM, Ecanow DB, Jeske JM. Axillary staging of breast cancer: what the radiologist should know. Radiographics. 2013;33(6):1589–612.
7. Erguvan-Dogan B, Whitman GJ, Kushwaha AC, Phelps MJ, Dempsey PJ. BI-RADS-MRI: a primer. AJR Am J Roentgenol. 2006;187(2):W152–60.
8. Giess CS, Yeh ED, Raza S, Birdwell RL. Background parenchymal enhancement at breast MR imaging: normal patterns, diagnostic challenges, and potential for false-positive and false-negative interpretation. Radiographics. 2014;34(1):234–47.
9. Yitta S, Joe BN, Wisner DJ, Price ER, Hylton NM. Recognizing artifacts and optimizing breast MRI at 1.5 and 3 T. AJR Am J Roentgenol. 2013;200(6):W673–82.
10. Hochman MG, Orel SG, Powell CM, Schnall MD, Reynolds CA, White LN. Fibroadenomas: MR imaging appearances with radiologic-histopathologic correlation. Radiology. 1997;204(1):123–9.
11. Mack M, Chetlen A, Liao J. Incidental Internal Mammary Lymph Nodes Visualized on Screening Breast MRI. AJR Am J Roentgenol. 2015;205(1):209–14.
12. Saslow D, Boetes C, Burke W, Harms S, Leach MO, Lehman CD, et al. American Cancer Society guidelines for breast screening with MRI as an adjunct to mammography. CA Cancer J Clin. 2007;57(2):75–89.
13. Buchanan CL, Morris EA, Dorn PL, Borgen PI, Van Zee KJ. Utility of breast magnetic resonance imaging in patients with occult primary breast cancer. Ann Surg Oncol. 2005;12(12):1045–53.
14. Stomper PC, Waddell BE, Edge SB, Klippenstein DL. Breast MRI in the Evaluation of Patients with Occult Primary Breast Carcinoma. Breast J. 1999;5(4):230–4.
15. Argus A, Mahoney MC. Indications for breast MRI: case-based review. Am J Roentgenol. 2011;196(3 Suppl):WS1–14.
16. American College of Radiology. ACR Manual on Contrast Media 2021 [Available from: https://www.acr.org/-/media/ACR/Files/Clinical-Resources/Contrast_Media.pdf.
17. Greenberger PA, Patterson R. The prevention of immediate generalized reactions to radiocontrast media in high-risk patients. J Allergy Clin Immunol. 1991;87(4):867–72.
18. D'Orsi CJ., Sickles EA., Mendelson EB., Morris EA. ACR BI-RADS® Atlas, Breast imaging reporting and data system. 5th rev. ed ed. Reston, VA: American College of Radiology; 2013.
19. Giuliano AE, Edge SB, Hortobagyi GN. Eighth Edition of the AJCC Cancer Staging Manual: Breast Cancer. Ann Surg Oncol. 2018;25(7):1783–5.
20. Couch FJ, Nathanson KL, Offit K. Two decades after BRCA: setting paradigms in personalized cancer care and prevention. Science. 2014;343(6178):1466–70.
21. ACR–SPR Practice Parameter for the Safe and Optimal Performance of Fetal Magnetic Resonance Imaging (MRI) 2020. Available from: https://www.acr.org/-/media/ACR/Files/Practice-Parameters/mr-fetal.pdf.
22. Expert Panel on MRS, Kanal E, Barkovich AJ, Bell C, Borgstede JP, Bradley WG Jr, et al. ACR guidance document on MR safe practices: 2013. J Magn Reson Imaging. 2013;37(3):501–30.

Interventional Procedures

6

Bo Li, Nina Capiro, Craig Wilsen, Puja Shahrouki,
Parsa Asachi, and Lucy Chow

B. Li (✉) · N. Capiro · C. Wilsen · P. Shahrouki · P. Asachi · L. Chow
Department of Radiology, David Geffen School of Medicine at UCLA,
Los Angeles, CA, USA
e-mail: BoLi@mednet.ucla.edu; NCapiro@mednet.ucla.edu;
CWilsen@mednet.ucla.edu; pshahrouki@mednet.ucla.edu;
pasachi@mednet.ucla.edu; lchow@mednet.ucla.edu

1a. A 55-year-old female presents for new calcifications in the right breast on screening mammogram. A diagnostic mammogram is shown. What is the next best step in management?

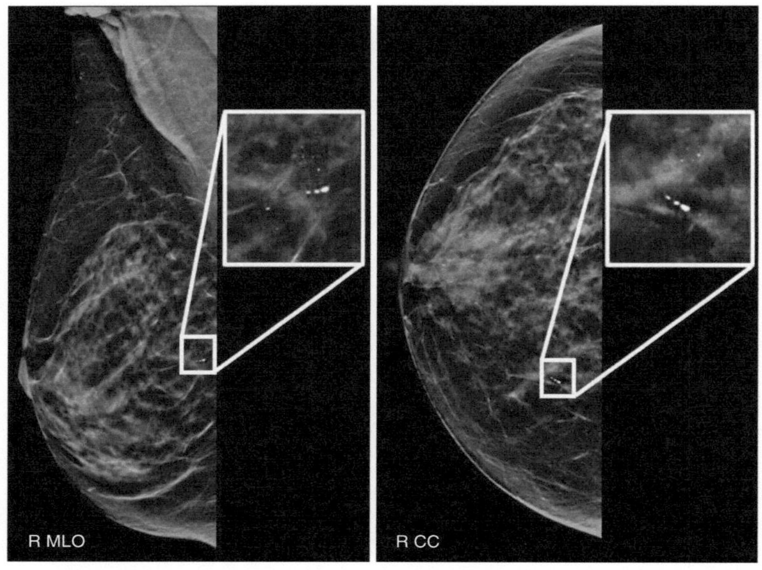

(a) Ultrasound-guided biopsy.
(b) Stereotactic biopsy.
(c) MRI-guided biopsy.
(d) Surgical excision.

1b. What is the best approach for stereotactic biopsy?
(a) Medial.
(b) Lateral.
(c) Superior.
(d) Inferior.

1c. A stereotactic-guided biopsy was performed. This post-fire diagram of the stereotactic biopsy demonstrates the location of the needle in relation to the biopsy target. What type of error do these diagrams demonstrate?

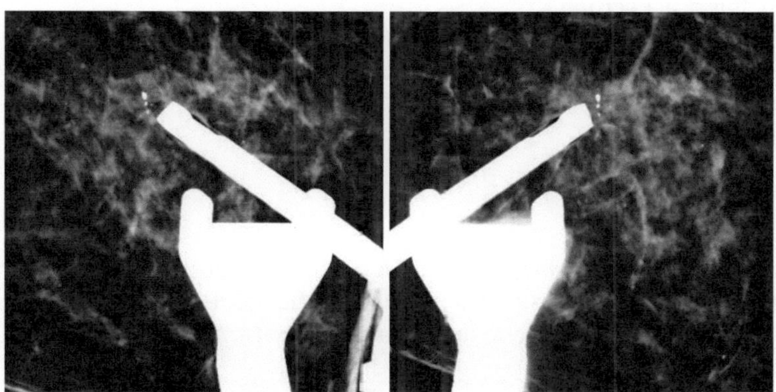

(a) None, the needle is in good position.
(b) *X*-axis error.
(c) *Y*-axis error.
(d) Z-axis error.

2a. An 80-year-old female presents with a palpable abnormality in the left breast. Diagnostic mammogram demonstrates an irregular mass in the left breast. No sonographic correlate is identified on diagnostic breast ultrasound. What is the next best step in management?

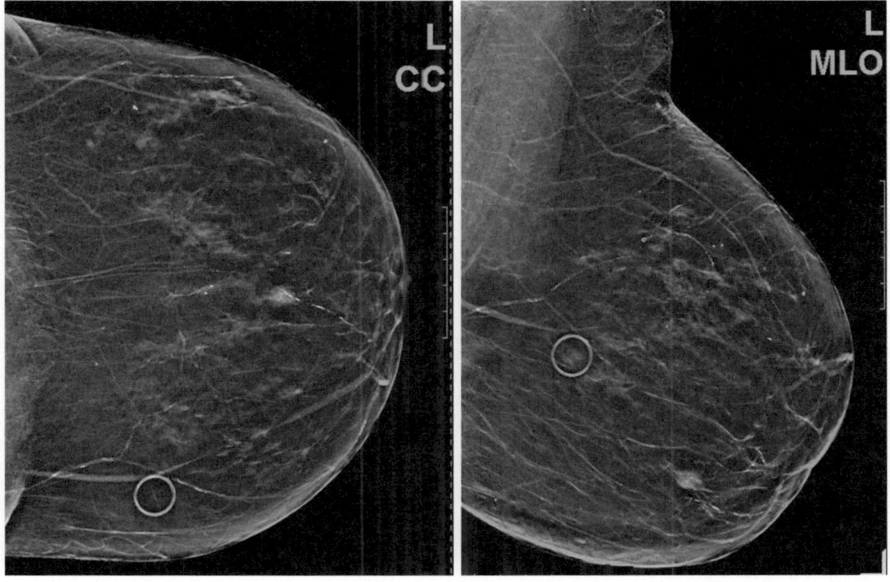

    (a) Ultrasound-guided biopsy.
    (b) Stereotactic biopsy.
    (c) Breast MRI.
    (d) Surgical excision.

2b. What is the best approach for stereotactic biopsy?
    (a) Medial.
    (b) Lateral.
    (c) Superior.
    (d) Inferior.

2c. A stereotactic guided biopsy was performed. These post-fire images of the stereotactic biopsy demonstrate the location of the needle in relation to the biopsy target. What type of error do these images demonstrate?

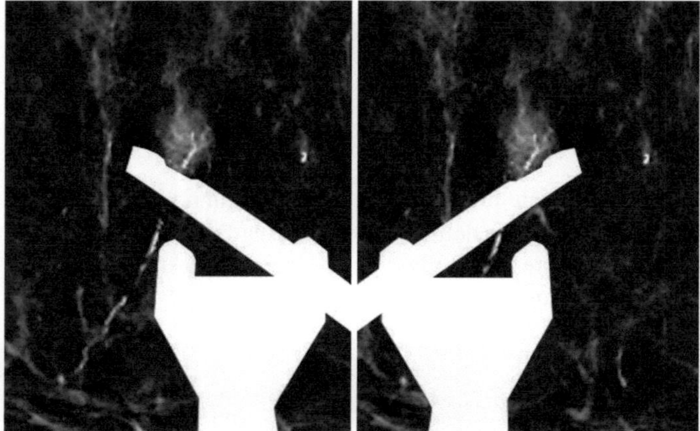

    (a) Y-axis and Z-axis error.
    (b) X-axis error.
    (c) Y-axis error.
    (d) Z-axis error.

3. A 53-year-old female has a new left breast mass seen on screening mammogram. Diagnostic mammogram (image on the left) demonstrates a suspicious mass (circled) in the superior breast, and a presumed sonographic correlate was visualized (BI-RADS 4). Ultrasound-guided core needle biopsy was performed and a biopsy microclip was placed. Post-procedure mammogram (image on the right) demonstrates post-biopsy changes and biopsy microclip. The originally seen suspicious mass is circled in both images. What is the next best step?

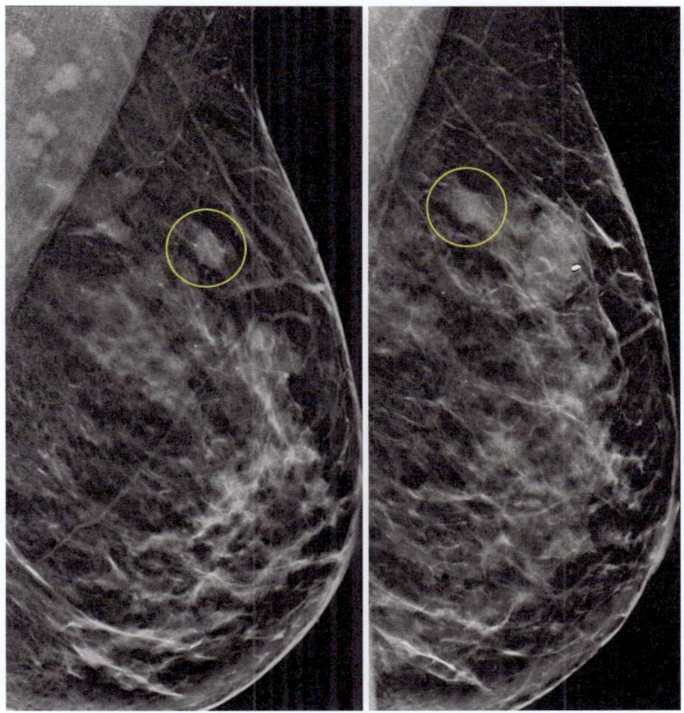

(a) Await pathology results as findings are related to clip migration.
(b) Repeat ultrasound-guided core needle biopsy.
(c) Perform stereotactic biopsy of the mammographic finding.
(d) Perform wire localization targeting the microclip.

4a. A 48-year-old female underwent diagnostic mammogram and ultrasound for a palpable abnormality in the right breast at 9 o'clock. Diagnostic mammogram demonstrates a spiculated mass, and a correlate mass is seen on diagnostic breast ultrasound. What is the next best step in management?

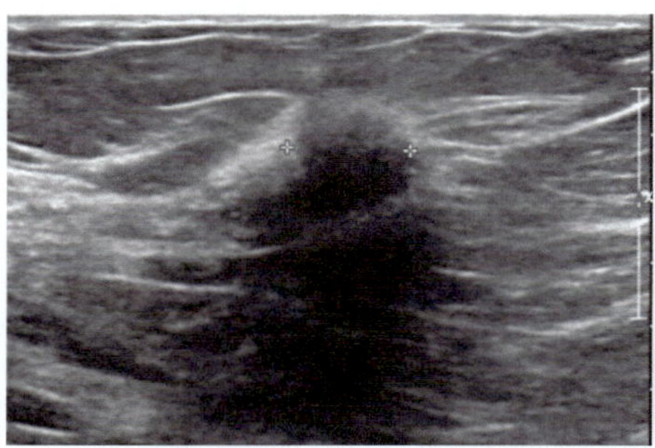 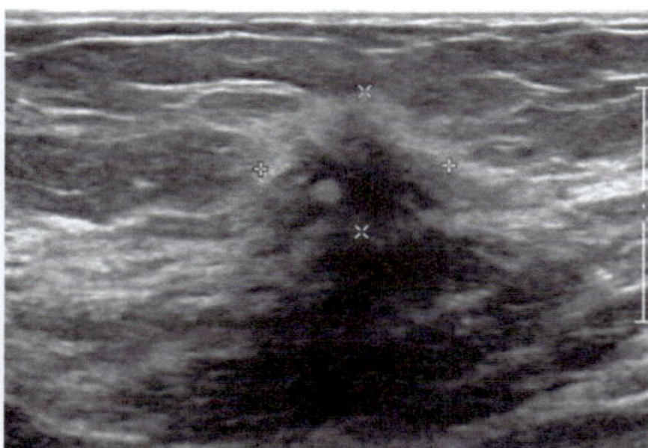

    (a) Fine-needle aspiration.
    (b) Ultrasound-guided core needle biopsy.
    (c) Stereotactic biopsy.
    (d) Breast MRI.

4b. What is the best approach for ultrasound-guided biopsy?
    (a) Medial.
    (b) Lateral.
    (c) Superior.
    (d) Inferior.

4c. What area should be targete.d at the time of biopsy?

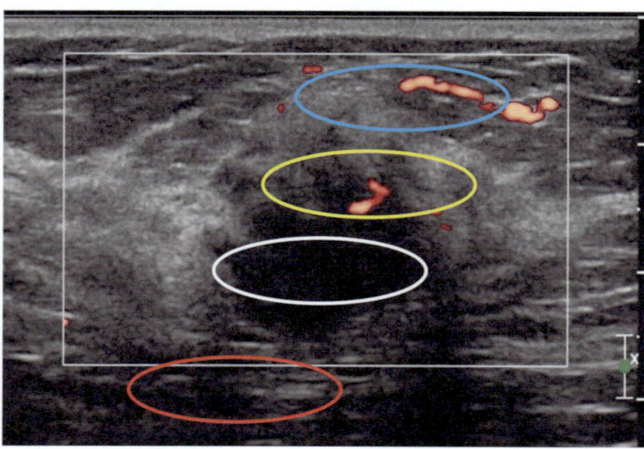

    (a) Blue circle.
    (b) Yellow circle.
    (c) White circle.
    (d) Red circle.

5a. A 28-year-old female presents with a palpable abnormality in the right breast. Diagnostic breast ultrasound demonstrates a complicated cyst. The cyst was aspirated to completion and clear fluid was obtained. What is the next best step?

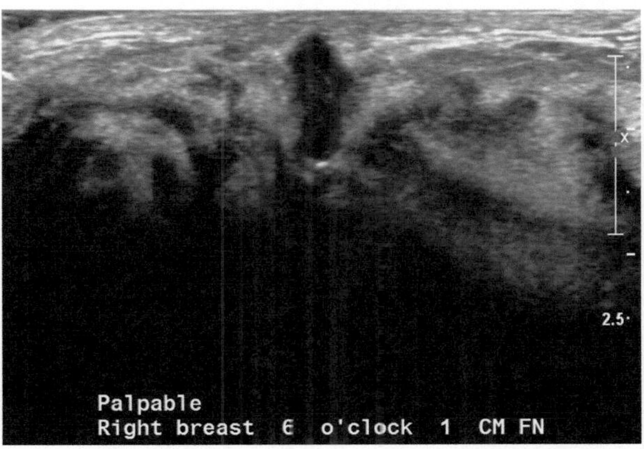

 (a) Discard fluid.
 (b) Send fluid for culture.
 (c) Place a microclip and send fluid for cytology.
 (d) Perform ultrasound-guided core needle biopsy.

5b. If cyst aspiration had yielded bloody fluid, what would be the next best step?
 (a) Nothing.
 (b) Send fluid for culture.
 (c) Place a biopsy microclip and send fluid for cytology.
 (d) Perform ultrasound-guided core needle biopsy.

5c. If the finding did not fully resolve following aspiration, what would be the next best step?
 (a) Nothing.
 (b) Send fluid for culture.
 (c) Place a microclip and send fluid for cytology.
 (d) Perform ultrasound-guided core needle biopsy.

6a. A 32-year-old breastfeeding female with a strong family history of breast cancer presents with 3 days of pain, warmth, and redness of the left breast with an associated palpable abnormality. Diagnostic breast ultrasound was performed. What is the most likely diagnosis?

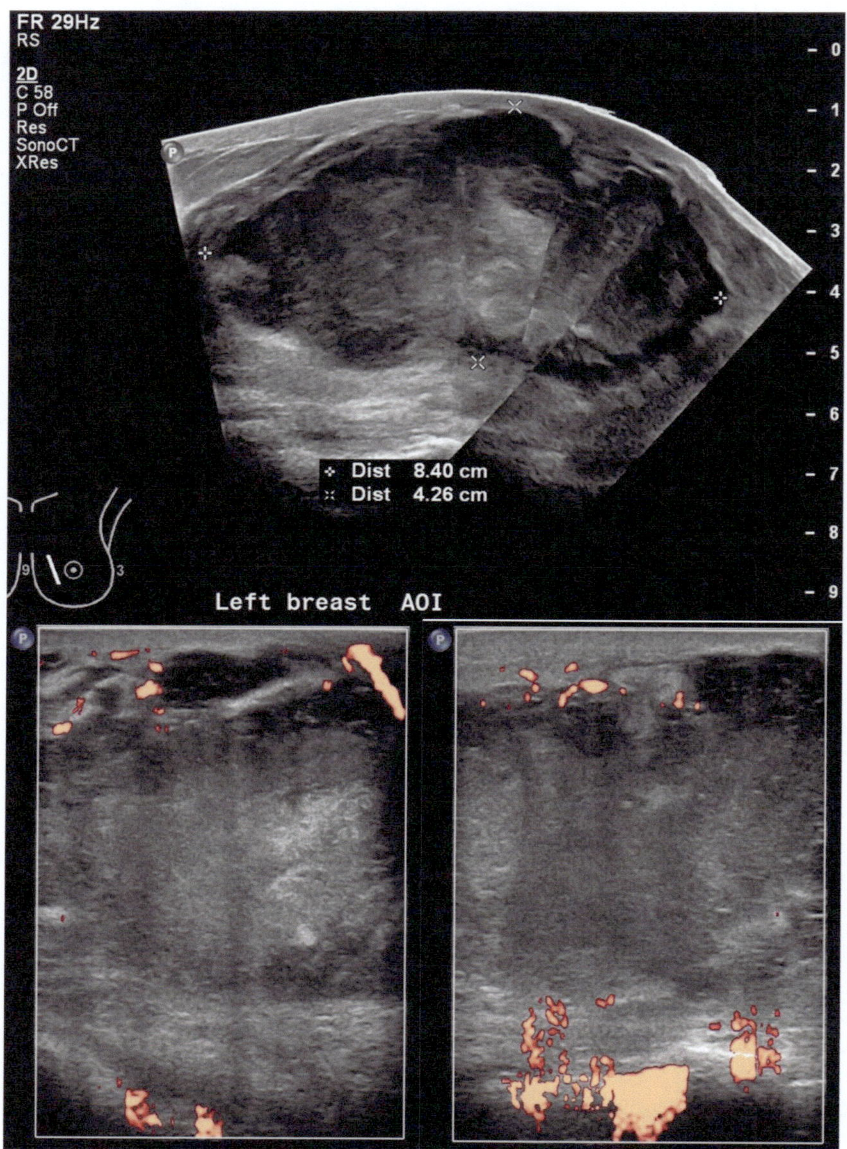

(a) Invasive ductal carcinoma.
(b) Breast abscess.
(c) Complicated cyst.
(d) Simple cyst.

6b. What is the next best step?
   (a) Ultrasound-guided core-needle biopsy.
   (b) Ultrasound-guided drainage.
   (c) Six-month follow-up ultrasound.
   (d) Clinical follow-up. No follow-up imaging is required.

6c. Following multiple aspirations and several courses of antibiotics, the patient continues to report a painfully palpable abnormality in the left breast. What is the next best step?
   (a) Ultrasound-guided core-needle biopsy and surgical consultation.
   (b) Ultrasound-guided drainage.
   (c) Six-month follow-up ultrasound.
   (d) Clinical follow-up. No follow-up imaging required.

7a. A 53-year-old female with left breast cancer underwent breast MRI for surgical planning. A focus of enhancement was seen in the lateral right breast (circled). At the time of MRI-guided biopsy, the suspicious focus of enhancement is not seen on post-contrast images. What is the appropriate step to take following nonvisualization of an MRI finding during MRI biopsy?

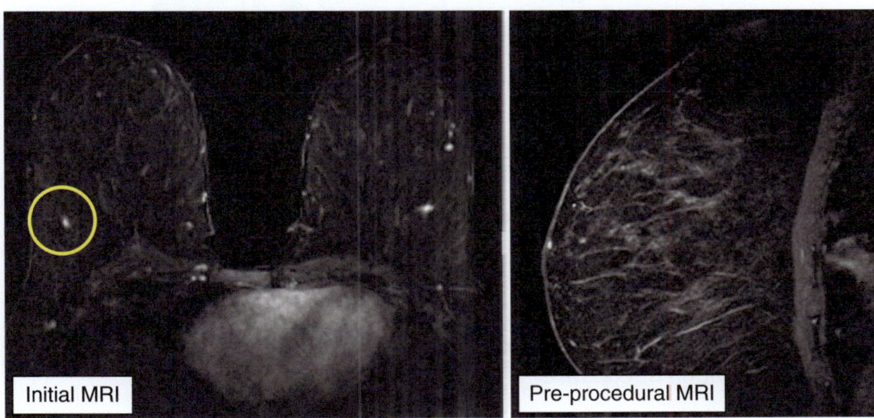

   (a) Verify grid positioning.
   (b) Obtain delayed post-contrast images.
   (c) Decrease compression.
   (d) All of the above.

7b. The finding was not visualized after all appropriate steps were taken (as noted in the above question). What is the next best step?
   (a) Return to screening breast MRI.
   (b) Short term interval follow-up breast MRI.
   (c) Decrease compression.
   (d) All of the above.

8. A 49-year-old female with left bloody nipple discharge undergoes a ductography. Which of these best describes the finding seen on ductography?

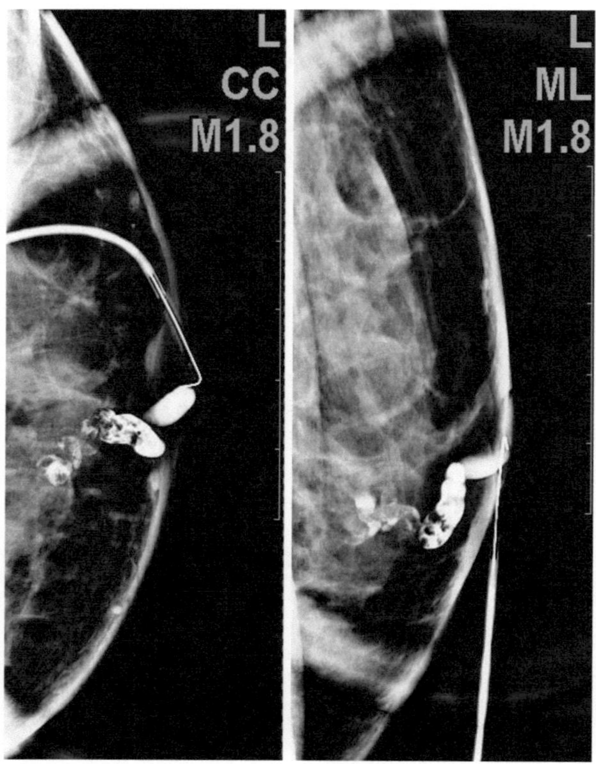

(a) Normal duct without filling defect.
(b) Duct ectasia without filling defect.
(c) Multiple intraductal filling defects.
(d) Extravasation of contrast.

9a. A 58-year-old female underwent stereotactic biopsy of suspicious calcifications in the lower inner quadrant of the left breast, with pathology consistent with invasive ductal carcinoma. A microclip was placed at the time of biopsy (circle). Post-procedure mammogram demonstrated accurate microclip placement without clip migration. Pre-surgery wire-free localization using a reflector device is planned under mammographic guidance. If the microclip is to be targeted at time of wire-free localization, which approach should be taken?

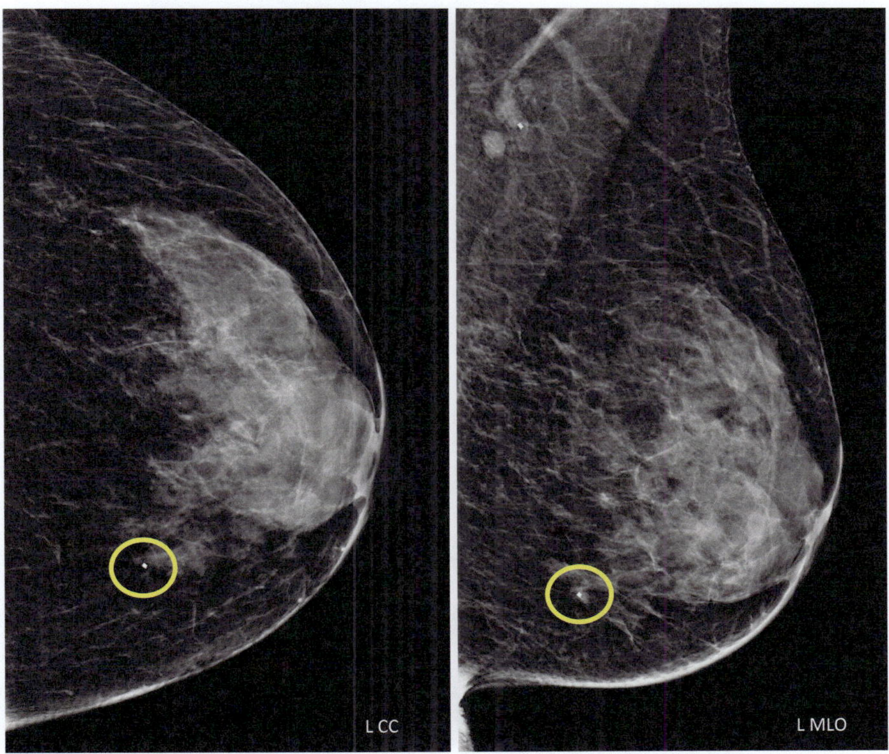

(a) Medial.
(b) Lateral.
(c) Superior.
(d) Oblique.

9b. A reflector device is placed from a medial approach. Prior to deployment, a craniocaudal mammogram is performed to confirm position. What is the next best step?

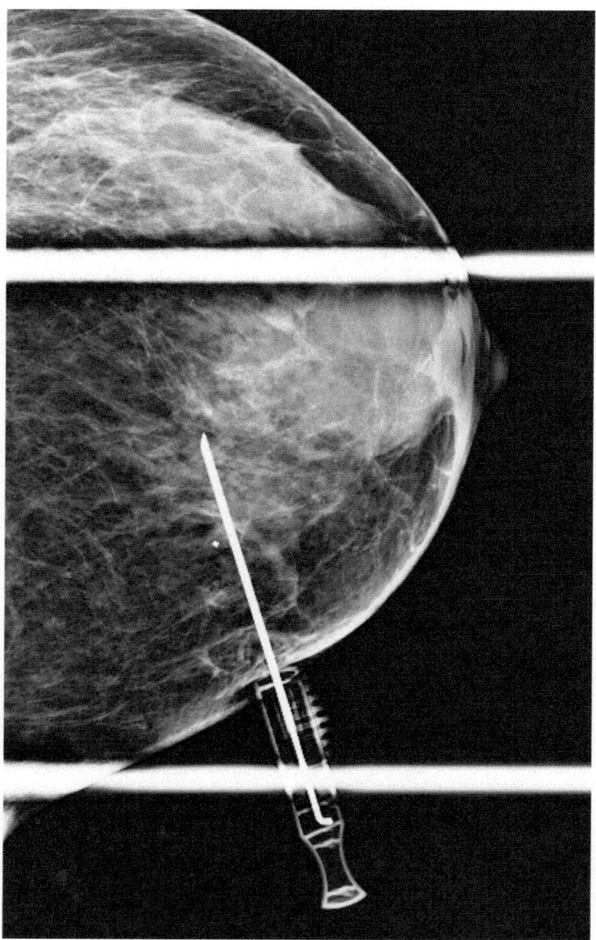

(a) Deploy the reflector.
(b) Pull back the deployment device and repeat craniocaudal view mammogram to confirm position.
(c) Advance the reflector deployment device and repeat craniocaudal view mammogram to confirm position.
(d) Remove the reflector deployment device and repeat placement via the inferior approach.

9c. Following surgical excision, a specimen radiograph is obtained. What should
be communicated to the surgeon?

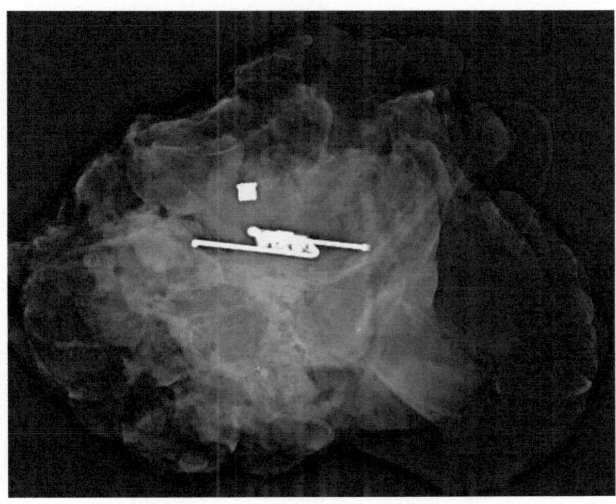

(a) Biopsy microclip is seen within the specimen.
(b) Reflector is seen within the specimen.
(c) Both a and b.
(d) None of the above.

9d. What is an advantage of wire-free localization?
(a) Improved patient experience.
(b) Device can be placed prior to day of surgery.
(c) Potential for removal of smaller amount of nontargeted tissue.
(d) All of the above.

10a. A 33-year-old female underwent a stereotactic biopsy for an architectural distortion noted on diagnostic mammogram. There was 10-mm lateral migration of the biopsy clip (yellow circle) relative to the architectural distortion (red circle) noted on the post-biopsy mammogram. Pathology demonstrated radial scar. What finding should be targeted at time of pre-surgery wire localization?

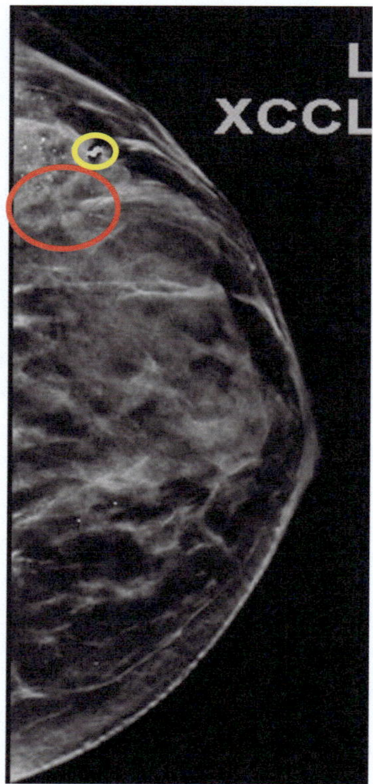

(a) Architectural distortion with associated calcifications.
(b) Biopsy microclip.
(c) Biopsy microclip and calcifications.
(d) None of the above.

10b. The architectural distortion and associated calcification were targeted at time of pre-surgery wire localization. A specimen radiograph is performed following surgical excision. What should be communicated to the operating room?

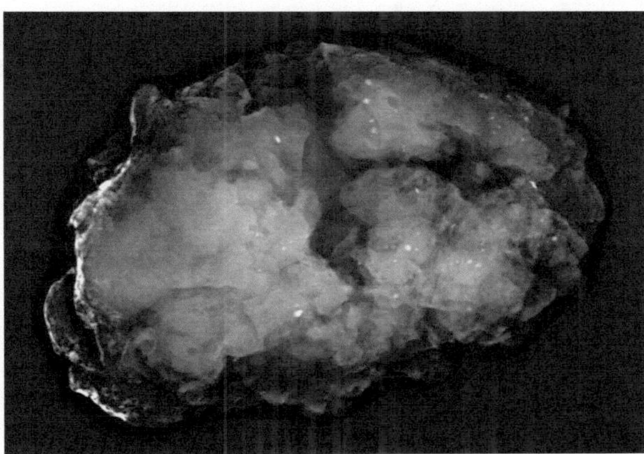

(a) The biopsy microclip is seen within the specimen.
(b) The biopsy microclip is not seen within the specimen and more tissue should be excised in order to remove the target.
(c) The biopsy microclip is not seen within the specimen, which is expected as the microclip was not the localization target.

11a. A 71-year-old female underwent stereotactic biopsy for an architectural distortion in the right breast. Post-procedure mammogram demonstrated accurate placement of the biopsy microclip. Pathology demonstrates atypical ductal hyperplasia, and surgical excision is recommended. Pre-surgery needle-wire localization is performed under mammographic guidance. Using the biopsy microclip as a target, needle-wire localization is performed from a medial approach. What are the closest coordinates to the target?

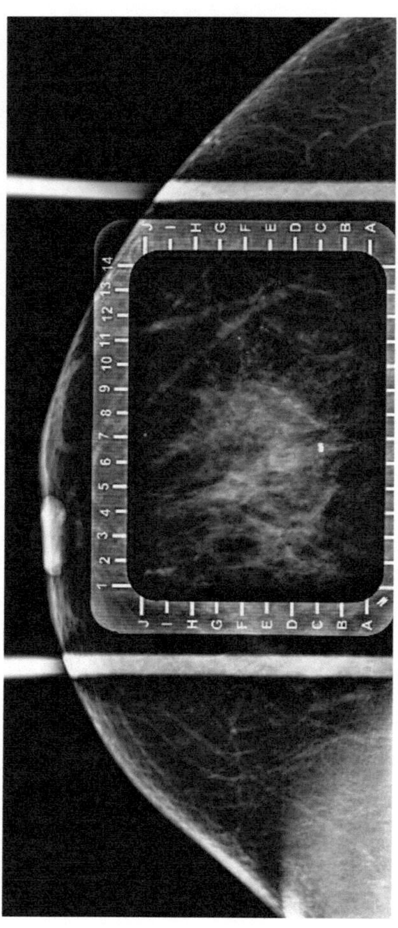

(a) A14.
(b) C6.
(c) F3.
(d) J10.

11b. Using the biopsy microclip as a target, needle-wire localization is performed from a medial approach. What is the next best step?

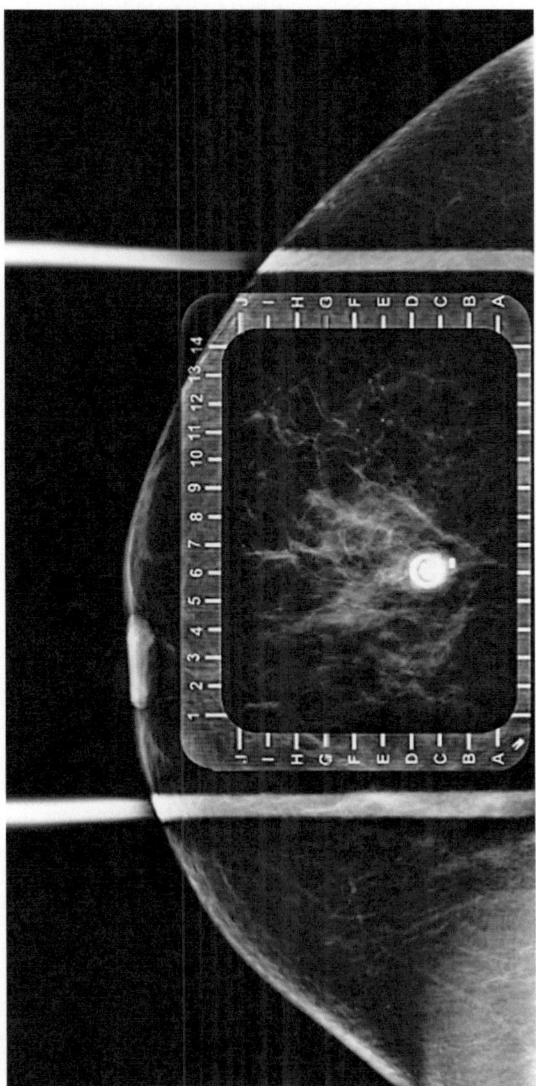

(a) Obtain a craniocaudal mammogram to confirm positioning.
(b) Deploy needle in the current position.
(c) Remove needle and re-position over the microclip.
(d) Remove needle and attempt from a superior approach.

12a. A 62-year-old female presents with a palpable abnormality in the left breast
     1 week after stereotactic biopsy for suspicious calcifications. The lump is
     located in the area of her recent biopsy. The following finding is seen in the
     area of concern on diagnostic breast ultrasound. What is the most likely
     finding?

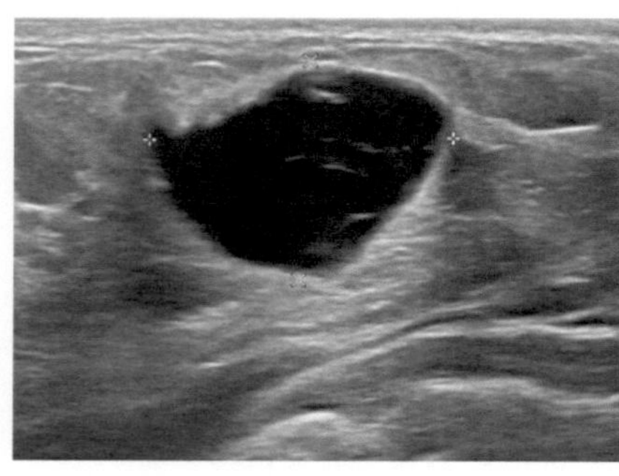 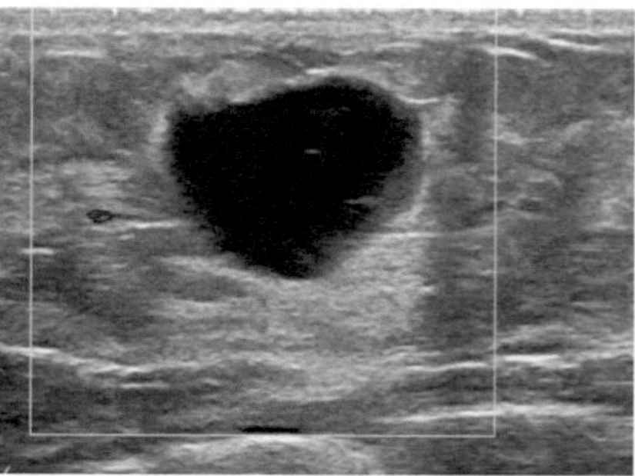

   (a) Abscess.
   (b) Fibroadenoma.
   (c) Invasive ductal carcinoma.
   (d) Hematoma.

12b. What steps can be taken if excessive bleeding is noted during image-
     guided biopsy?
   (a) Administer additional lidocaine with epinephrine.
   (b) Maintain manual compression against a hard surface in the plane of nee-
       dle insertion for 10–20 minutes.
   (c) Apply a pressure dressing to maintain continuous pressure.
   (d) Obtain surgical consultation if excessive bleeding persists.
   (e) All of the above.

Answers

1a. b. Stereotactic biopsy.

Magnification views show grouped coarse heterogeneous calcifications.
According to BI-RADS fifth edition [1], grouped coarse heterogeneous calcifications are BI-RADS 4b. Category 4b lesions have a 10–50% likelihood of
malignancy. As a result, biopsy should be recommended. For suspicious findings seen only on mammography, stereotactic biopsy should be performed to
obtain tissue diagnosis.

1b. a. Medial.

Suspicious calcifications are seen in the right breast at 3 o'clock. The biopsy approach should be made based on the projection that provides the best visualization of the finding and the shortest distance from the skin entry site to the target [2, 3]. In this case, the shortest distance for biopsy would be via a medial approach.

1c. d. Z-axis error.

For stereotactic biopsies, a scout image demonstrating the target lesion is acquired. Then, two images are acquired at $+15°$ and $-15°$ angles to form the stereo pair. Another stereo pair image is acquired after firing the biopsy needle mechanism to confirm needle placement. In this example, the needle and target are aligned on the x-axis and y-axis, however, the needle has not reached the target on the z-axis, consistent with a z-axis error [4, 5]. A z-axis error corresponds to an error in depth positioning. If the needle is too deep to the target, the needle needs to be pulled back and re-imaged to ensure the target is in the trough. If the needle is too shallow to the target, the needle needs to be pushed further in.

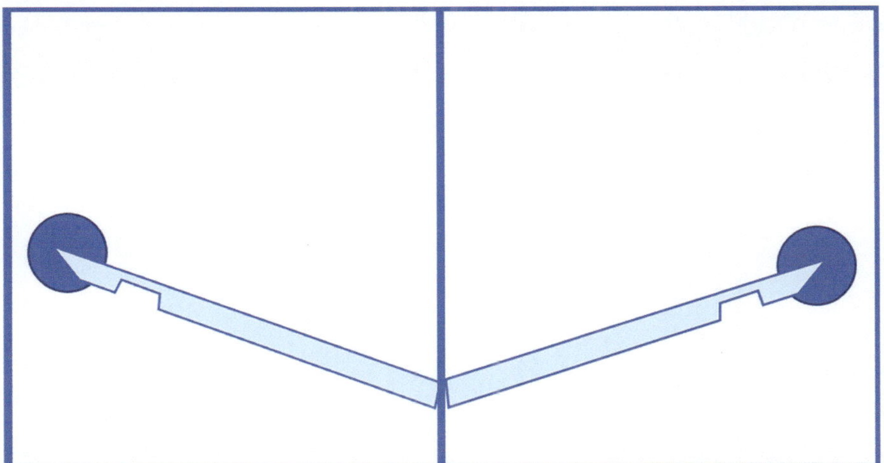

Z-axis error

2a. b. Stereotactic biopsy.

Given the presence of an irregular mass seen on mammogram, biopsy should be recommended. If no sonographic correlate is identified, stereotactic biopsy should be performed to obtain tissue diagnosis.

2b. d. Inferior.

An irregular mass is seen in the left breast at 6 o'clock. The shortest distance for biopsy would be via an inferior approach.

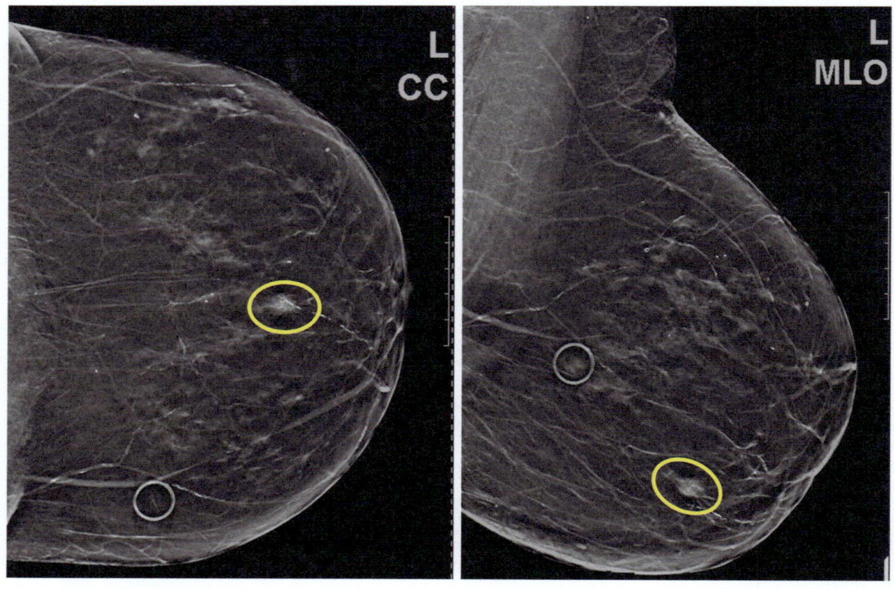

2c. c. *Y*-axis error.

In this example, the needle and target are aligned on the *x*-axis and *z*-axis, however, the needle is below the target on the *y*-axis, consistent with a *y*-axis error [4, 5]. A *y*-axis error corresponds to an error in vertical positioning, with the needle either below or above the target. Either re-targeting or sampling more above or below the needle can help correct the error.

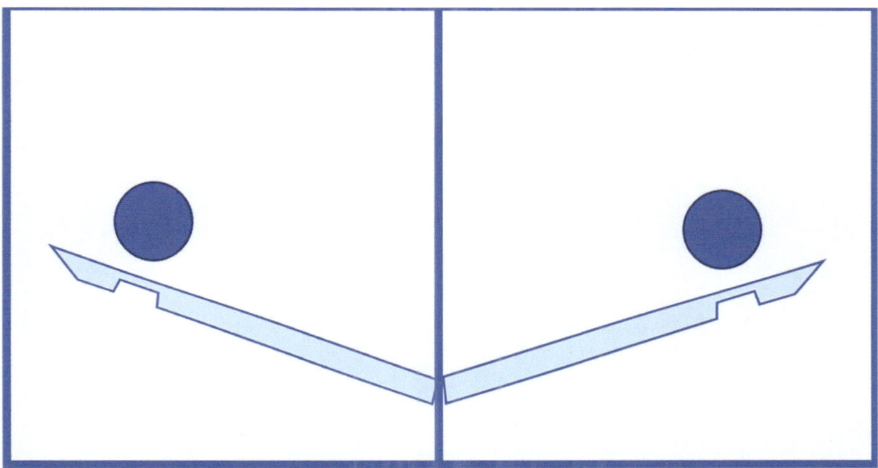

Y-axis error

An *x*-axis error corresponds to an error in horizontal positioning, with the needle either too far to the right side or left side of the target.

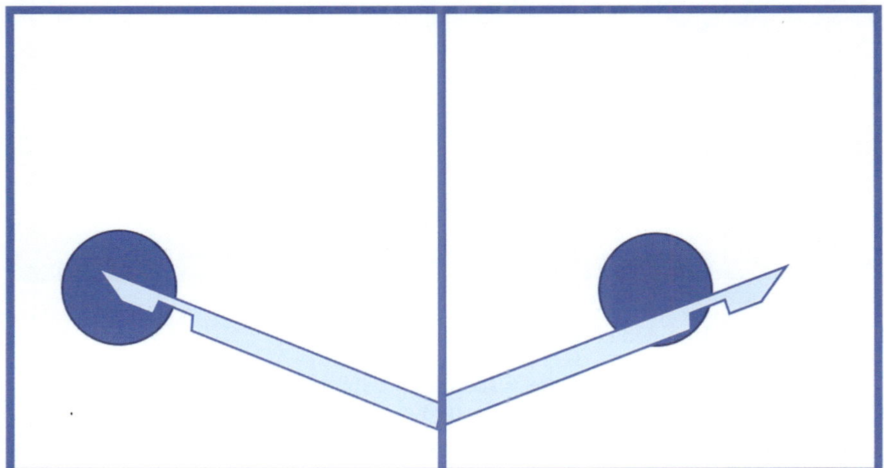

X-axis error

3. c. Perform stereotactic biopsy of the mammographic finding.

Post-procedure mammogram following ultrasound-guided biopsy is needed to confirm biopsy microclip placement. It is also used to confirm that the biopsied sonographic finding correlates to the original mammographic area of interest. If the sonographic biopsy target does not correlate with the mammographic finding, a re-biopsy using stereotactic guidance should be performed. Note that in the annotated images, the microclip and hematoma (red circle) are located anterior to the biopsy target (yellow circle).

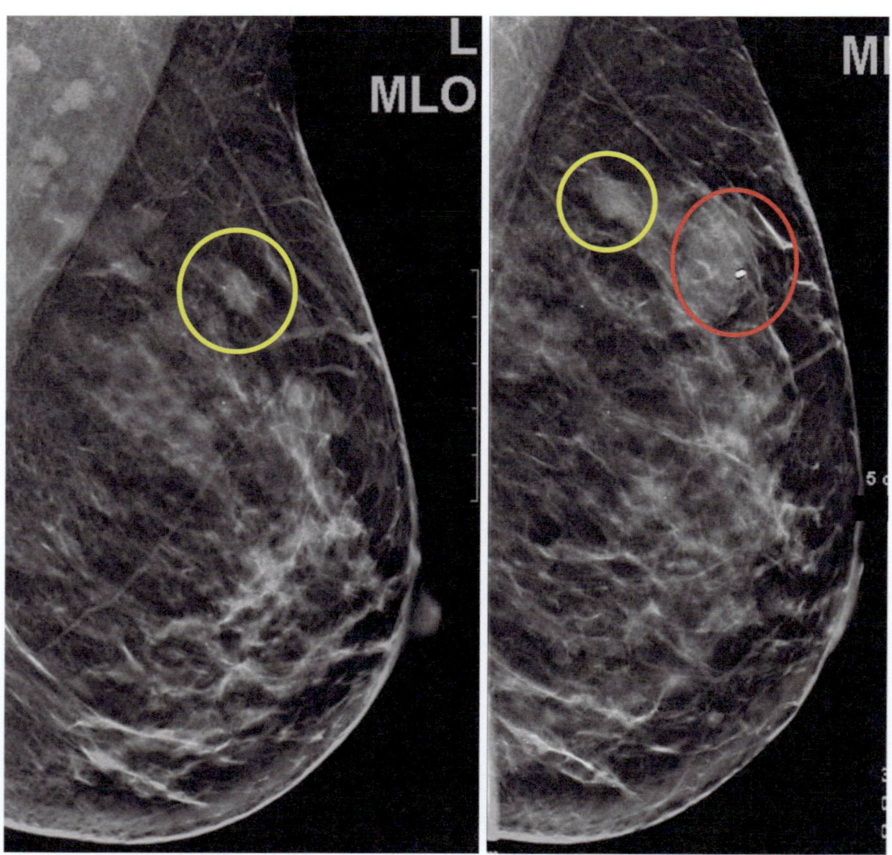

4a. b. Ultrasound-guided core needle biopsy.

When a sonographic correlate is seen for a mammographically detected abnormality, ultrasound-guided core needle biopsy should be performed for tissue diagnosis. Benefits of ultrasound-guided biopsy when compared to stereotactic biopsy include lack of radiation exposure, greater patient comfort and real-time visualization [6, 7]. Although fine-needle aspiration was previously utilized, better specimen quality is obtained with core needle biopsy [2].

4b. b. Lateral.

The suspicious mass is seen in the right breast at 9 o'clock. A lateral approach would provide the shortest distance to the lesion while avoiding the nipple and interference from the contralateral breast.

4c. c. White circle.

When performing an ultrasound-guided biopsy, care should be taken to avoid vascularity [8] surrounding a mass (blue circle) and within the mass (yellow circle). Targeting the central portion of the mass with the least vascularity (white circle) will ensure adequate sampling and decreased bleeding risk.

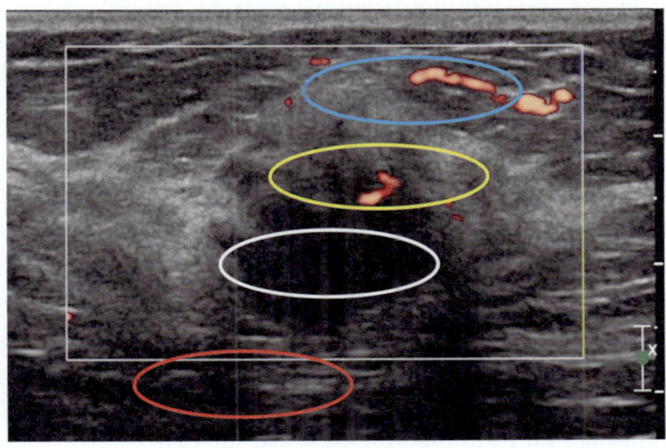

5a. a. Discard fluid.

If cyst aspiration yields non-bloody clear fluid and the cyst collapses following the procedure, the fluid may be discarded [2]. Routine follow-up is recommended.

5b. c. Place a biopsy microclip and send fluid for cytology.

If a cyst aspiration yields bloody fluid, the fluid should be sent for cytology in order to rule out occult malignancy [2]. A biopsy microclip should be placed as the lesion will likely resolve following aspiration.

5c. d. Perform ultrasound-guided core needle biopsy.

A failed cyst aspiration suggests that the finding is a solid mass [9]. Given the suspicious imaging features, ultrasound-guided core needle biopsy should be performed to obtain tissue diagnosis.

6a. b. Breast abscess.

In a lactating patient, a breast abscess can occur as a complication of mastitis. Patients can present clinically with focal pain, warmth, and redness of the affected breast with associated palpable abnormality, as well as systemic symptoms such as fever [10]. On ultrasound, an abscess can present as a hypoechoic collection with mobile internal debris. Abscesses lack internal color Doppler flow; however, the surrounding soft tissues may appear hyperemic.

6b. b. Ultrasound-guided drainage.

Patients with mastitis or breast abscesses should be prescribed a course of oral antibiotics. For treatment of breast abscesses, ultrasound-guided percutaneous drainage may be performed using an 18-gauge needle. The material obtained should be sent for cultures in order to determine the pathogen and antibiotic sensitivity. Antibiotics can be adjusted as needed [11].

6c. a. Ultrasound-guided core-needle biopsy and surgical consultation.

If symptoms of mastitis and/or breast abscess persist despite appropriate management, an ultrasound-guided core needle biopsy or skin punch biopsy should be performed to rule out malignancy, such as inflammatory breast cancer. Surgical consultation is also recommended for patients with breast abscesses that fail to resolve after multiple ultrasound-guided drainages [10, 11].

7a. d. All of the above.

Target nonvisualization at time of MRI-guided biopsy occurs in approximately 12% of cases [12]. Grid positioning should be verified in order to ensure that the target is not outside of the field of view. Obtaining delayed post-contrast sequences and decreasing compression of the breast will allow for better vascular perfusion [13]. If there is persistent nonvisualization of the target, hormonal changes in the breast may be the cause of the initial MRI finding.

7b. b. Short-term interval follow-up breast MRI.

If nonvisualization of the target occurs at time of MRI-guided biopsy, short-term follow-up MRI should be performed in order to rule out malignancy [2]. In this case, the focus of enhancement was not seen on the six-month follow-up MRI.

8. c. Multiple intraductal filling defects.

Ductography can be used for evaluation of unilateral spontaneous nipple discharge arising from a single pore. At the time of procedure, discharge is elicited using periareolar pressure. The discharging pore is then cannulated using a 30-gauge blunt-tipped catheter, and 0.2–0.3 mL of iodinated contrast is slowly administered through the catheter via extension tubing. The cannula can then be removed or secured in place using paper tape. Craniocaudal and 90-degree mediolateral magnification views of the subareolar breast are then obtained in order to visualize the contrast-opacified duct [14].

9a. a. Medial.

The biopsy microclip is in the lower inner quadrant of the left breast. Of the answer choices provided, the shortest distance for pre-surgery localization would be via a medial approach. Although an inferior approach would also provide a short distance to the target, performing the procedure from the inferior breast can be technically challenging for the radiologist.

9b. b. Pull back the deployment device and repeat craniocaudal view mammogram to confirm position.

For accurate wire-free localization, the tip of the needle device should be placed at the target prior to deployment. In this image, the tip of the reflector deployment device needs to be pulled back, so that the tip is at the target. A repeat craniocaudal mammogram should be performed to confirm positioning, as was in this case. The reflector was then deployed, with post-deployment craniocaudal mammogram demonstrating appropriate reflector placement.

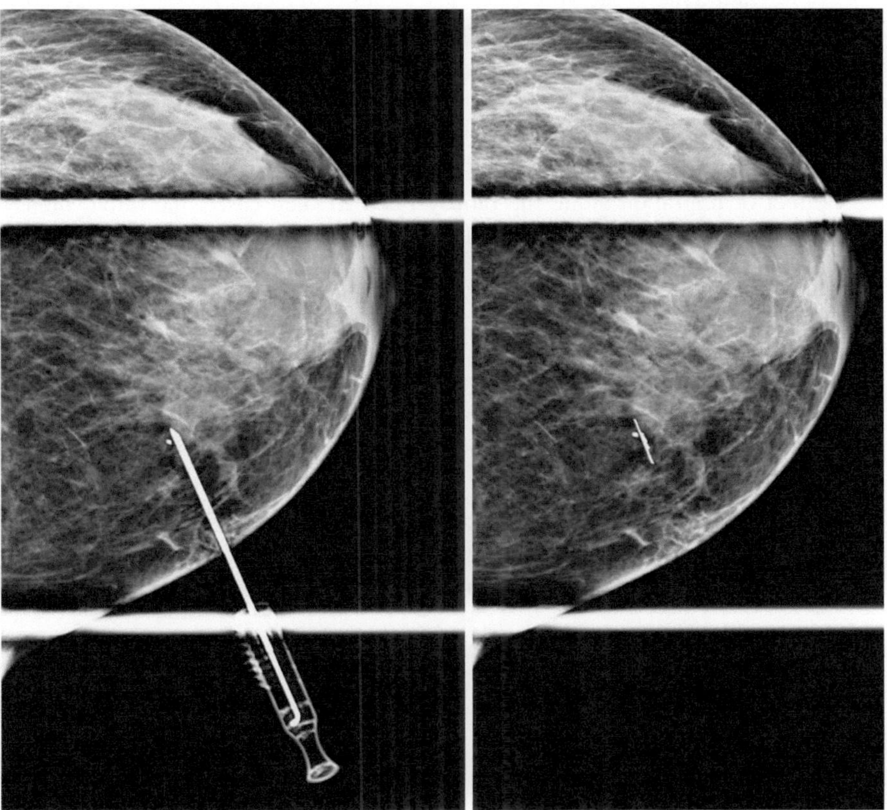

9c. c. Both a and b.

Specimen radiographs are obtained following excision to confirm that the target was excised. If a wire localization was performed, the wire and localization target should be seen within the specimen radiograph. If wire-free localization was performed, the wire-free device (in this case a reflector) and target should be seen within the specimen radiograph. Findings should be reported to the operating room as soon as possible in order to confirm adequate surgical excision.

9d. d. All of the above.

Wire localizations are typically performed just prior to surgical excision. Wire-free localization, however, may be performed days to months before the day of surgery. Since there is no need for patients to have a wire protruding from the breast while waiting in the pre-operative area, the overall patient experience is improved and patient anxiety is reduced with wire-free localization. Additionally, the wire-free device allows for continuous intraoperative reorientation in relation to the target, which gives the potential for removal of a smaller amount of nontargeted breast tissue.

10a. a. Architectural distortion with associated calcifications.

Following stereotactic biopsy, clip migration may occur due to accordion effect or migration along the biopsy tract. In such cases, the initial biopsy target should be localized rather than the biopsy microclip.

10b. c. The biopsy microclip is not seen within the specimen, which is expected as the microclip was not the localization target.

If the biopsy microclip was not targeted at time of pre-surgery localization, the microclip is not expected to be seen within the specimen radiograph.

11a. b. C6.

The grid overlying the area of localization target is used to determine accurate placement of the localization needle [15]. In this case, using the biopsy microclip as the target, the localization needle should be placed at approximately C6.

11b. c. Remove needle and re-position over the microclip.

On initial images following needle placement during mammographic localization, the needle should overlap the localization target, which in this case is the biopsy microclip. Once the needle is in appropriate position, an orthogonal view is obtained in order to determine needle position relative to the target. Once positioning is confirmed, the localization wire may be deployed [16].

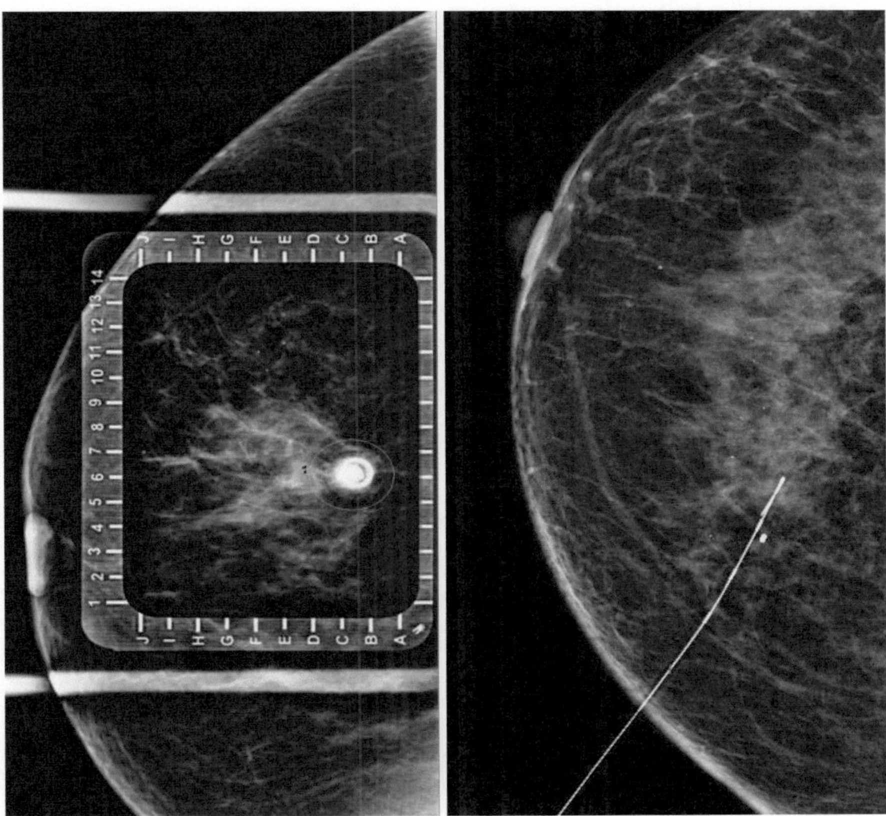

12a. d. Hematoma.

A post-biopsy hematoma can present as a hypoechoic fluid collection or as a complex cystic and solid mass, depending on the amount of clotted versus free blood within the cavity [11]. Most hematomas resolve within 2–4 weeks.

12b. e. All of the above.

If excessive bleeding is encountered during image-guided biopsy, additional lidocaine with epinephrine may be administered in order to cause vasoconstriction. Additionally, manual compression should be applied and a pressure dressing may be utilized. If excessive bleeding cannot be controlled, a surgical consultation should be obtained [11].

References

1. D'Orsi CJ, Sickles EA, Mendelson EB, Morris EA, et al. ACR BI-RADS® atlas. VA, American College of Radiology: Breast Imaging Reporting and Data System. Reston; 2013.
2. Mahoney MC, Newell MS. Breast intervention: how I do it. Radiology. 2013;268(1):12–24. https://doi.org/10.1148/radiol.13120985.
3. Carr JJ, Hemler PF, Halford PW, Freimanis RI, Choplin RH, Chen MY. Stereotactic localization of breast lesions: how it works and methods to improve accuracy. Radiographics. 2001;21(2):463–73. https://doi.org/10.1148/radiographics.21.2.g01mr11463.
4. Huang ML, Adrada BE, Candelaria R, Thames D, Dawson D, Yang WT. Stereotactic breast biopsy: pitfalls and pearls. Tech Vasc Interv Radiol. 2014;17(1):32–9. https://doi.org/10.1053/j.tvir.2013.12.006.
5. Chesebro AL, Chikarmane SA, Ritner JA, Birdwell RL, Giess CS. Troubleshooting to overcome technical challenges in image-guided breast biopsy. Radiographics. 2017;37(3):705–18. https://doi.org/10.1148/rg.2017160117.
6. Tomkovich KR. Interventional radiology in the diagnosis and treatment of diseases of the breast: a historical review and future perspective based on currently available techniques. AJR Am J Roentgenol. 2014;203(4):725–33. https://doi.org/10.2214/AJR.14.12994.
7. Youk JH, Kim EK, Kim MJ, Lee JY, Oh KK. Missed breast cancers at US-guided core needle biopsy: how to reduce them. Radiographics. 2007;27(1):79–94. https://doi.org/10.1148/rg.271065029.
8. Rocha RD, Pinto RR, Aquino Tavares DBP, Aires Gonçalves CS. Step-by-step of ultrasound-guided core-needle biopsy of the breast: review and technique. Radiol Bras. 2013;46(4):234–41. https://doi.org/10.1590/S0100-39842013000400010.
9. Ciatto S, Cariaggi P, Bulgaresi P. The value of routine cytologic examination of breast cyst fluids. Acta Cytol. 1987;31(3):301–4.
10. Trop I, Dugas A, David J, et al. Breast abscesses: evidence-based algorithms for diagnosis, management, and follow-up. Radiographics. 2011;31(6):1683–99. https://doi.org/10.1148/rg.316115521.
11. Mahoney MC, Ingram AD. Breast emergencies: types, imaging features, and management. AJR Am J Roentgenol. 2014;202(4):W390–9. https://doi.org/10.2214/AJR.13.11758.
12. Neal CH. Lesion nonvisualization at MRI-guided breast biopsy: now what? Acad Radiol. 2018;25(9):1099–100. https://doi.org/10.1016/j.acra.2018.06.001.
13. Pinnamaneni N, Moy L, Gao Y, et al. Canceled MRI-guided breast biopsies due to nonvisualization: follow-up and outcomes. Acad Radiol. 2018;25(9):1101–10. https://doi.org/10.1016/j.acra.2018.01.016.
14. Slawson SH, Johnson BA. Ductography: how to and what if? Radiographics. 2001;21(1):133–50. https://doi.org/10.1148/radiographics.21.1.g01ja15133.
15. Kapoor MM, Patel MM, Scoggins ME. The wire and beyond: recent advances in breast imaging preoperative needle localization. Radiographics. 2019;39(7):1886–906. https://doi.org/10.1148/rg.2019190041.
16. Esserman LE, Cura MA, DaCosta D. Recognizing pitfalls in early and late migration of clip markers after imaging-guided directional vacuum-assisted biopsy. Radiographics. 2004;24(1):147–56. https://doi.org/10.1148/rg.241035052.

Pathology

Stephanie Histed Chung, Natalie Cain,
and Antionette Roth

S. H. Chung
Department of Diagnostic Radiology, Cooper University Hospital,
Camden, NJ, USA
e-mail: Chung-Stephanie@cooperhealth.edu

N. Cain
Department of Radiology, David Geffen School of Medicine at UCLA, Los Angeles,
CA, USA
e-mail: ncain@mednet.ucla.edu

A. Roth (⊠)
Department of Radiology, Olive View-UCLA Medical Center, Sylmar, CA, USA
e-mail: aroth@dhs.lacounty.gov

L. Chow, B. Li (eds.), *Absolute Breast Imaging Review*,
https://doi.org/10.1007/978-3-031-08274-0_7

1. A 35-year-old woman presented with a palpable mass. The ultrasound-guided biopsy results showed fibroadenoma, which was thought to be concordant with imaging. Six months after the biopsy, the patient reported significant growth of the mass. On ultrasound exam, the mass had doubled in size compared to prior. The patient underwent a localized surgical excision.

   At surgical excision, the pathology showed malignant Phyllodes tumor. Which of the following is true regarding radiology–pathology correlation? Radiology–pathology correlation should be performed on the following biopsy cases:
   (a) Cases with malignancy pathology.
   (b) Cases with benign pathology.
   (c) Cases when surgery is recommended.
   (d) Cases where the patient will return to screening mammography.
   (e) All cases.

2. The radiology–pathology correlation statement that is placed on a benign biopsy should include the following:
   (a) A statement of concordance or discordance.
   (b) A clear recommendation for follow-up or return to screening.
   (c) A BIRADS classification.
   (d) a and b.
   (e) All of the above.

3. One of the main reasons for performing radiology–pathology correlations is:
   (a) To prevent unnecessary surgery.
   (b) To decide when to order an MRI.
   (c) To limit the number of false negatives.
   (d) To increase the true positive rate.

4. Which of the following is (are) true regarding false negatives?
   (a) False negative is defined as a test result that wrongly indicates that a patient does not have a disease.
   (b) Is a type I error.
   (c) Is a type II error.
   (d) A and B.
   (e) A and C.

5. Which of the following is (are) an example(s) of a false-negative result?
   (a) An invasive ductal carcinoma diagnosed in a mass that was previously biopsied two years ago and had yielded a benign result.
   (b) An invasive ductal carcinoma diagnosed in the ipsilateral breast 10 months after a benign biopsy.
   (c) A benign biopsy that was deemed discordant with imaging and excision was recommended. On excision, the pathology showed invasive carcinoma.
   (d) A biopsy result showed ductal carcinoma in situ that underwent surgical excision. On excision, the mass was found to be invasive carcinoma.
   (e) All of the above.

6a. A 60-year-old woman with no available prior mammograms was called back from screening mammogram for calcifications in the right lower inner quadrant. Diagnostic images of grouped amorphous calcifications among benign secretory calcifications are submitted below. The diagnostic mammogram was given a BIRADS 4B and a stereotactic biopsy was recommended. The pathology showed atypical ductal hyperplasia.

When performing radiology–pathology correlation for biopsied calcifications, what is required to conclude the pathology result is concordant with imaging findings?

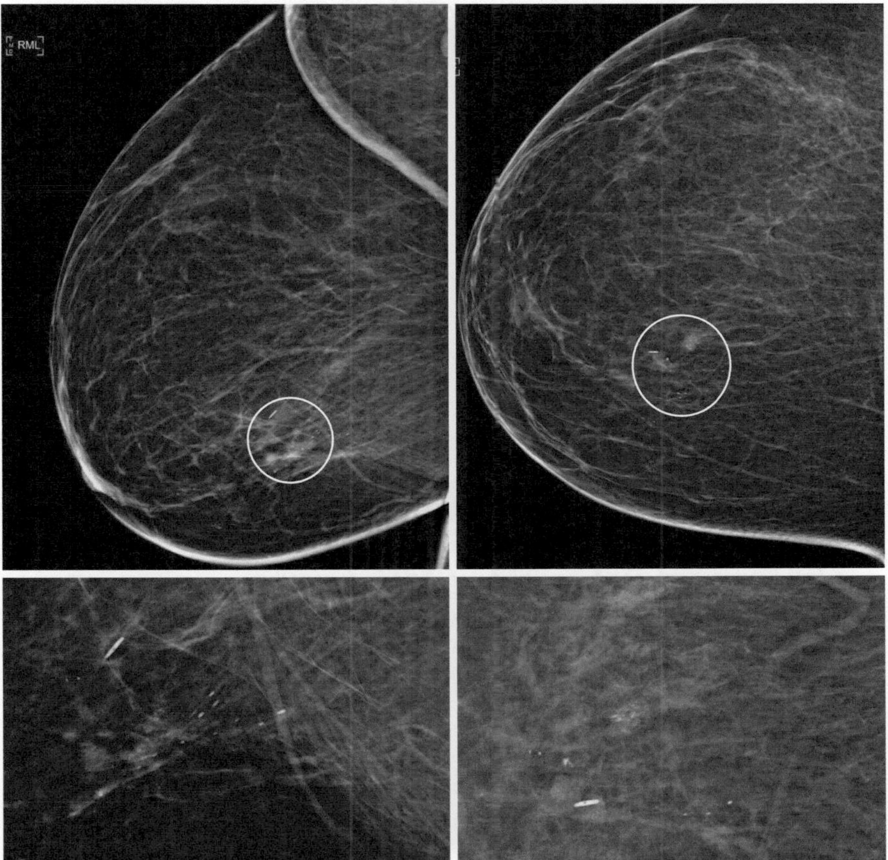

(a) A review of imaging to confirm that the histologic diagnosis explains the imaging findings.
(b) That the specimen radiographs of a stereotactic biopsy specimen contain calcifications from the cluster identified on diagnostic mammogram.
(c) There are post-biopsy changes and a decrease in the number of calcifications in the area of concern on post-procedure mammogram.
(d) All of the above.

6b. The following images are images from the stereotactic biopsy specimen and post-clip placement mammogram. What is your radiology–pathology correlation statement?

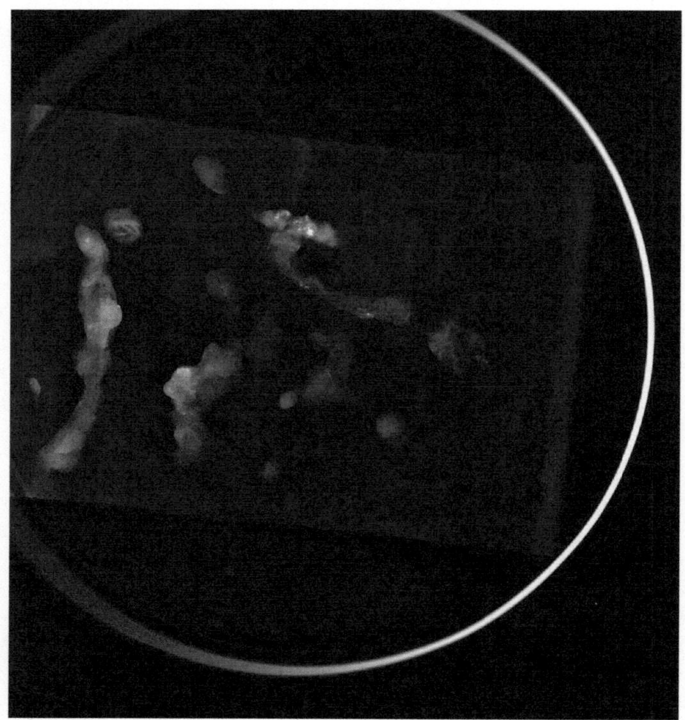

(a) Concordant, follow-up mammogram in 6 months.
(b) Concordant, recommend MRI.
(c) Concordant, recommend surgical excision.
(d) Discordant, recommend excision.

7. All the following are examples of high-risk pathology for which surgical excision should be recommended except:
(a) Sclerosing adenosis.
(b) Atypical ductal hyperplasia.
(c) Radial scar with atypia.
(d) Flat epithelial atypia.
(e) Atypical papillary lesion.

8. The biopsy technique that has the highest rate of false negatives is:
(a) Ultrasound core biopsy.
(b) Stereotactic core biopsy.
(c) MRI core biopsy.
(d) Excisional biopsy.

9a. A 35-year-old breast-feeding female presents with breast erythema and tenderness in the peri-areolar region. Her ultrasound is shown below. What is the next best step?

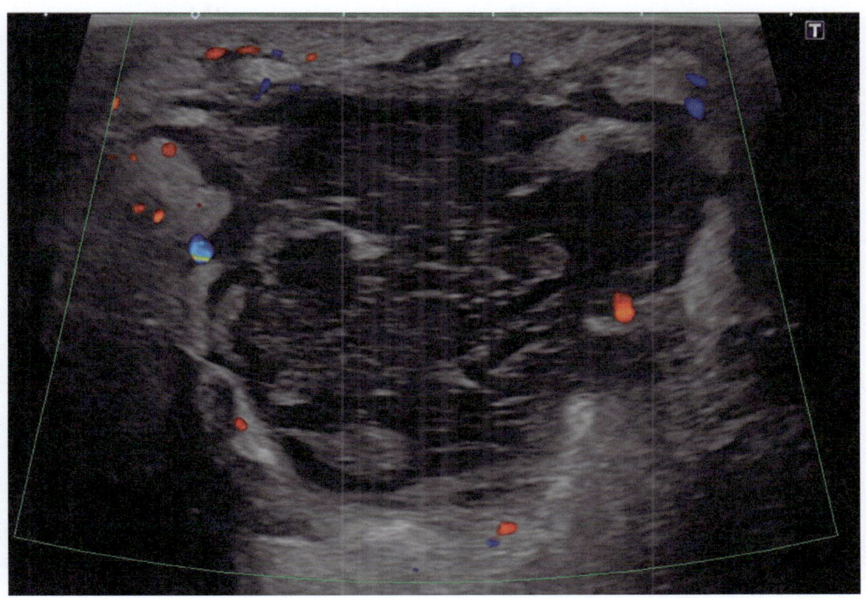

(a) Close follow up (in 6 months).
(b) Mammogram.
(c) Ultrasound-guided biopsy.
(d) Ultrasound-guided drainage and antibiotics.

9b. The most common bacteria causing breast abscess is:
(a) *Staphylococcus epidermidis.*
(b) *Streptococcus pyogenes.*
(c) *Staphylococcus aureus.*
(d) *Peptostreptococcus.*
(e) *Bacteroides.*

10a. A 35-year-old, non-breastfeeding woman presents with redness and pain in her right breast. Mammogram and ultrasound imaging is shown below. What is the differential diagnosis for this patient?

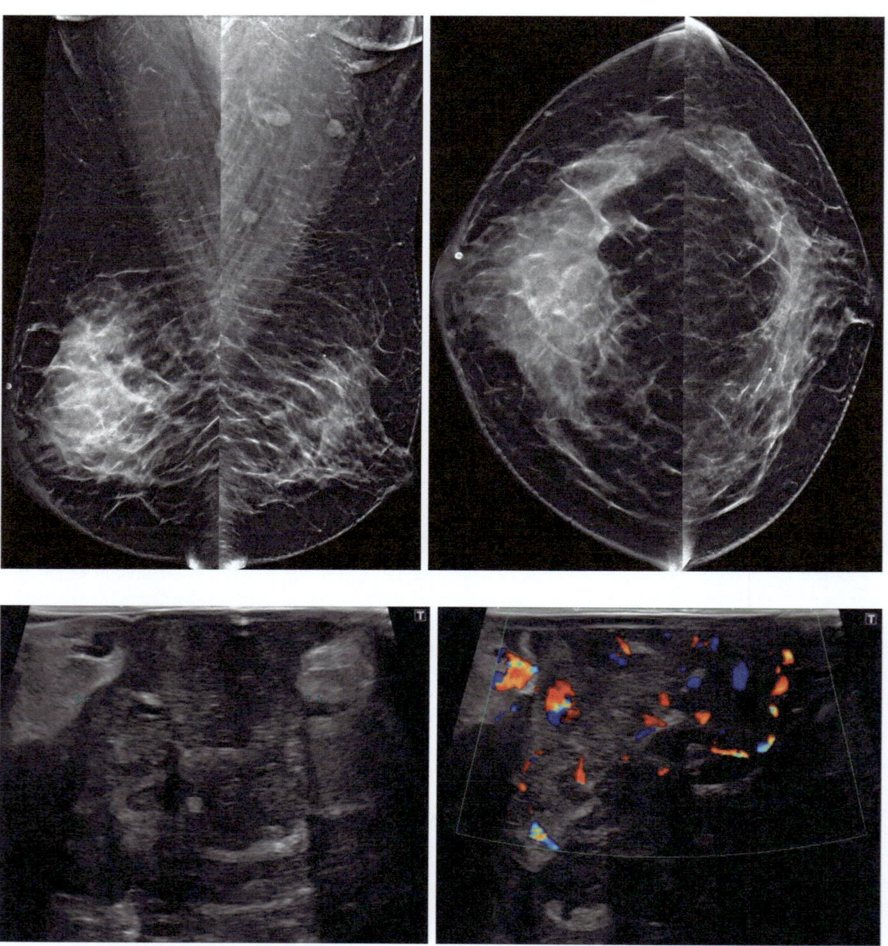

   (a) Infectious breast abscess.
   (b) Idiopathic granulomatous mastitis.
   (c) Inflammatory breast cancer.
   (d) Diabetic mastitis.
   (e) All of the above.

10b. Percutaneous aspiration was attempted, and no fluid could be obtained. A biopsy was performed showing idiopathic granulomatous mastitis. Which of the following are true regarding this pathologic diagnosis?
 (a) Most commonly occurs in pre-menopausal women.
 (b) The etiology is unknown.
 (c) Imaging features can mimic malignancy.
 (d) Pathology shows chronic granulomatous inflammation composed of giant cells.
 (e) Has a high recurrence rate.
 (f) All of the above.

11a. A 55-year-old woman presented with a growing palpable breast mass. Ultrasound images are shown.
 Ultrasound core biopsy pathology showed malignant phyllodes tumor. What is your radiology–pathology correlations statement for this lesion?

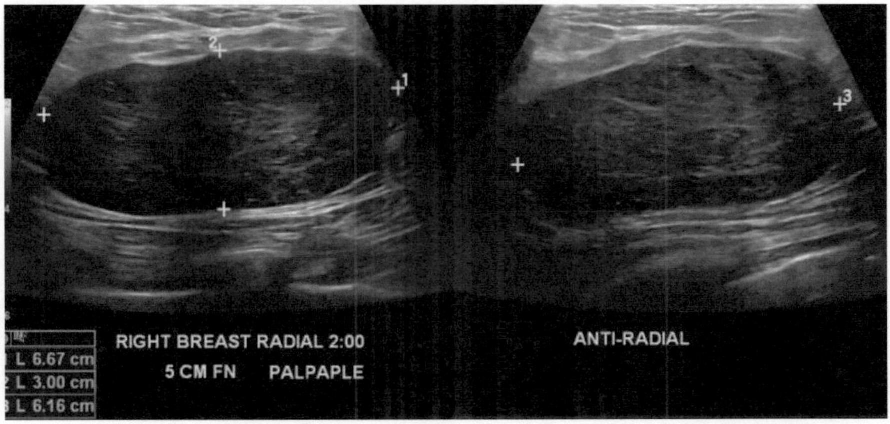

 (a) Concordant— recommend ultrasound in 6 months.
 (b) Concordant—recommend excision.
 (c) Discordant—recommend excision.
 (d) Discordant—recommend MRI.

11b. What is the method of metastasis for phyllodes tumors?
 (a) Hematogenous.
 (b) Lymphangitic.
 (c) Direct extension.
 (d) None of the above.

11c. What is the most common location of metastasis of phyllodes tumor?
    (a) Axillary lymph nodes.
    (b) Bone.
    (c) Lungs.
    (d) None of the above.

11d. If the pathology was benign phyllodes, what would be your concordance statement?
    (a) Concordant—recommend ultrasound in 6 months.
    (b) Concordant—recommend excision.
    (c) Discordant—recommend excision.
    (d) Discordant—recommend MRI.

11e. What imaging characteristics are used to characterize benign from malignant phyllodes tumors?
    (a) There are no imaging characteristics that differentiate benign from malignant phyllodes.
    (b) Size.
    (c) Margins.
    (d) Internal cystic spaces.
    (e) Interval growth pattern.

12a. A 61-year-old woman presents for biopsy of the mammographic findings below. Her pathology returned as ductal carcinoma in situ. What is the most common mammographic finding if this was high-grade DCIS?

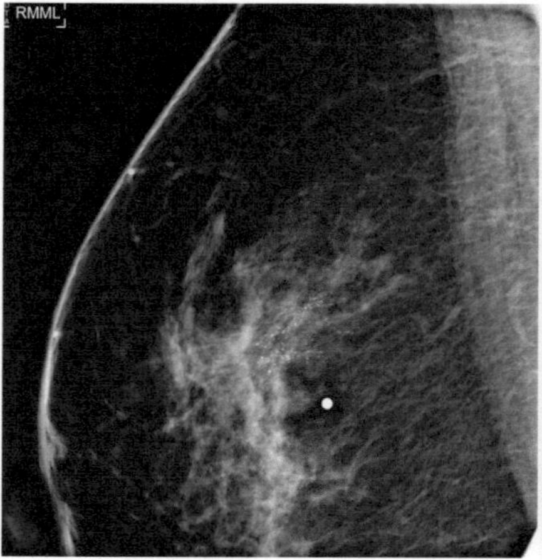
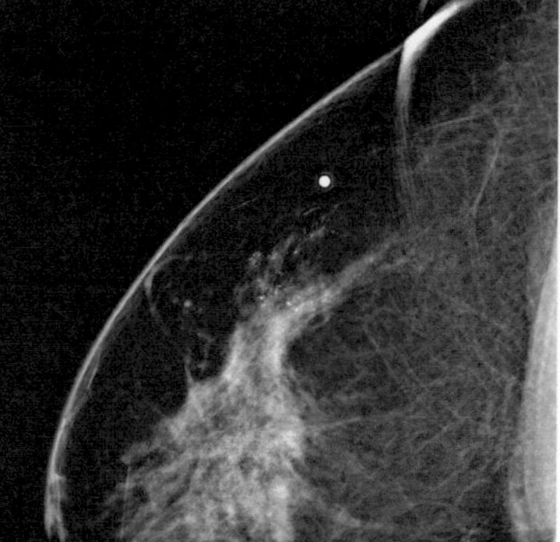

    (a) Non-calcified mass.
    (b) Architectural distortion.
    (c) Skin thickening and nipple retraction.
    (d) Fine pleomorphic or fine linear-branching calcifications.

12b. What grading system is used to classify DCIS?
    (a) TNM classification.
    (b) Van Nuys classification.
    (c) Luminal Subtype.
    (d) Molecular Subtype.

12c. What is the typical MRI enhancement pattern of this lesion?
    (a) Enhancing mass.
    (b) Focal enhancement in a regional distribution.
    (c) No enhancement.
    (d) Non-mass enhancement in a segmental distribution.

12d. What are the most important risk factors for disease recurrence in DCIS?
    (a) Hormone receptor-positive status.
    (b) Post-excision positive margins and synchronous foci that were not excised.
    (c) Male gender.
    (d) Morphology of the calcifications.

13a. A 20-year-old pregnant patient presents with a new palpable breast mass. Targeted ultrasound images are below. Which of the following is false regarding the evaluation of palpable breast masses in pregnancy?

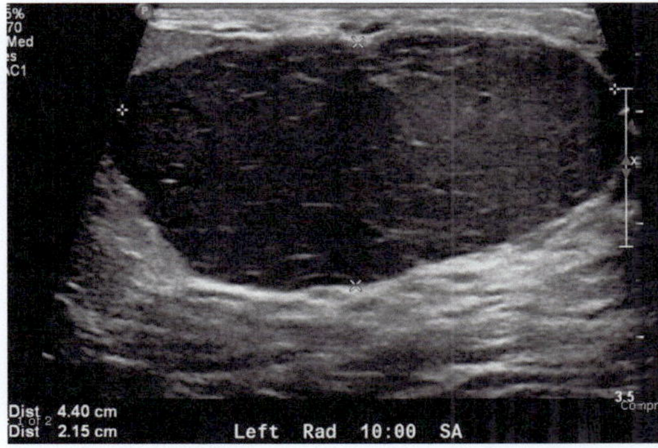
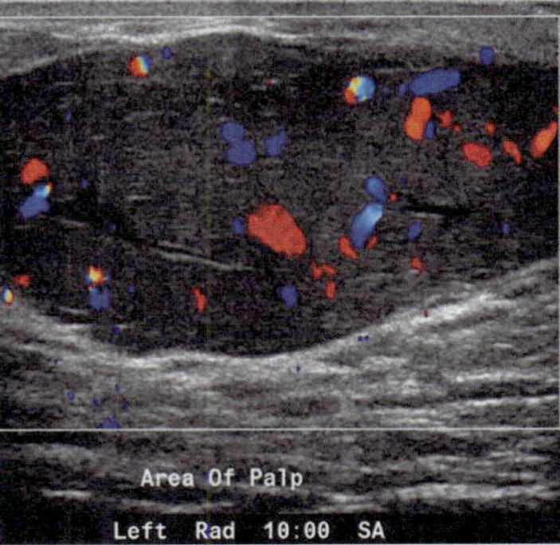

    (a) Benign masses are more common than malignant masses.
    (b) Mammogram is contraindicated in pregnancy.
    (c) Most pregnancy-related malignancy is invasive ductal cancer.
    (d) Masses suspicious for malignancy in pregnant/lactating women should be biopsied despite the risk of milk fistula.

13b. A biopsy of the above mass results in lactational adenoma. What is your radiology–pathology concordance statement for this biopsy?
    (a) Concordant—recommend surgical excision.
    (b) Concordant—recommend ultrasound follow up in 6 months.
    (c) Discordant—recommend MRI.
    (d) Discordant—recommend surgical excision.

13c. Which of the following are false regarding lactational adenomas?
 (a) Usually presents as a palpable mass.
 (b) Ultrasound characteristics are commonly a circumscribed hypoechoic mass.
 (c) Can have imaging characteristics of a fibroadenoma.
 (d) The presence of interval growth during pregnancy necessitates excision.

14a. A 73-year-old woman was called back for further evaluation from an abnormal screening mammogram. Spot mammogram and ultrasound images are provided below. This mass was biopsied. The pathology results were reported as papilloma with atypia. What is your radiology–pathology correlations statement?

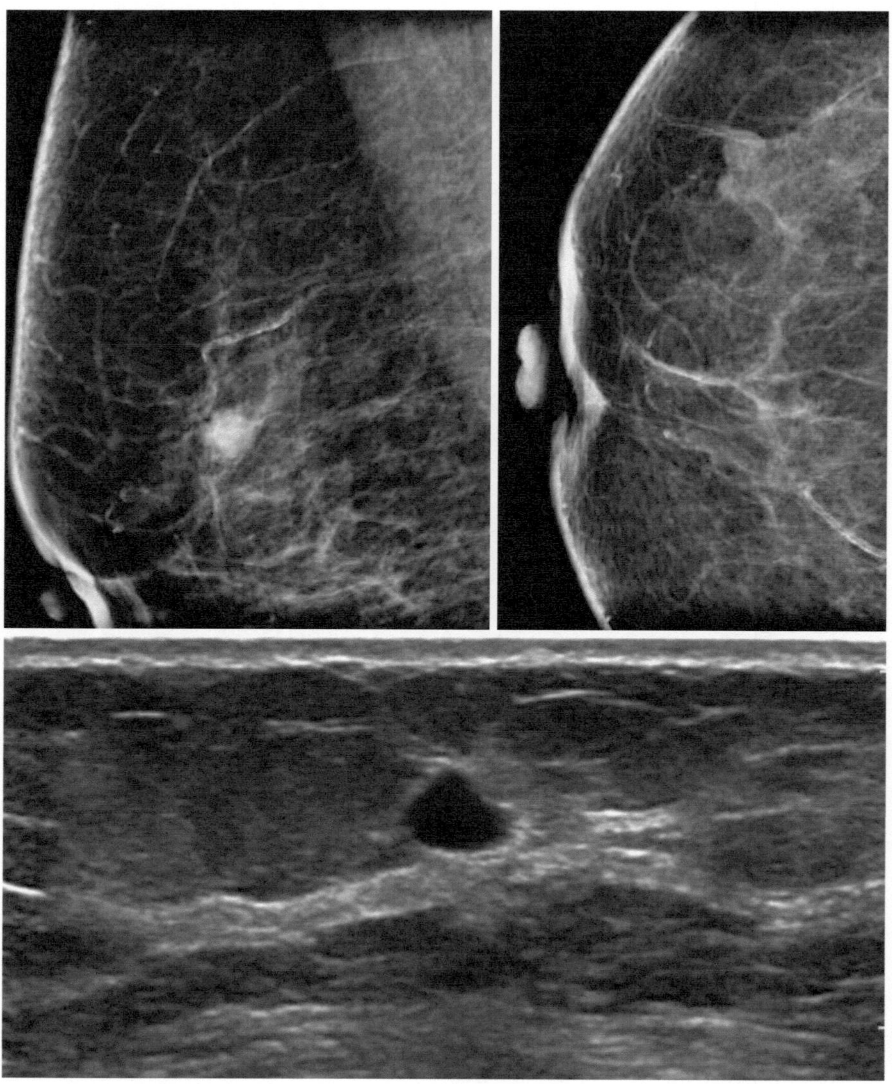

    (a) Concordant—recommend surgical excision.
    (b) Concordant—recommend 6-month follow-up diagnostic mammogram.
    (c) Discordant—recommend MRI.
    (d) Discordant—recommend surgical excision.

14b. This biopsied lesion underwent wire localization and excision. The excisional biopsy upstaged the pathology to 4 mm low-grade ductal carcinoma in situ, papillary and micropapillary types. No invasive component was identified. All margins were negative. Based on these pathology results, what TNM stage is the patient?

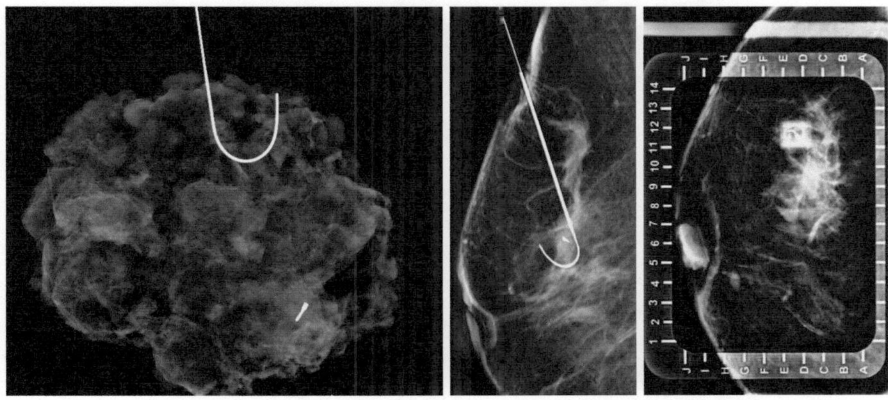

    (a) Stage 0.
    (b) Stage 1A.
    (c) Stage 2A.
    (d) Unable to determine.

15a. A 59-year-old woman called back for a screening mammogram for architectural distortion in the right breast. MLO and CC tomosynthetic 2D images are below respectively.

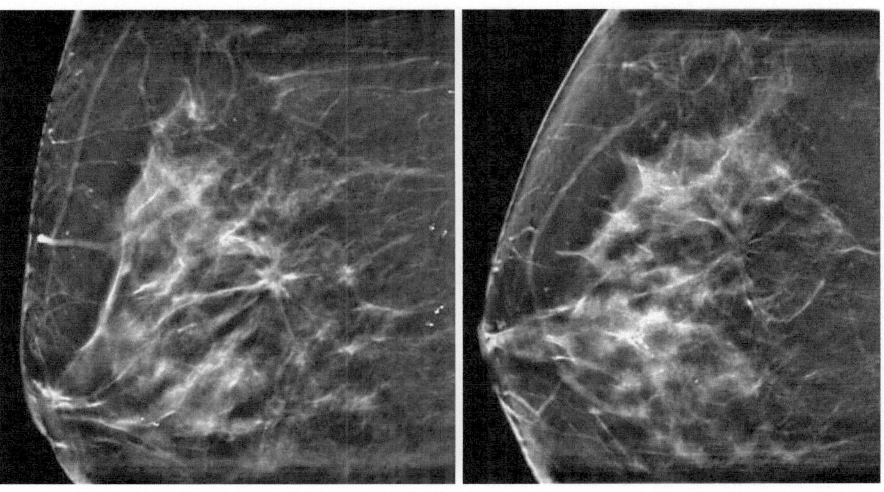

No sonographic correlation was identified. BIRADS 4 was given to the diagnostic workup, and a stereotactic core needle biopsy was performed. No specimen radiograph was obtained. Post-procedure mammograms are submitted below.

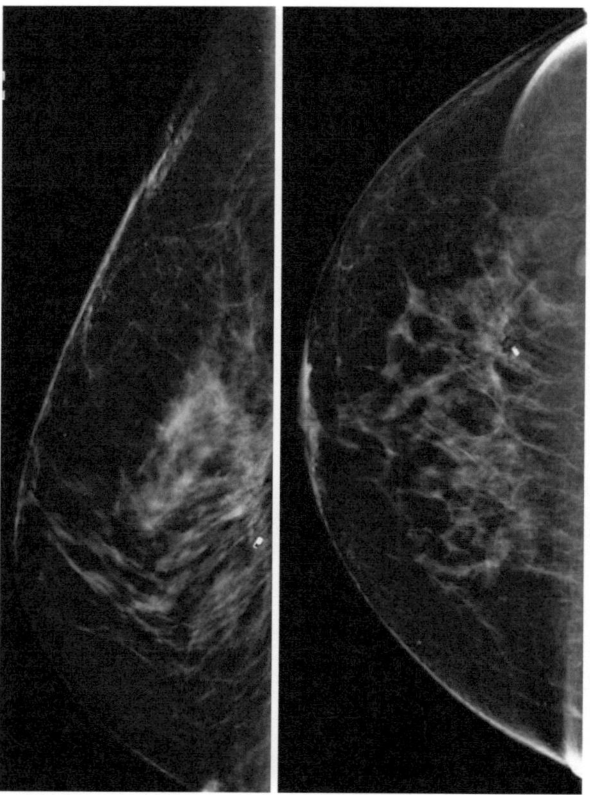

Pathology results showed focal microcalcifications in association with benign ducts. The radiology–pathology correlation for this biopsy is:
(a) Concordant—recommend mammogram in 6 months.
(b) Concordant—recommend mammogram and ultrasound in 6 months.
(c) Discordant—recommend MRI.
(d) Discordant—recommend surgical excision.

15b. An excisional biopsy was performed showing invasive ductal carcinoma with lobular features. All of the following may explain architectural distortion on mammogram and be considered concordant except?
(a) Radial scar.
(b) Lobular carcinoma.
(c) Post-surgical scar.
(d) Ductal Carcinoma In situ.
(e) Papilloma.

16a. A 73-year-old woman was called back from screening mammogram for a new mass in the right breast. Diagnostic mammogram images and ultrasound are provided below. The below diagnostic workup was given a BIRADS 5—Highly suspicious and the mass underwent core needle biopsy. Pathology reported invasive lobular carcinoma. Of the mammographic findings below, what is the most common conventional mammographic finding of this pathology?

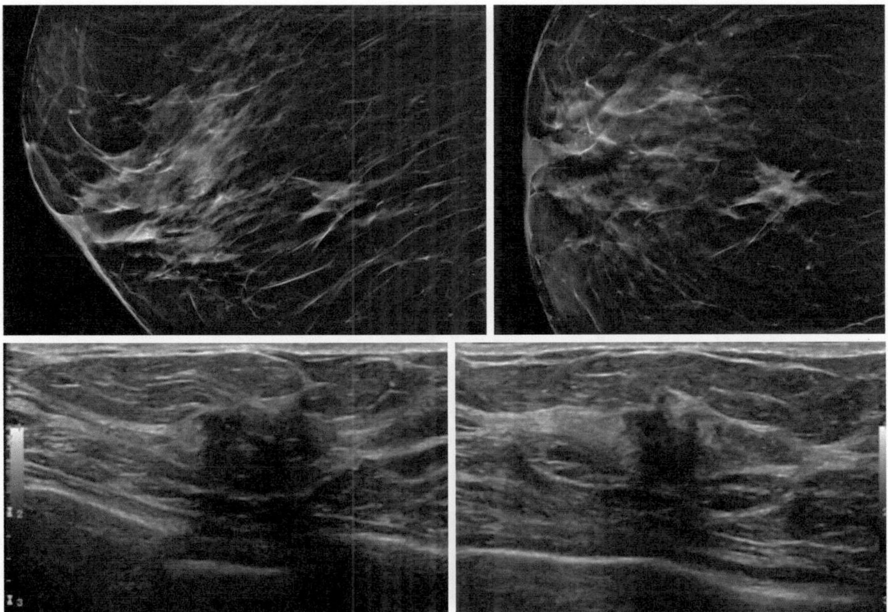

    (a) Irregular mass.
    (b) Pleomorphic calcifications.
    (c) Course, heterogeneous calcifications.
    (d) Circumscribed mass.

16b. What is the most common ultrasound finding of invasive lobular carcinoma?
    (a) Dermal thickening with an ill-defined heterogeneous echogenicity.
    (b) An anechoic cystic mass with a vascular papillary projection from its wall.
    (c) An irregular mass with angular margins, hypoechoic, heterogeneous internal echoes, and posterior acoustic shadowing.
    (d) A circumscribed, isoechoic mass with no posterior acoustic features.

16c. What is the next best step?
    (a) Lumpectomy with sentinel node biopsy.
    (b) MRI.
    (c) Neoadjuvant therapy.

17. Which of the following description and associated BIRADS has the highest likelihood of a discordant pathology?
    (a) A stereotactic biopsy of heterogeneous calcifications (BIRADS 4) with pathology result of fibroadenoma.
    (b) An MRI biopsy of non-mass enhancement (BIRADS 4) with pathology result of DCIS.
    (c) An ultrasound mass with angulated margins (BIRADS 5) with pathology result of fibroadenoma.
    (d) A circumscribed mass on ultrasound (BIRADS 4) with pathology result of medullary carcinoma.

18. Which of the following biomarkers are not routinely tested for on breast cancer biopsy specimens and excision specimens?
    (a) ER.
    (b) PR.
    (c) HER2.
    (d) PD-L1.
    (e) Ki-67 antigen.

19. A 45-year-old woman with BRCA1 mutation underwent screening and diagnostic mammogram and screening breast MRI with images shown below. Because of the abnormalities, a stereotactic biopsy was performed. Based on the imaging findings, what is the most likely grade of her cancer?

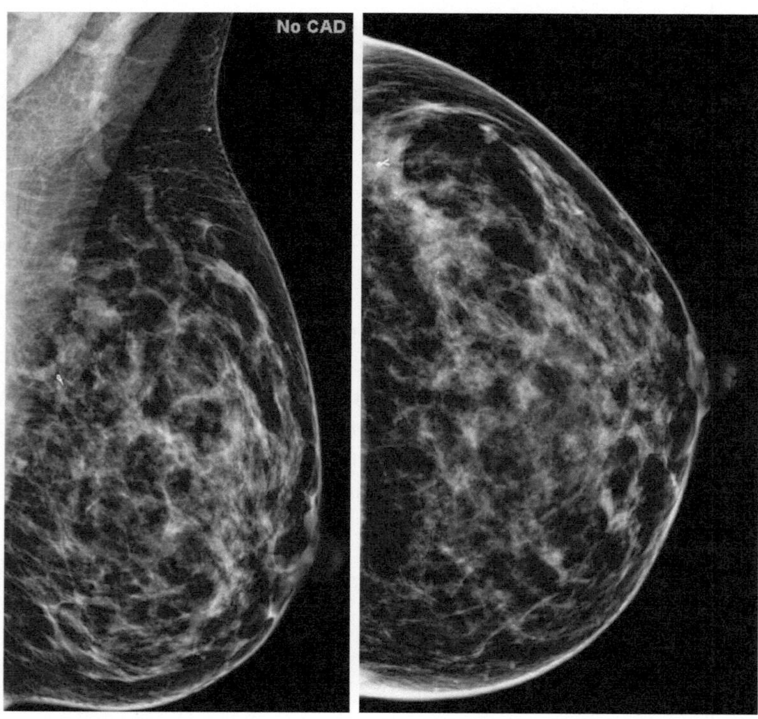

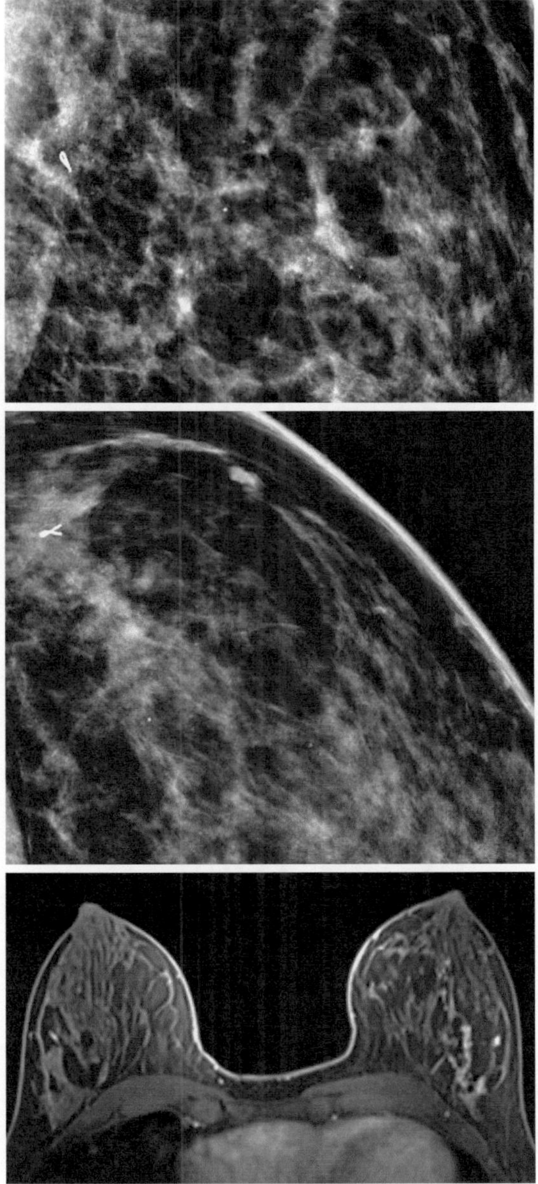

(a) Low grade.
(b) Intermediate grade.
(c) High grade.
(d) Benign findings.

20. In BRCA 1 and BRCA 2 mutation carriers, what is the lifetime risk of developing breast cancer?
    (a) 20%.
    (b) 50%.
    (c) 85%.
    (d) 99%.

21a. A 34-year-old female presenting with a new right breast palpable mass. Targeted ultrasound image is below:
     What proportion of malignant lesions are isoechoic on ultrasound?

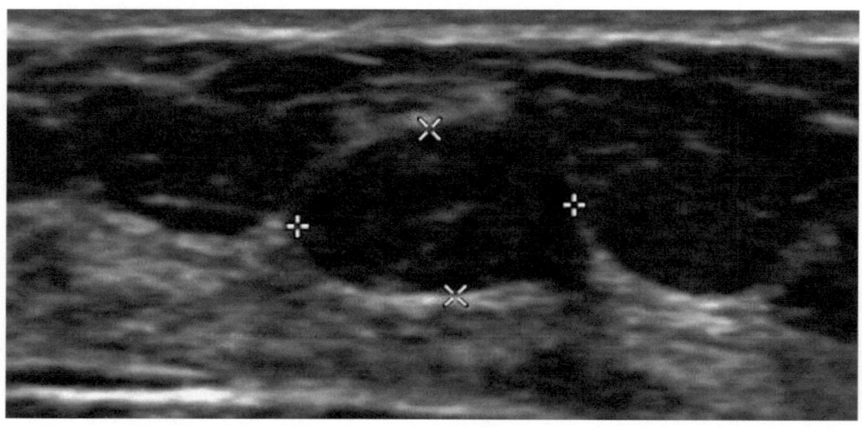

    (a) 1/8.
    (b) 3/4.
    (c) 1/2.
    (d) 1/3.

21b. The echogenicity of a lesion on ultrasound is determined relative to what structure in the breast?
     (a) Fat.
     (b) Fibroglandular tissue.
     (c) Surrounding tissue.
     (d) Muscle.

21c. If a mass in the patient's fatty breast tissue was depicted on mammography but not detected on ultrasound, what is the next best step to assist in ultrasound visualization
     (a) Contrast-enhanced mammography.
     (b) MRI.
     (c) Tissue harmonic imaging.
     (d) Widen the dynamic range on ultrasound.

22a. A 58-year-old woman who was called back from an abnormal screening mammogram. Diagnostic mammogram and ultrasound images are provided below. Which of the following pathologies can present as a circumscribed mass on imaging?

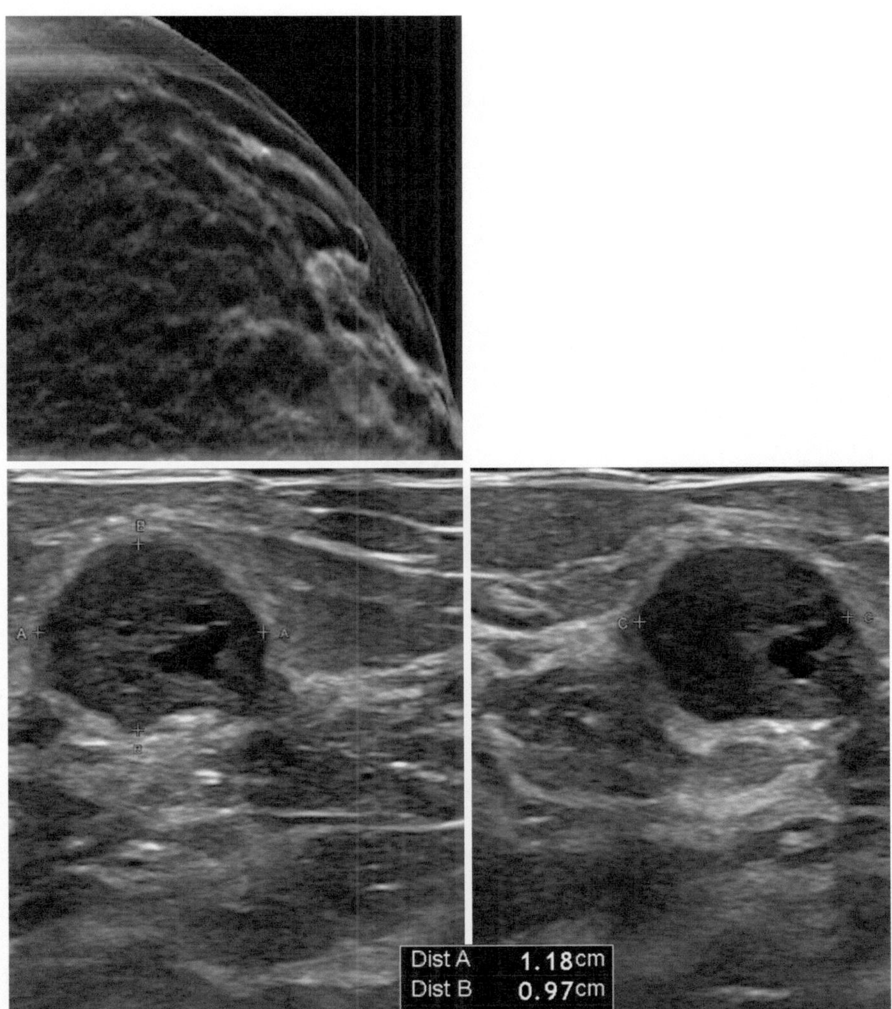

(a) Mucinous carcinoma.
(b) Medullary carcinoma.
(c) Papillary carcinoma.
(d) Invasive ductal carcinoma not otherwise specified.
(e) All of the above.

22b. The circumscribed mass above was biopsied and showed a circumscribed carcinoma composed of poorly differentiated cells. If the tumor were to show
rapid growth over time, which subtype of circumscribed ductal carcinomas
would this most likely be?
(a) Mucinous carcinoma.
(b) Medullary carcinoma.
(c) Papillary carcinoma.
(d) Invasive ductal carcinoma not otherwise specified.
(e) None of the above.

23a. A 45-year-old female presents for screening mammography shown below,
which showed a rapidly growing focal asymmetry in the right breast upper
outer quadrant.

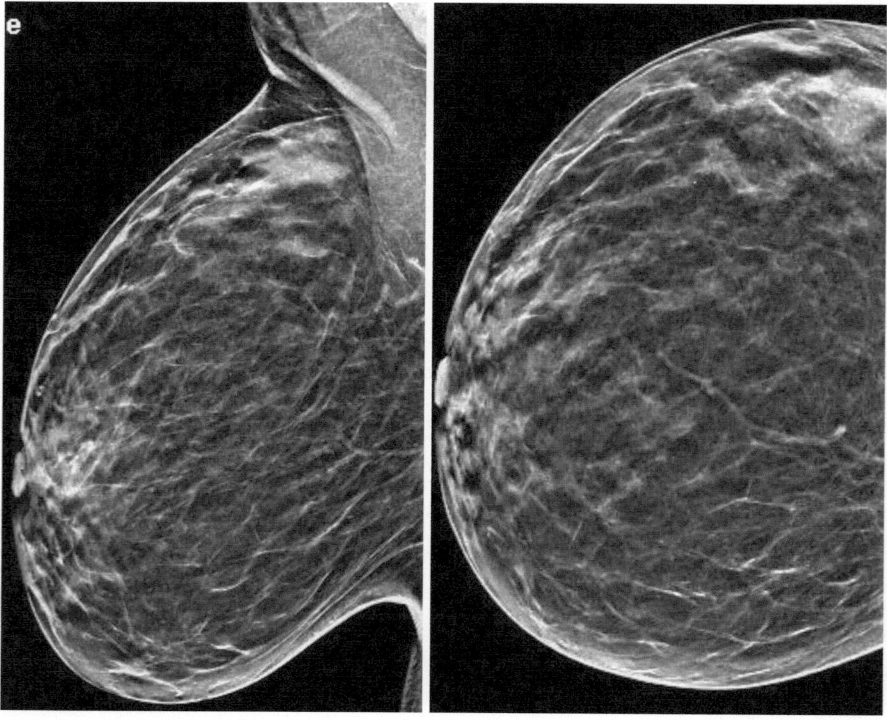

Additional magnification views and ultrasound were performed, as shown below.

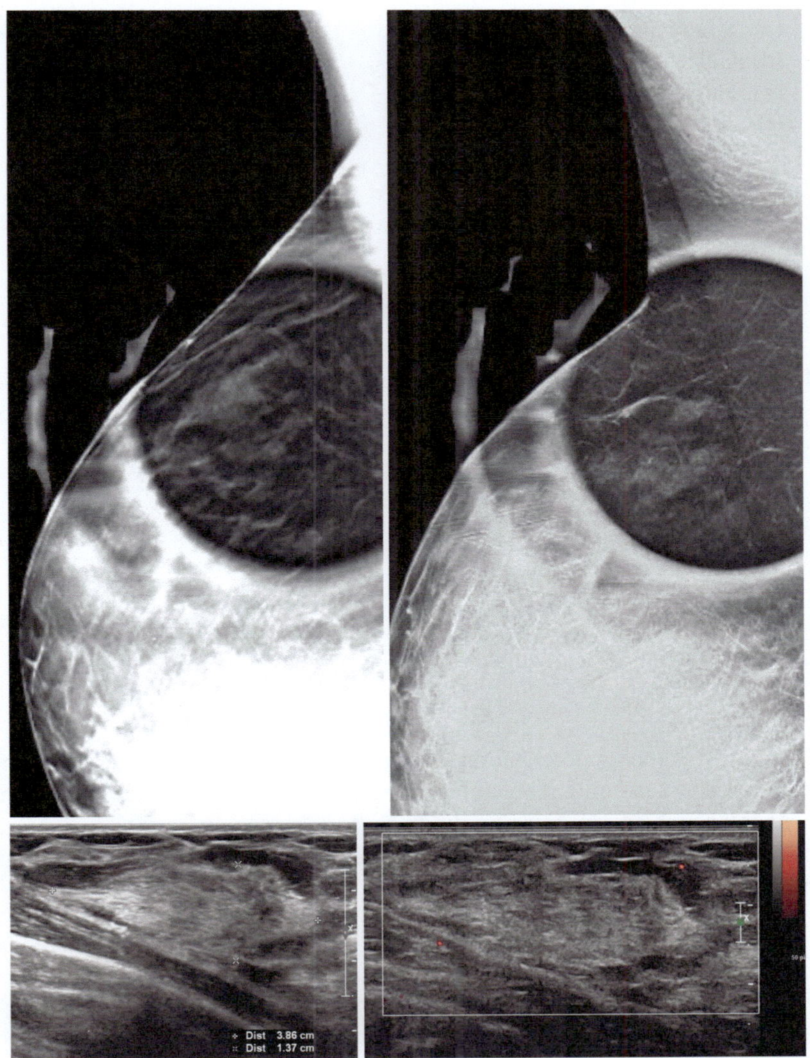

Which of the following is false regarding hyperechoic breast masses?

(a) An echogenic breast mass that is radiolucent on mammography is benign and does not need biopsy.
(b) Most hyperechoic breast masses are benign.
(c) Hyperechogenicity on ultrasound alone is enough to exclude malignancy.
(d) The differential for hyperechoic breast masses includes benign and malignant etiologies.
(e) None of the above.

23b. Which of the following benign lesions can be hyperechogenic at ultrasound?
    (a) Lipoma.
    (b) Hematoma.
    (c) Silicone granuloma.
    (d) Galactocele.
    (e) Fat necrosis.
    (f) All of the above.

23c. Based on the images above, what is the most likely diagnosis
    (a) PASH.
    (b) Phyllodes tumor.
    (c) Hamartoma.
    (d) Fibroadenoma.

23d. The patient underwent biopsy of the lesion, which demonstrated PASH. When performing your radiology-pathology correlation, in which situations would surgical excision be recommended?
    (a) All cases of PASH should be excised.
    (b) PASH with atypia.
    (c) Rapidly growing in size.
    (d) Size greater than 5 cm.
    (e) B and C.

Answers

1. e. All cases.

   Radiology–Pathology correlation is required in all cases of percutaneous biopsy performed by a radiologist regardless of pathology or treatment plan. Determining concordance between imaging findings and histologic results is important because it guides the treatment plan, including the need to recommend surgical excision or short-term follow-up [1].

2. d (A and B).

   Radiology–pathology statement is included in the percutaneous biopsy report performed by the radiologist. In this statement, both concordance and a follow-up recommendation are required. A BIRADS assessment is not part of the radiology–pathology correlation statement [2].

3. c. To limit the number of false negatives.

   There are multiple reasons to perform radiology-pathology correlation, including regulatory compliance and data gathering for practice parameters. One of the main reasons to perform radiology-pathology correlation is limiting the number of false-negative biopsy results. A false negative result as defined by the National Cancer Institute is a test result that indicates a person does not have a specific disease or condition when the person does have the disease or condition. An example of this would be a benign biopsy result when the patient has cancer [3].

4. e (A and C).

A false-negative test in interventional breast radiology is a breast biopsy that is initially histologically determined to be benign and later proven to be carcinoma at the same site. Type II error is a statistical term used to describe the acceptance of a null hypothesis that is in reality true. A type II error produces a false negative [3].

5. b. An invasive ductal carcinoma diagnosed in the ipsilateral breast 10 months after a benign biopsy.

A False-Negative (FN) is tissue diagnosis of cancer within 1 year of a negative or benign examination. A false negative does not include cases with discordant or underestimation of disease if excisional biopsy is performed and cancer is identified without significant delay in diagnosis [4].

6a. d. All of the above.

Radiology–Pathology correlation of calcifications requires all of the above [3].

6b. c. Concordant, recommend surgical excision.

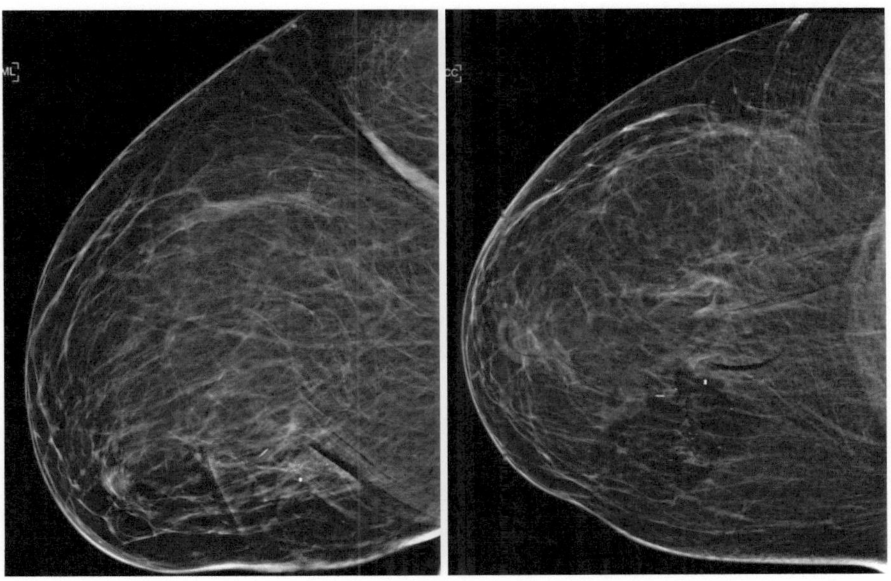

Atypical ductal hyperplasia (ADH) is a high-risk lesion, meaning it can underestimate the associated presence of underlying cancer. Up to 44% of ADH lesions diagnosed with a 14-gauge stereotactic biopsy turned out to be cancer on excisional biopsy [3]. Of the upgraded cases, 25% are associated with invasive carcinomas, and the remaining 75% are any grade DCIS [3]. In the above case, pathology was upgraded to DCIS upon surgical excision.

7. a. Sclerosing adenosis.

High-risk lesions are pathologic diagnoses on core needle biopsy that are not malignant but can underestimate the presence of an associated cancer. They occur in approximately 10% of percutaneous biopsies and may require surgical excision [3]. For atypical ductal hyperplasia (ADH), a meta-analysis showed a pooled upgrade rate higher than 2%, and therefore excision is often recommended and pursued [5]. Although the management recommendations for radial scar and papillary lesions can be complex, the presence of atypia in the pathology specimen warrants excision [3].

8. b. Stereotactic core biopsy.

One of the most important measures of biopsy accuracy is the false-negative rate. The literature reports a 4.0–22.2% false-negative rate for stereotactic core-needle biopsy using a 14-gauge needle vs. 0–3.3% for an 11-gauge needle [6]. Therefore, in stereotactic biopsies, it may be helpful to use an 11-guage needle or larger with vacuum assist [6]. MRI biopsy false negative rates have been reported as 0.6–2.4% [7, 8]. Ultrasound core biopsy false-negative rate is 2.4% [9]. Excisional biopsy has a 2.0% false-negative rate [6].

9a. d. Ultrasound-guided drainage and antibiotics.

In a 35-year-old female patient who is lactating and has ultrasound findings typical for a breast abscess, it is appropriate to perform percutaneous drainage and treat with antibiotics.

There are many advantages to ultrasound-guided intervention:

– Performed rapidly with local anesthesia in the ambulatory setting.
– Lower rates of milk fistula.
– No need to interrupt lactation.
– Percutaneous drainage results in minimal to no scarring. US-guided drainage has a complication rate similar to or lower than surgical incision and drainage [10].

9b. *Staphylococcus aureus.*

Most abscesses occur due to secondary bacterial infection from skin contamination. The most common pathogen by far is *Staphylococcus aureus.* Other bacterial causes include *S. pyogenes*, *S. epidermidis*, *Peptostreptococcus*, and Bacteroides. Less commonly, breast abscesses can occur from fungi, parasites, and mycobacterium including Tuberculosis, especially in certain geographic settings and patient populations. When you aspirate the collection, the fluid should be sent for gram stain and culture [10].

10a. e. All of the above.

Common symptoms of breast infection include pain, redness, and warmth. However, it is important to consider the many causes of breast pain and erythema with these imaging findings, especially in non-lactating and older women. The differential includes breast abscess, inflammatory carcinoma, and noninfectious inflammatory processes including diabetic mastopathy, chronic idiopathic granulomatous mastitis, and immunologic diseases such as Churg-Strauss syndrome, amyloidosis, Wegener granulomatosis, and sarcoidosis [10].

10b. f. All of the above.

Granulomatous mastitis is a rare disease that occurs in parous, premenopausal women with a history of lactation and is often associated with hyperprolactinemia. The exact etiology is unknown, but it has been postulated to stem from a local inflammatory response in connective tissue and has been shown to be associated with multiple factors, with established connections to pregnancy, lactation, and hyperprolactinemia. The most common presentation is a tender, palpable mass, with imaging features often mimicking malignancy thus biopsy is frequently performed. On ultrasound, findings include irregular masses, focal regions of inhomogeneity with hypoechoic or tubular/nodular structures, or parenchymal hypoechogenicity with posterior acoustic shadowing. Mammographic findings usually show a focal or global asymmetry, ill-defined breast masses, or negative findings; calcifications are rarely seen. Pathology shows noncaseating granulomatous inflammation centered in the lobules, with associated giant cells, leukocytes, macrophages, abscesses, and epithelioid cells. Infection, including mycobacterial and fungal pathogens, should be excluded. Treatment is controversial and varies by institution, ranging from surveillance in mild cases to oral steroid therapy, methotrexate or bromocriptine, and even surgery which is typically reserved for refractory or recurrent disease. Up to 50% of cases will recur, which can be reduced by immunosuppressive treatment until complete remission [3, 11].

11a. b. Concordant—recommendation excision.

Phyllodes tumor classically presents as a rapidly enlarging mass in a woman in her fifth decade. It is a high-risk breast lesion and wide surgical excision is the preferred treatment. Incomplete excision of either a benign or malignant phyllodes tumor can result in local recurrence 15% of the time. Approximately 25% of phyllodes tumors are malignant [3].

11b. a. Hematogenous.

Metastatic disease is common in phyllodes tumors. Metastatic disease has been reported in 13–40% of patients with phyllodes tumors. Unlike most other breast cancers, the method of spread is hematogenous [3].

11c. c. Lungs.
The most common location for metastasis to occur from phyllodes tumor is the lungs [12, 13].

11d. b. Concordant—recommend excision.

Phyllodes tumors of the breast account for 0.3%–1% of all primary breast tumors and constitute 2.5% of fibroepithelial tumors [3]. Phyllodes tumors are graded according to recommendations by the World Health Organization as benign, borderline, or malignant based on the presence of stromal cellularity, atypia, mitotic activity, and stomal overgrowth [14]. Surgical excision is required for all types of phyllodes tumors [3].

11e. a. There are no imaging characteristics that differentiate benign from malignant phyllodes.

12a. d. Fine pleomorphic or fine linear-branching calcifications.

Microcalcifications are found in 50–75% of DCIS [15]. Low-grade DCIS lesions are more likely than high-grade lesions to demonstrate non-calcified abnormalities on mammography, including asymmetry and mass. Fine pleomorphic or fine linear-branching calcifications have been noted in high-grade DCIS according to the WHO system of classification [15].

12b. b. Van Nuys classification.

The Van Nuys classification system is the simplest and most reproducible classification system for classifying DCIS. It identifies three groups of DCIS lesions, differentiated first according to nuclear grade (low, intermediate, or high grade) and then with presence or absence of necrosis [15].

12c. d. Non-mass enhancement in a segmental distribution.

Non-mass enhancement is the most common MRI finding of DCIS and is seen in 60–80% of cases [15]. A segmental distribution of this non-mass enhancement is the most common pattern and accounts for 33–77% of cases of DCIS [15]. Ductal, linear or regional distribution of non-mass enhancement are other commonly reported MRI findings. An enhancing mass is seen in 14–34% of cases and focal enhancement is seen in 1–12% [16].

12d. b. Post-excision positive margins and synchronous foci that were not excised.

In DCIS, the most important risk factors for disease recurrence are post excision positive margins and synchronous foci that were not removed. In the National Surgical Adjuvant Breast Project, B-06 protocol, patients treated with excision followed by radiation therapy had a 6.9% recurrence, whereas those who did not undergo radiation therapy had a 22.7% rate of recurrence [16]. Gender and hormone receptor-positive status are not risk factors for disease recurrence. Adjuvant endocrine therapy has been shown to decrease the rate of recurrence by up to 50% in ER-positive tumors [17].

13a. b. Mammogram is contraindicated in pregnancy.

Most masses that occur in pregnancy are benign and include benign lactational adenoma, fibroadenoma, galactocele, and abscess [3]. According to

ACR appropriateness criteria, while ultrasound is the first indicated examination for pregnant and lactating women with palpable concerns, mammography is not contraindicated in pregnancy and the dose to the fetus is negligible (4-view mammogram is <0.03 mGy) [18]. NCCN guidelines state that mammogram with shielding can be done safely in pregnant women [18]. As always, discussion of risk and benefit should be performed with the patient prior to proceeding with mammogram. Also, lactation is not a contraindication for mammogram. Mammography in a diagnostic workup is important to identify findings of breast cancer such as microcalcifications. Milk fistula is an uncommon condition that occurs when there is an abnormal connection that forms between the skin surface and the duct in the breast of a lactating woman. This is more commonly associated with surgical intervention than percutaneous biopsy but can occur [19, 20]. However, 3% of breast cancers are coincident with pregnancy or lactation [3]. Therefore, if suspicious image findings are identified, a biopsy should be performed.

13b. b. Concordant—recommend ultrasound follow up in 6 months.

Benign concordant lesions can be false-negative. For this reason, meticulous radiology-pathology concordance must occur by the radiologist performing the biopsy, with confirmation of appropriate sampling, correlation with clinical symptoms and breast cancer risk, and lesion radiologic features prior to biopsy with correlating pathologic results [3]. Recent studies have indicated routine screening is appropriate if the biopsy is benign and concordant [21]. Imaging follow-up can be performed at the discretion of the radiologist on the same imaging modality that guided the biopsy. This may occur more frequently in younger patients who would not be expected to have routine breast imaging if <40 years or if not on a high-risk screening schedule. If the lesion increases in size at follow-up, repeat biopsy or surgical excision can be considered [21].

13c. d. The presence of interval growth during pregnancy necessitates excision.

Lactating adenoma is a solid, benign tumor diagnosed during pregnancy. It typically presents as a firm, painless palpable lump late in pregnancy or during lactation. On ultrasound, it has some similarities to fibroadenoma and appears as a well-circumscribed, hypoechoic mass that may contain echogenic bands (which are fibrotic bands seen on pathology). Interval growth is common and may represent change stimulated by hormonal alterations [3].

14a. a. Concordant—recommend surgical excision.

The management of papilloma found on biopsy is controversial. In contrast to central papillomas, papillomas in the periphery of the breast are associated with epithelial proliferation, which can have atypical features. Atypia is thought to increase the risk of malignancy [3]. Papillary lesions without atypia have recently been shown in a prospective study to have an upgrade rate of just 1.7%, below the 2% threshold for probably benign findings and therefore if concordant imaging findings, may be considered safe to follow [22]. It is generally agreed that any papillary lesion with atypia, regardless of location, should undergo excision.

14b. a. Stage 0.

Anatomic stage is based on the extent of cancer using T (extent of tumor), N (nodal disease), and M (distant metastasis) categories. When the primary tumor does not invade the basement membrane and only ductal carcinoma in situ is found, it is stage 0, or Tis, N0M0 [23].

15a. d. Discordant—recommend surgical excision.

Architectural distortion is defined as distortion of the normal breast parenchyma architecture with no definite mass. It can be seen in both benign and malignant entities [3]. Architectural distortion has a high positive predictive value for malignancy in both screening and diagnostic 2D mammography, 10–67% and 60–83%, respectively [24]. The pathology of benign ducts does not explain the mammographic findings. Therefore, the radiology–pathology is discordant, and excision should be recommended secondary to the high positive predictive value of architectural distortion [24].

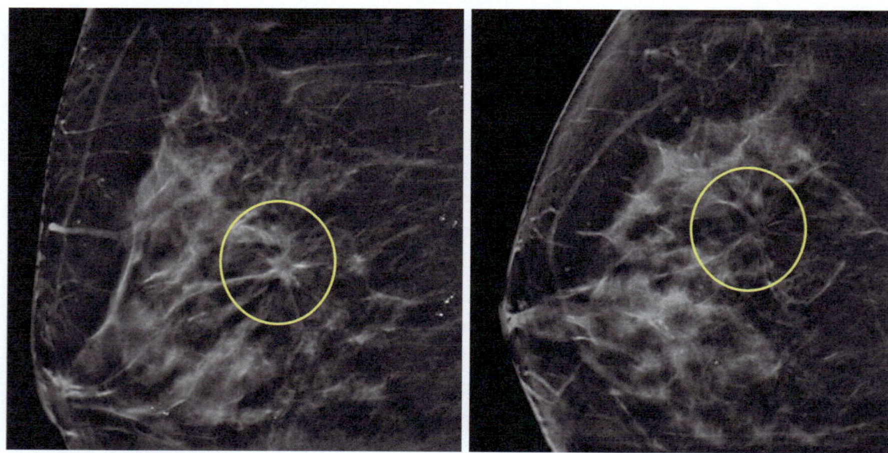

15b. e. Papilloma.

Architectural distortion can be caused by invasive carcinoma, DCIS, radial scar, sclerosing adenosis, post-surgical scar, and post-radiation change. On mammography, papilloma can demonstrate a markedly dilated duct extending into the breast from the nipple with or without an associated mass. Ultrasound usually shows a solid mass within fluid-filled, dilated ducts. Solitary architectural distortion is not associated with papilloma [3].

16a. a. Irregular mass.

Invasive lobular carcinoma (ILC) most commonly manifests as a mass with spiculated or indistinct margins on mammography (44–65%) [25]. Much less commonly, these cancers will present as round or circumscribed masses (1–3%) [25]. Architectural distortion is the second most common manifestation of invasive lobular carcinoma (10–34%) [25]. Reported microcalcifications associated with invasive lobular carcinoma vary (0–24%), however, is known to be less than with invasive ductal carcinoma [25].

16b. c. An irregular mass with angular margins, hypoechoic, heterogenous internal echoes, and posterior acoustic shadowing.

Ultrasound is superior to mammography in identifying multicentric and multifocal diseases. The most common ultrasound manifestation of invasive lobular carcinoma is an irregular mass with indistinct, angular or spiculated margins, hypoechoic and heterogeneous internal echoes, and posterior acoustic shadowing. Other less common findings include circumscribed masses, focal shadowing without a discrete mass, and sonographically occultlesions [25].

16c. b. MRI.

MRI should be performed in biopsy proven invasive-lobular carcinoma because it has been found to affect clinical management in 50% of cases, leading to changes in surgical management in 28% [25]. MRI is able to detect additional ipsilateral disease in 32% of cases and contralateral disease in 7% of cases that were not detected on mammography or ultrasonography [25].

17. c. An ultrasound mass with angulated margins (BIRADS 5) with pathology result of fibroadenoma.

Ultrasound findings suggestive of cancer include an irregular shape, noncircumscribed margins (angular, indistinct, microlobulated, and spiculated), thick echogenic rim or halo, duct extension, or surrounding tissue changes, microcalcifications (in or out of a mass or intraductal), non-parallel orientation, or posterior shadowing. These descriptors are included in the ACR BI-RADS ultrasound lexicon. A fibroadenoma should have circumscribed margins without suspicious features [3].

18. d. PD-L1.

ER, PR, HER2, and Ki-67 antigen are biomarkers that are tested consistently in invasive breast carcinoma due to their potential effect on prognosis and clinical management [17].

19. c. High grade.

Linear enhancement is seen on MRI and calcifications on mammography most often correspond to high-grade carcinoma [26].

20. c. 85%.

The lifetime breast cancer risk is as high as 85% for BRCA1 and BRCA2 mutation carriers. They also have a 50% risk of developing breast cancer by the age of 50 years [26].

21a. d. 1/3.

Isoechogenicity is not classified as a suspicious finding for malignancy but is considered an indeterminate finding. It can be seen in both benign and malignant lesions. About one-third of breast carcinomas are isoechoic on ultrasound. Isoechogenicity can also be seen in usual ductal hyperplasia, atypical ductal hyperplasia, papillary apocrine metaplasia, adenosis, debris/cellularity in fibrocystic and benign proliferative conditions, fibroadenoma, and papilloma. In the above patient, ultrasound-guided core biopsy confirmed fibroadenoma, benign, and concordant [27].

21b. a. Fat.

The echogenicity of a mass is assessed by its relationship to the echogenicity of fat in the breast [27].

21c. c. Tissue harmonic imaging.

When a lesion is seen on mammogram in the fatty tissues but not identified on standard ultrasound, it is likely an isoechoic lesion. Tissue harmonic imaging uses nonlinear sound propagation that allows the processing of only the returned high-frequency harmonic signals and rejects echoes from fundamental frequencies. This technique improves lesion conspicuity on ultrasound by increasing tissue contrast and lateral resolution. Widening the dynamic range on ultrasound is not the next best step because a wide range allows isoechoic lesions to persist and remain undetectable. Contrast-enhanced mammography and MRI may be helpful but are not the next best step in evaluation [27]. Shown here is an example of the same finding with and without harmonics.

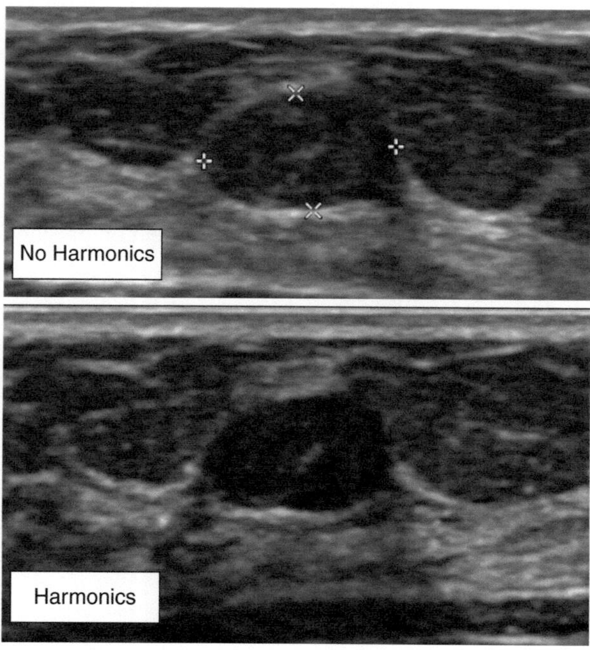

22a. e. All of the above.

The well-differentiated invasive ductal carcinomas including mucinous, medullary, and papillary, can have a relatively circumscribed appearance on imaging. Invasive ductal carcinoma not otherwise specified can also present as a circumscribed mass, but typically has a poorer prognosis. Other circumscribed cancers of the breast include triple-negative breast cancer adenoid cystic carcinoma and malignant phyllodes tumor [28].

22b. b. Medullary carcinoma.

Medullary carcinoma accounts for less than 2% of breast cancers [28]. It occurs more frequently in younger women and is characterized by rapid growth, often manifesting clinically with a palpable mass. The other lesions described above grow slowly in comparison to medullary carcinoma [28].

23a. c. Hyperechogenicity on ultrasound alone is enough to exclude malignancy.

Echogenic breast masses are defined as a lesion that is hyperechoic in comparison with subcutaneous fat at ultrasound, in accordance with the BI-RADS ultrasound lexicon. On ultrasound, up to 5.6% of breast masses are reported to be echogenic of which most are benign [29]. Both benign and malignant etiologies can be echogenic. If a hyperechoic mass correlates with a well-delineated radiolucent mass at mammography, it does not need biopsy. One large study found that of 1849 lesions that were malignant, 9 (0.5%) were hyperechoic [30]. Therefore, although the vast majority of echogenic breast masses are benign, hyperechogenicity at US alone does not exclude malignancy [29].

23b. f. All of the above.

The differential for hyperechoic breast masses is extensive.

Benign lesions that can be hyperechoic include:

Lipoma, angiolipoma, hematoma, seroma, fat necrosis, silicone granuloma, sebaceous or epidermal inclusion cyst, abscess, pseudoangiomatous stromal hyperplasia (PASH), galactocele or lactating adenoma, ductal ectasia, and apocrine metaplasia [29].

Malignant lesions that can be hyperechoic on ultrasound include:

Invasive ductal carcinoma, invasive lobular carcinoma, metastasis, lymphoma, and angiosarcoma [29].

23c. a. PASH.

Pseudoangiomatous stromal hyperplasia (PASH) is a benign breast mass of unknown etiology. It usually presents in pre-menopausal women or post-menopausal women on hormone therapy, and can rapidly grow in size. On ultrasound, it appears as a mixed or hypoechoic mass with ill-defined borders but can also be hyperechoic. Mammography will demonstrate an oval mass, sometimes with well-circumscribed borders [3].

23d. e. B and C.

A histological diagnosis of pseudoangiomatous stromal hyperplasia (PASH) is considered safe to manage conservatively with imaging follow-up. Because low-grade angiosarcoma can mimic PASH on biopsy, surgical excision is recommended in PASH with atypia and in cases of PASH with interval growth [3].

References

1. Ho CP, et al. Interactive case review of radiologic and pathologic findings from breast biopsy: are they concordant? How do I manage the results? Radiographics. 2013;33(4):E149–52.
2. Bassett LW, Mahoney MC, Apple SK. Interventional breast imaging: current procedures and assessing for concordance with pathology. Radiol Clin N Am. 2007;45:881–94.
3. Ikeda DM. Breast imaging: the requisites. 2nd ed. ELSEVIER MOSBY; 2004.
4. D'Orsi CJ, Sickles EA, Mendelson EB, Morris EA, et al. ACR BI-RADS® atlas, breast imaging reporting and data system. 5th ed. American College of Radiology; 2013.
5. Schiaffino S, et al. Upgrade rate of percutaneously diagnosed pure atypical ductal hyperplasia: systematic review and meta-analysis of 6458 lesions. Radiology. 2020;294(1):76–86.
6. Jackman RJ, Marzoni FA, Rosenberg J. False-negative diagnoses at stereotactic vacuum-assisted needle breast biopsy: long-term follow-up of 1,280 lesions and review of the literature. Am J Roentgenol. 2009;192(2):341–51.
7. Hayward JH, Ray KM, Wisner DJ, Joe BN. Follow-up outcomes after benign concordant MRI-guided breast biopsy. Clin Imaging. 2016;40(5):1034–9.
8. Huang ML, Speer M, Dogan BE, Rauch GM, Candelaria RP, Adrada BE, Hess KR, Yang WT. Imaging-concordant benign MRI-guided vacuum-assisted breast biopsy may not warrant MRI follow-up. Am J Roentgenol. 2017;208(4):916–22.
9. Hyun Youk J, Kim EK, Kim MJ, Oh KK. Sonographically guided 14-gauge Core needle biopsy of breast masses: a review of 2,420 cases with long-term follow-up. Am J Roentgenol. 2008;190(1):202–7.
10. Trop I, et al. Breast abscesses: evidence-based algorithms for diagnosis, management, and follow-up. Radiographics. 2011;31:1683–99.
11. Pluguez-Turull CW, Nanyes JE, Quintero CJ, Alizai H, Mais DD, Kist KA, Dornbluth NC. Idiopathic granulomatous mastitis: manifestations at multimodality imaging and pitfalls. Radiographics. 2018;38(2):330–56.
12. Chaney AW, et al. Primary treatment of cystosarcoma phyllodes of the breast. Cancer. 2000;89(7):1502.
13. Barrio AV, et al. Clincopathologic features and long-term outcomes of 293 phyllodes tumors of the breast. Ann Surg Oncol. 2007;14:2961.
14. Tan PH, et al. Fibroepithelial tumors: WHO classification of tumors of the breast. Int Agency Res Cancer. 2012;4:414–147.
15. Yamada, et al. Radiologic-pathologic correlation of ductal carcinoma in situ. Radiographics. 2010;30:1183–98.
16. Mossa-Basha M, et al. Ductal carcinoma in situ of the breast: MR imaging findings with histopathologic correlation. Radiographics. 2010;30:1673–87.
17. Tirada N, et al. Breast cancer tissue markers, genomic profiling, and other prognostic factors: a primer for radiologists. Radiographics. 2018;38:1902–20.
18. diFlorio-Alexander RM, Slanetz PJ, Moy L, Baron P, Didwania AD, Heller SL, Holbrook AI, Lewin AA, Lourenco AP, Mehta TS, Niell BL, Stuckey AR, Tuscano DS, Vincoff NS, Weinstein SP, Newell MS. ACR appropriateness criteria® breast imaging of pregnant and lactating women. J Am Coll Radiol. 2018;15(11S):S263–75.

19. Schackmuth EM, Harlow CL, Norton LW. Milk fistula: a complication after core breast biopsy. Am J Roentgenol. 1993;161(5):961–2.
20. Larson KE, Valente SA. Milk fistula: diagnosis, prevention, and treatment. Breast J. 2015;22(1):111–2.
21. Monticciolo DL, Hajdik RL, Hicks MG, Winford JK, Larkin WR, Vasek JV Jr, Ashton BM. Six-month short-interval imaging follow-up for benign concordant Core needle biopsy of the breast: outcomes in 1444 cases with long-term follow-up. Am J Roentgenol. 2016;207(4):912–7.
22. Nakhlis F, Baker GM, Pilewskie M, et al. The incidence of adjacent synchronous invasive carcinoma and/or ductal carcinoma in situ in patients with intraductal papilloma without atypia on Core biopsy: results from a prospective multi-institutional registry (TBCRC 034). Ann Surg Oncol. 2021;28(5):2573–8.
23. Kalli S, et al. American joint committee on Cancer's staging system for breast cancer, eighth edition: what the radiologist needs to know. Radiographics. 2018;38(7):1921–33.
24. Alshafeiy TI, et al. Outcome of architectural distortion detected only at breast tomosynthesis versus 2D mammography. Radiology. 2018;288(1):38–46.
25. Lopez JK, Bassett LW. Invasive lobular carcinoma of the breast: Spectrum of mammographic, US, and MR imaging findings. Radiographics. 2009;29:165–76.
26. Causer PA, et al. Breast cancers detected with imaging screening in the BRCA population: emphasis on MR imaging with histopathologic correlation. Radiographics. 2007;27:S165–82.
27. Kim MJ, et al. How to find an isoechoic lesion with breast US. Radiographics. 2011;31:663–76.
28. Harvey JA. Unusual breast cancers: useful clues to expanding the differential diagnosis. Radiology. 2007;242:683–94.
29. Gao Y, Slanetz PJ, Eisenberg RL. Echogenic breast masses at US: to biopsy or not to biopsy? Radiographics. 2013;33:419–34.
30. Linda A, Zuiani C, Lorenzon M, et al. Hyperechoic lesions of the breast: not always benign. Am J Roentgenol. 2011;196(5):1219–24.

Male Breast

Cheryce Poon Fischer, Bo Li, Steven R. Plimpton,
and Lucy Chow

C. P. Fischer (✉) · B. Li · S. R. Plimpton · L. Chow
Department of Radiology, David Geffen School of Medicine at UCLA,
Los Angeles, CA, USA
e-mail: CPFischer@mednet.ucla.edu; boli@mednet.ucla.edu; splimpton@mednet.ucla.edu;
lchow@mednet.ucla.edu

© The Author(s), under exclusive license to Springer Nature
Switzerland AG 2022
L. Chow, B. Li (eds.), *Absolute Breast Imaging Review*,
https://doi.org/10.1007/978-3-031-08274-0_8

1a. A 90-year-old male presented with 1 month of left breast periareolar pain and possible palpable mass. A marker was placed in the area of the palpable abnormality. What is the dominant abnormality?

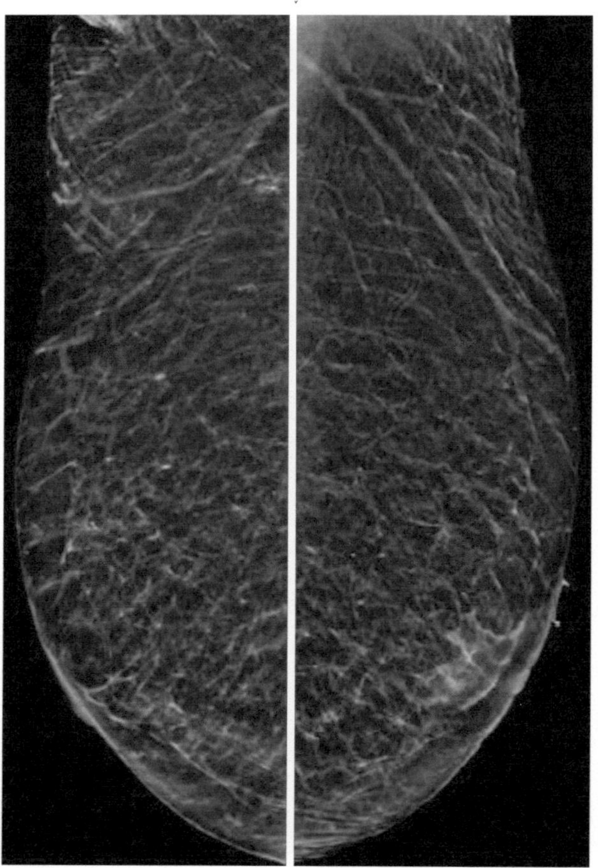

   (a) Bilateral calcifications.
   (b) Asymmetry in the left subareolar breast.
   (c) Asymmetry in the right subareolar breast.
   (d) Architectural distortion in the left breast.
   (e) No abnormality.

1b. What is the next step?
   (a) Ultrasound.
   (b) MRI.
   (c) Biopsy.
   (d) No additional workup.

1c. What is your assessment and recommendation?
    (a) BI-RADS 1—Negative.
    (b) BI-RADS 2—Benign.
    (c) BI-RADS 3—Probably Benign.
    (d) BI-RADS 4—Suspicious.

2. Which of the following is not a cause of gynecomastia?
    (a) Testosterone.
    (b) Marijuana.
    (c) Cirrhosis.
    (d) Renal Failure.
    (e) Hypothyroidism.

3. Which of the following is not a pattern of gynecomastia?
    (a) Nodular.
    (b) Interstitial.
    (c) Dendritic.
    (d) Diffuse Glandular.

4a. A 74-year-old male presented with firm, immobile right breast mass which has reportedly been enlarging for the past two years. What mammographic finding is most concerning for malignancy in this patient?

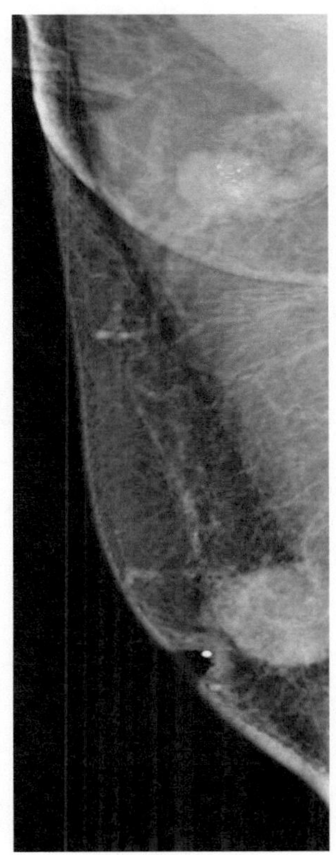

    (a) Subareolar mass.
    (b) Lipoma.
    (c) Nipple inversion.
    (d) Gynecomastia.
    (e) A and C.

4b. What is the next step?
    (a) Ultrasound.
    (b) MRI.
    (c) CT.
    (d) PET.

5. Which of the following is not considered a risk factor for male breast cancer?
    (a) Gynecomastia.
    (b) BRCA2 Mutation.
    (c) Cirrhosis.
    (d) Klinefelter syndrome.
    (e) Crypto-orchidism.

6. A 67-year-old male presented with a left breast palpable abnormality. An ultrasound was performed. What is the next best step for this patient?

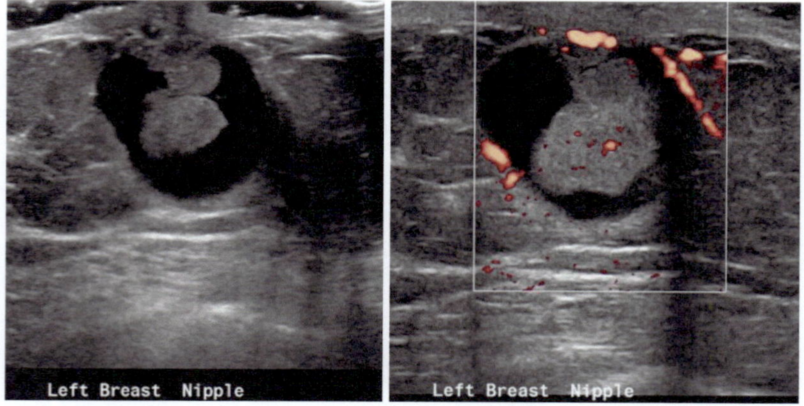

    (a) Short-term US follow-up.
    (b) Mammographic evaluation.
    (c) MRI.
    (d) Biopsy/Aspiration.

7. A 53-year-old male patient presented with low-grade fever. Targeted ultrasound evaluation of the chest wall was performed. What is the most likely etiology of the finding in the male breast?

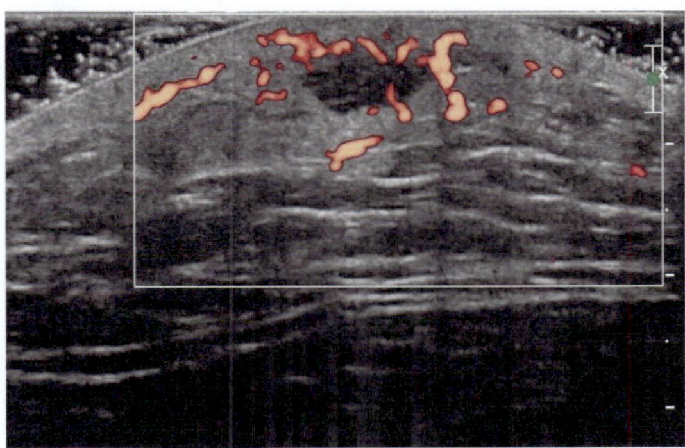

   (a) Infectious.
   (b) Neoplastic.
   (c) Endocrine.
   (d) Traumatic.

8. A 30-year-old male presented with a palpable abnormality in the right axilla. Mammogram and ultrasound were performed. What is the next step for the following mammographic and ultrasound findings corresponding to the palpable abnormality?

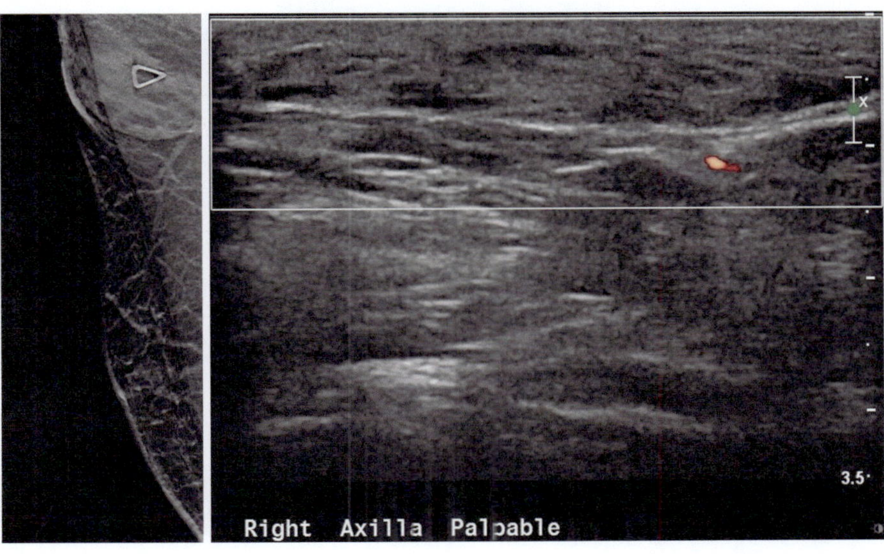

   (a) MRI.
   (b) Stereotactic biopsy.
   (c) US biopsy.
   (d) No further workup.

9. Mammographic images of a 50-year-old transfeminine patient (male-to-female) are provided below. Which of the following patients may be appropriate or are usually appropriate for screening mammography?

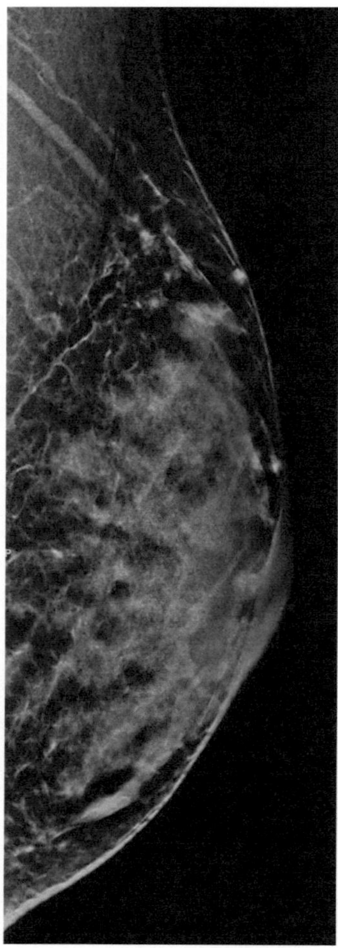

   (a) A 55-year-old transfeminine (male-to-female) patient with current hormone use of 7 years.

   (b) A 63-year-old transfeminine (male-to-female) patient with no current or past hormone.

   (c) A 37-year-old transmasculine (female-to-male) patient with history of bilateral mastectomies.

   (d) A 45-year-old transmasculine (female-to-male) patient with no history of chest surgery.

   (e) A and D.

10. A 55-year-old male presents with a palpable abnormality. A BB marker is placed in the area of the palpable abnormality. What is the BI-RADS for the palpable mammographic finding? CC views, with and without magnification are provided.

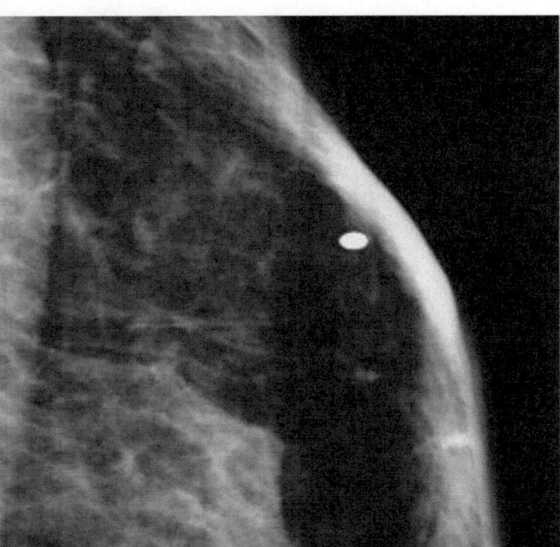

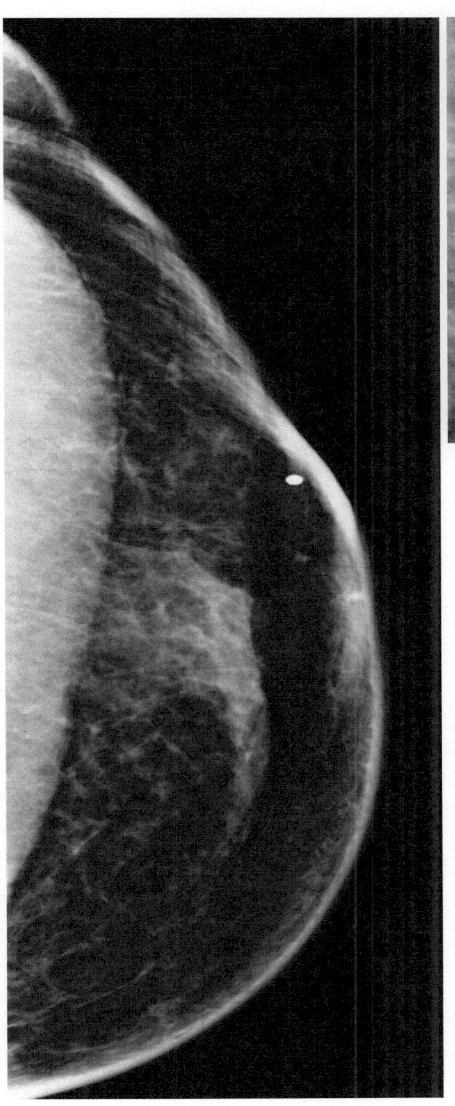

(a) BI-RADS 1—Negative.
(b) BI-RADS 2—Benign.
(c) BI-RADS 3—Probably Benign.
(d) BI-RADS 4—Suspicious.

11. A 45-year-old male presented with a painful, palpable abnormality in his right breast. What is the most appropriate management of the ultrasound lesion?

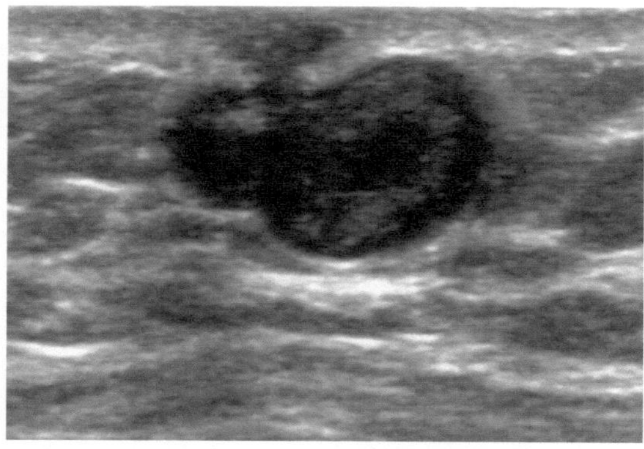

    (a) Image-guided biopsy.
    (b) MRI.
    (c) Clinical follow-up.
    (d) Mammogram.

12. A 70-year-old male presented with a growing palpable abnormality in the peri-areolar region of his breast. An irregular mass was identified. A biopsy was performed and the pathology demonstrated an invasive ductal carcinoma. Which statement regarding male breast cancer is false?

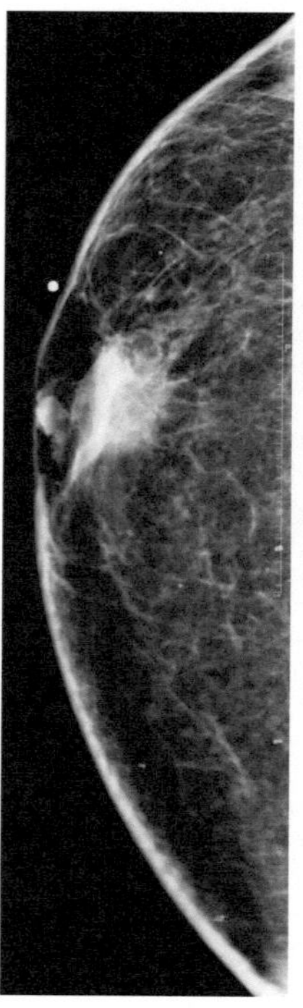

(a) The most common histologic subtype is invasive ductal carcinoma (IDC).
(b) The majority of male breast cancers are hormone positive.
(c) The tumor grade correlates with overall survival.
(d) The disease-free survival and overall survival at 10 years with breast cancer are less in males than that of stage-matched females.

13. What is the least likely origin of male breast cancer?
  (a) Lobular.
  (b) Ductal.
  (c) Mucinous.
  (d) Tubular.

14. Mammographic and sonographic views of a palpable growing mass in an elderly male presenting for diagnostic evaluation. What imaging feature is most *inconsistent* with a benign process in the male breast?

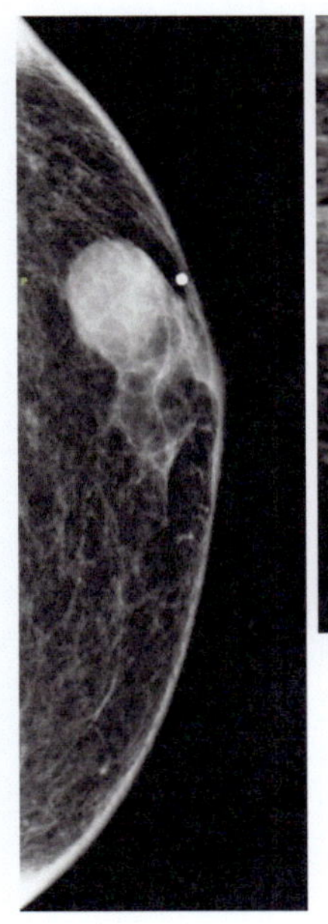
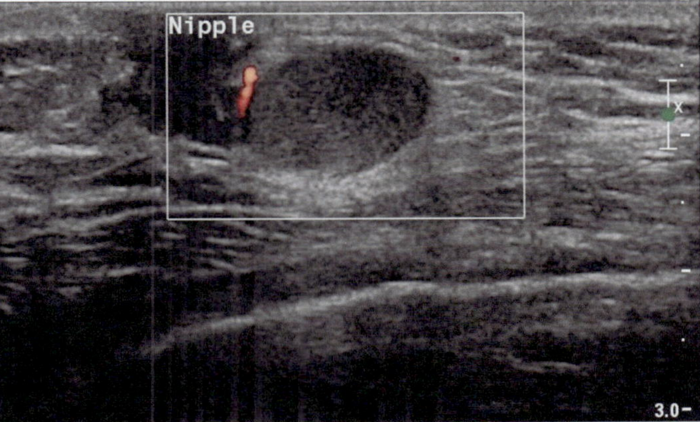

  (a) Density/Echogenicity.
  (b) Size.
  (c) Eccentricity to nipple.
  (d) Circumscribed margins.

Answers

1a. b. Asymmetry in the left subareolar breast.

There is an asymmetry in the left subareolar breast seen on the MLO view.

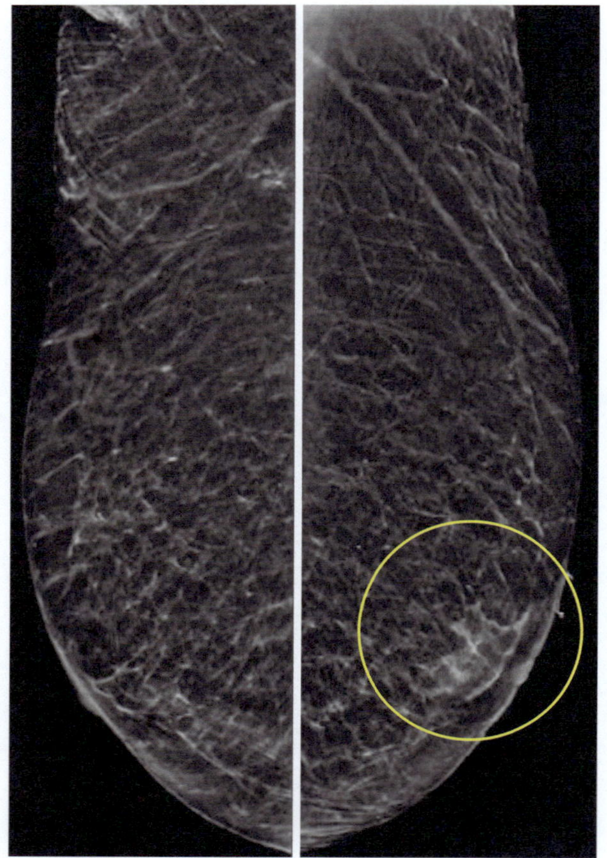

1b. d. No additional workup.

No additional workup is needed. This finding represents gynecomastia. Gynecomastia in the majority of patients appears unilaterally and/or asymmetrically.

1c. b. BI-RADS 2—Benign.

Though the differential includes breast cancer, the clinical presentation and mammographic findings are benign. Gynecomastia is a common diagnosis with at least 30% of men being affected in their lifetime. Gynecomastia results from an imbalance between estrogen and androgen. The causes are multifactorial and include iatrogenic and other underlying pathologies. Though the diagnosis may lead to anxiety or discomfort it is benign and does not require imaging workup or biopsy if a clinical diagnosis can be confidently made. However, if there is any concern for malignancy, the initial imaging exam should be mammography. If the diagnosis is made mammographically (majority of cases), no further imaging is warranted. Ultrasound is generally reserved if there are any suspicious findings or if the mammographic findings are indeterminate and should not be the first exam of choice for suspected gynecomastia. Gynecomastia has a pathognomonic appearance on mammography of increased subareolar glandular density, sometimes flame-shaped, and may be asymmetric and/or unilateral [1].

2. e. Hypothyroidism.

Increased testosterone exposure may lead to Leydig cell damage and inhibition resulting in elevation of estradiol. Marijuana has been shown to result in androgen receptor blockade. Cirrhosis may lead to increased androstenedione which is eventually converted to estradiol. Additionally, the liver is unable to clear adrenal androgens resulting in increased binding globulins and decreased free testosterone levels. Gynecomastia is seen in approximately 50% of dialysis patients which is thought to result from Leydig cell dysfunction as well as hormonal abnormalities, namely decreased testosterone and increased estradiol. Hyperthyroidism, not hypothyroidism, is associated with gynecomastia which is thought to result from direct stimulation of the enzyme aromatase and increased binding globulin resulting in increased concentration of estradiol and decreased free testosterone [2].

3. b. Interstitial.

There are three mammographic patterns of gynecomastia: nodular, dendritic, and diffuse glandular. Nodular pattern tends to be present in early stages of gynecomastia and manifests as a nodular subareolar density. Dendritic pattern appears in patients with gynecomastia for greater than 1 year and owes its appearance to fibrosis. This often appears as a dendritic subareolar density with linear projections radiating into the surrounding tissue. Diffuse glandular is commonly seen in patients receiving estrogen supplementation and presents as enlargement and diffusely increased density of the breast tissue with both dendritic and nodular features [3].

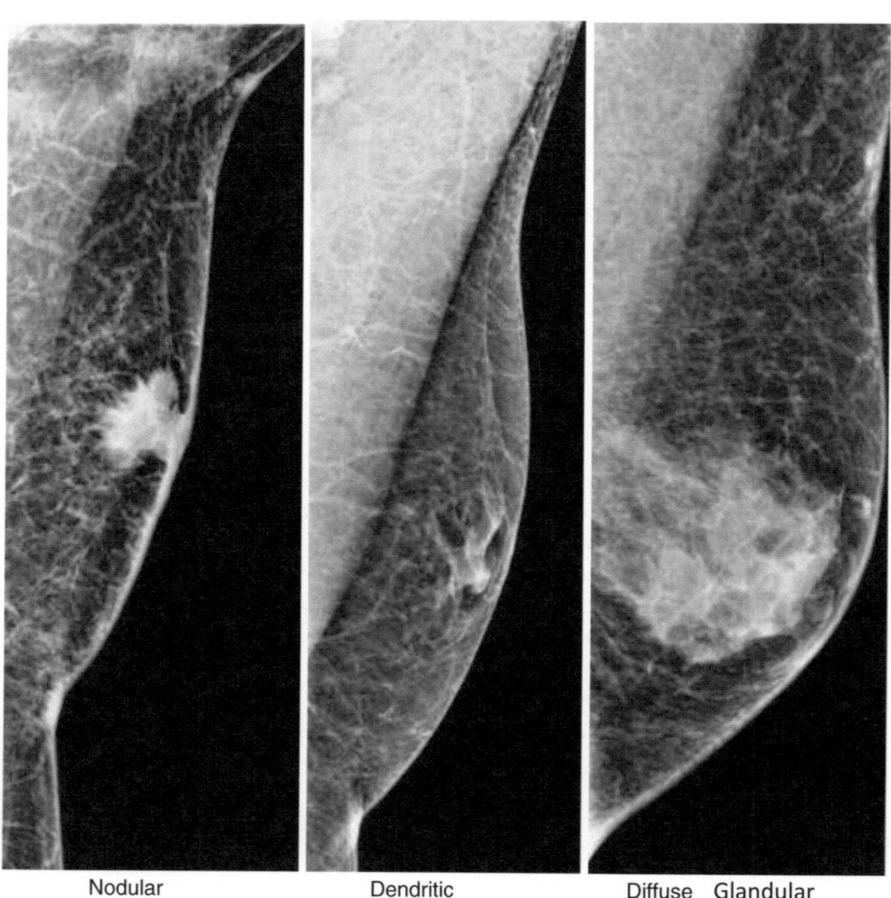

4a. e. a and c.

This patient has several suspicious findings on mammogram including a spiculated, irregular subareolar mass and an axillary mass with amorphous calcifications. Nipple inversion in the setting of an adjacent breast mass is malignancy until proven otherwise.

4b. a. Ultrasound.

Additional evaluation of the masses is warranted and best accomplished with ultrasound. Though the patient is a male, the next diagnostic steps are the same as in female patients. Male breast cancer is an uncommon but not entirely rare diagnosis and most commonly presents as a palpable lump [4]. Male breast cancers are most commonly invasive ductal carcinoma and present at a more advanced stage. Evaluation of the contralateral breast should also be performed given increased association of contralateral disease. Secondary features of malignancy are often common and may be evident on imaging including nipple retraction, skin thickening, skin ulceration, and axillary adenopathy.

5. a. Gynecomastia.

Gynecomastia does not inherently increase risk of male breast cancer. In fact, it is the most common benign entity of the male breast. BRCA2 gene mutation results in increased risk of breast cancer in males of approximately 50–80 per 10,000 men (relative to approximately 1 in 769 in the general male population) [5, 6]. Patients with Klinefelter syndrome have a 20-fold increased risk of breast cancer due to elevated estrogen-to-androgen ratio. Similarly, in crypto-orchidism and cirrhosis, relative hyperestrogenism predisposes to risk of breast cancer [2, 7].

6. d. Biopsy/Aspiration.

Cystic lesions in men commonly yield malignant pathologic findings. All cysts and complex masses in men should be considered potentially malignant. In particular, a mass with cystic components is suspicious for papillary ductal carcinoma in situ [8].

7. a. Infectious.

Ultrasound imaging demonstrates a heterogeneous fluid collection with marked increased peripheral vascularity, most consistent with abscess. There is also diffuse thickening of the overlying soft tissues and skin. Though rare, male breast abscess has been reported in numerous case reports. Cultures of aspirate often yield *S. aureus* and *S. epidermidis* as the dominant pathogens. Risk factors include malignancy, diabetes, smoking, vitamin A deficiency, and immuno-suppression [9].

8. d. No further workup.

The palpable abnormality in the patient's right axilla corresponds to accessory fibroglandular tissue. This is best confirmed on ultrasound which demonstrates heterogeneous tissue consistent with intermixed fat and glandular tissues. Accessory breast tissue is not entirely uncommon in male patients with a reported incidence of 1–3%. Approximately 2/3 of these cases present along the "milk line," commonly just caudal to the inframammary fold. The second most common location is the axilla, representing approximately 20% of cases. This tissue is at risk for the same pathologies as orthotopic breast tissue, but the incidence of breast cancer in ectopic breast tissue is low (approximately 0.3%) [10, 11].

9. e. a and d.

For the above options, ACR appropriateness criteria for transgender breast cancer screening published in 2021 states the following:

- Mammography may be appropriate in transfeminine (male-to-female) patients over 40 years of age with at least 5 years of past or current hormone use.
- Mammography is usually not appropriate for transmasculine (female-to-male) patients with history of bilateral mastectomies.
- Mammography is usually appropriate for transmasculine (female-to-male) patients older than 40 years of age with no history of chest surgery [12].

10. b. BI-RADS 2—Benign.

The mammographic finding corresponding to the palpable abnormality as indicated by the metallic marker demonstrates a circumscribed fat density mass. This is most consistent with a benign lipoma. Lipoma is the second most common benign lesion of the male breast.

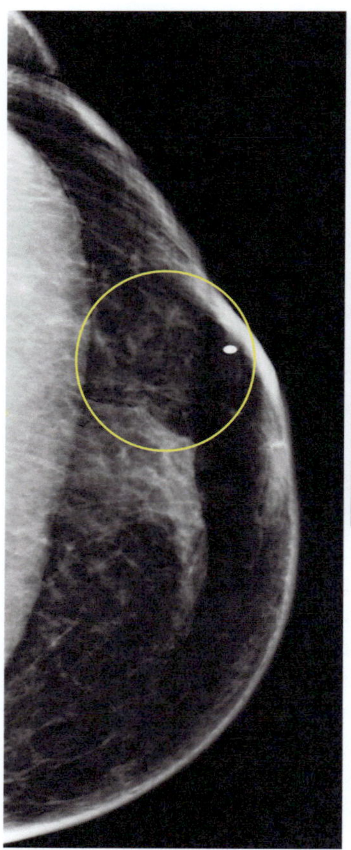
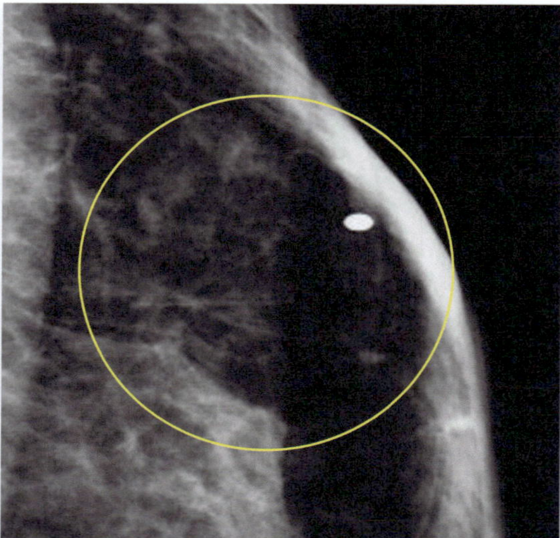

11. c. Clinical follow-up.

The ultrasound lesion is most consistent with an epidermal inclusion cyst or sebaceous cyst, the third most common benign lesion of the male breast. Most frequently, epidermal inclusion cysts present as a hypoechoic oval mass contiguous with the epidermis. Supporting sonographic features include increased through transmission, sinus tract to the skin (arrow), and the so-called claw-sign demarking epidermal origin.

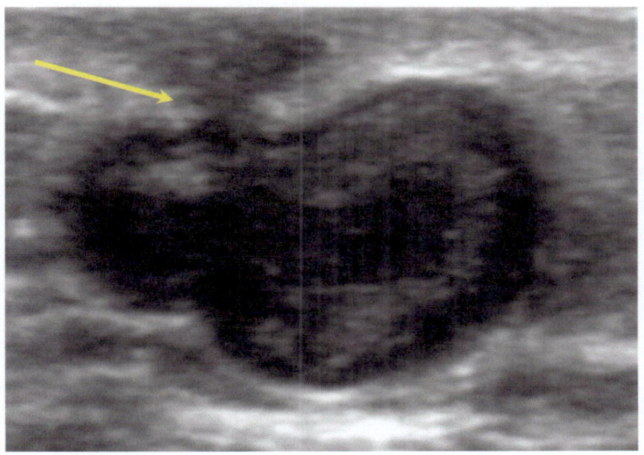

12. c. The tumor grade correlates with overall survival.

Tumor grade in male breast cancer has not been shown to correlate with survival as is the case in female breast cancer. The most common histologic subtype of male breast cancer is IDC, representing greater than 90% of cases. The majority of male breast cancer is hormone positive with greater than 90% estrogen receptor positive and greater than 80% progesterone receptor positive. Less than 0.5% of male breast cancers are triple negative. Stage-matched male breast cancers demonstrate a 10-year disease-free survival and overall survival of 40–52% and 32–71% respectively, as compared to 52–67% and 59–84% in women respectively [13].

13. a. Lobular.

The most common histologic subtype in the male breast is invasive ductal carcinoma not otherwise specified (NOS). Though mucinous and tubular breast cancers are exceedingly rare, lobular histology in male is even rarer. This is due to the inherent paucity of lobules in the male breast.

14. c. Eccentricity to Nipple.

The mammographic and sonographic images demonstrate a mass that is eccentric to the nipple. The most common benign entity in the male breast is gynecomastia, which is retroareolar in location. Any eccentricity of a mass to the nipple should be interpreted as inconsistent with a benign process.

References

1. Cooper RA, Gunter BA, Ramamurthy L. Mammography in men. Radiology. 1994;191:651–6.
2. Cuhaci N, Polat SB, Evranos B, Ersoy R, Cakir B. Gynecomastia: clinical evaluation and management. Indian J Endocrinol Metab. 2014;18:150.
3. Chau A, Jafarian N, Rosa M. Male Breast: Clinical and imaging evaluations of benign and malignant entities with histologic correlation. Am J Med. 2016;129(8):776–91. https://doi.org/10.1016/j.amjmed.2016.01.009. Epub 2016 Feb 1. PMID: 26844632.
4. Chen L, Chantra PK, Larsen LH, Barton P, Rohitopakarn M, Zhu EQ, Bassett LW. Imaging characteristics of malignant lesions of the male breast. Radiographics. 2006;26:993–1006.
5. Liede A, Karlan BY, Narod SA. Cancer risks for male carriers of germline mutations in BRCA1 or BRCA2: a review of the literature. J Clin Oncol. 2004;22:735–42.
6. Gao Y, Heller SL, Moy L. Male breast cancer in the age of genetic testing: an opportunity for early detection, tailored therapy, and surveillance. Radiographics. 2018;38:1289–311.
7. Johnson RE, Murad MH. Gynecomastia: pathophysiology, evaluation, and management. Mayo Clin Proc. 2009;84:1010–5.
8. Yang WT, Whitman GJ, Yuen EH, Tse GM, Stelling CB. Sonographic features of primary breast cancer in men. Am J Roentgenol. 2001;176:413–6.
9. Saber T, Backi SA, Ismail M, El Asmar A, El Khoury M. Management of recurrent idiopathic male breast abscess by nipple and areolar excision: 2 case reports. World J Surg Surg Res. 2019;2:1145.
10. Patel PP, Ibrahim AMS, Zhang J, Nguyen JT, Lin SJ, Lee BT. Accessory breast tissue. Eplasty. 2012;12:ic5.
11. Brandt SM, Swistel AJ, Rosen PP. Secretory carcinoma in the axilla. Am J Surg Pathol. 2009;33:950–3.
12. https://acsearch.acr.org/docs/3155692/Narrative/. Last accessed August 25, 2022.
13. Cardoso F, Bartlett JMS, Slaets L, et al. Characterization of male breast cancer: results of the EORTC 10085/TBCRC/big/NABCG international male breast cancer program. Ann Oncol. 2018;29:405–17.

Implants

9

Lucy Chow, Mikhail Roubakha, Puja Shahrouki, and Bo Li

L. Chow (✉) · M. Roubakha · P. Shahrouki · B. Li
Department of Radiology, David Geffen School of Medicine at UCLA,
Los Angeles, CA, USA
e-mail: lchow@mednet.ucla.edu; pshahrouki@mednet.ucla.edu;
boli@mednet.ucla.edu; mroubakha@mednet.ucla.edu

© The Author(s), under exclusive license to Springer Nature
Switzerland AG 2022
L. Chow, B. Li (eds.), *Absolute Breast Imaging Review*,
https://doi.org/10.1007/978-3-031-08274-0_9

1a. A 40-year-old female with a remote history of bilateral breast implants presents with right breast pain and subjective perception of change in right breast shape. What type of breast implant does this patient most likely have and what is the placement?

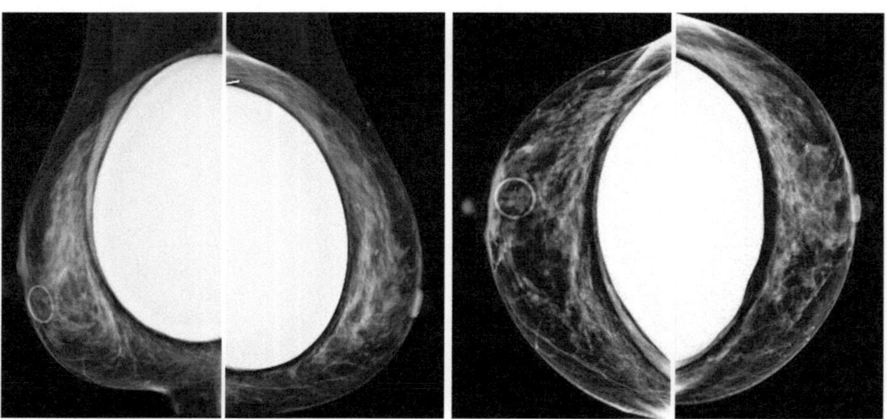

    (a) Silicone implant; subglandular.
    (b) Saline implant; subglandular.
    (c) Silicone implant; subpectoral.
    (d) Silicone implant; subcutaneous.

1b. What is the most appropriate next step given the patient's history?
    (a) Nothing, no evidence of rupture.
    (b) Repeat mammogram to obtain more views.
    (c) Ultrasound, followed by a non-contrast MRI if ultrasound is inconclusive.
    (d) Surgical removal of implant.

1c. The patient received an ultrasound with inconclusive results. The patient subsequently received an MRI without contrast. What is identified on the MRI? What named sign is observed?

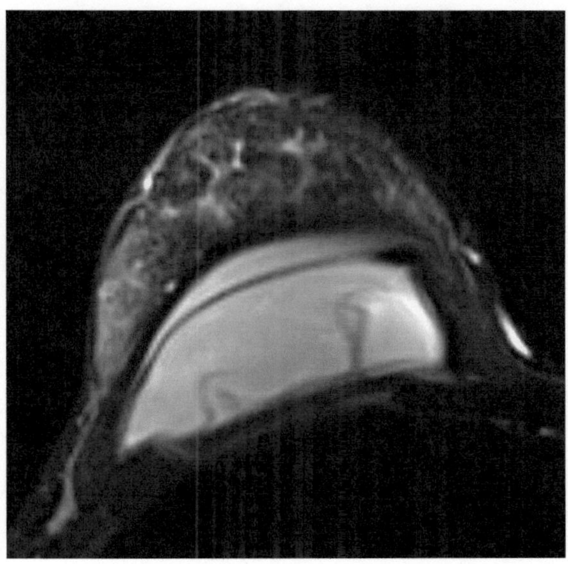

(a) Intracapsular rupture; subcapsular line sign.
(b) Intracapsular rupture; shell sign.
(c) Extracapsular rupture; keyhole sign.
(d) Extracapsular rupture; teardrop sign.

1d. If the patient's breast implant were imaged on ultrasound, what named sign would suggest the presence of intracapsular implant rupture?

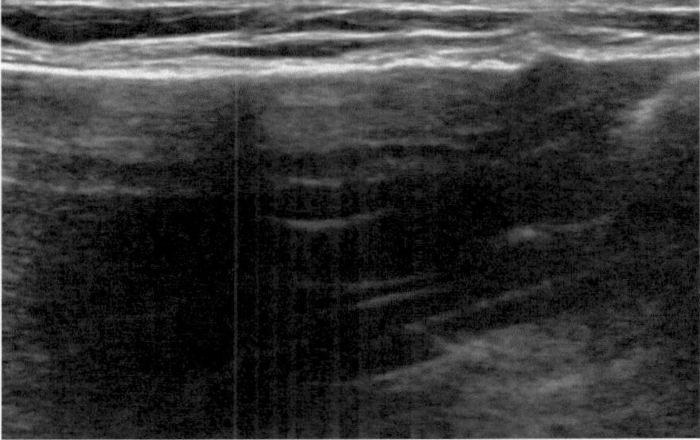

(a) Snowstorm sign.
(b) Stepladder sign.
(c) Shell sign.
(d) Shovel sign.

2. In a patient with silicone implants, what is demonstrated on this ultrasound?

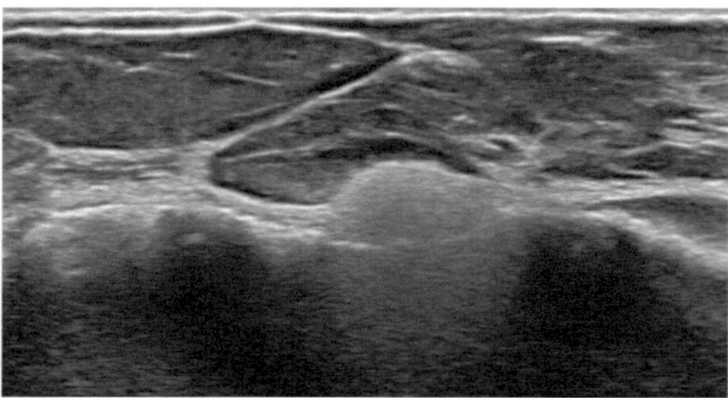

    (a) Donut sign.
    (b) Snowstorm sign.
    (c) Keyhole sign.
    (d) Shadowing sign.

3. A 32-year-old female with a remote history of bilateral breast implants presents complaining of subjective perception of change in left breast shape. Based on the mammographic findings, what is the diagnosis?

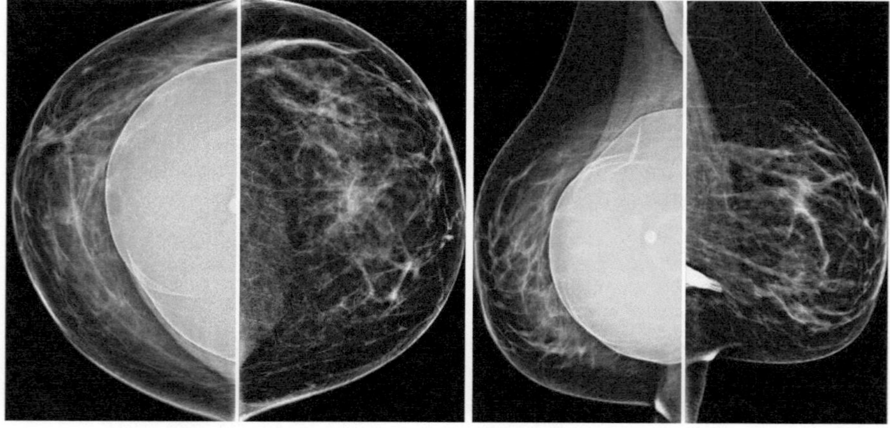

    (a) Left subpectoral saline implant rupture.
    (b) Left subglandular silicone implant rupture.
    (c) Left subglandular saline implant rupture.
    (d) Left subpectoral silicone implant rupture.

4a. A 53-year-old female with history of implants presents with left breast pain, firmness, and change in shape. CC and MLO views of the left breast are shown. What is the most likely diagnosis?

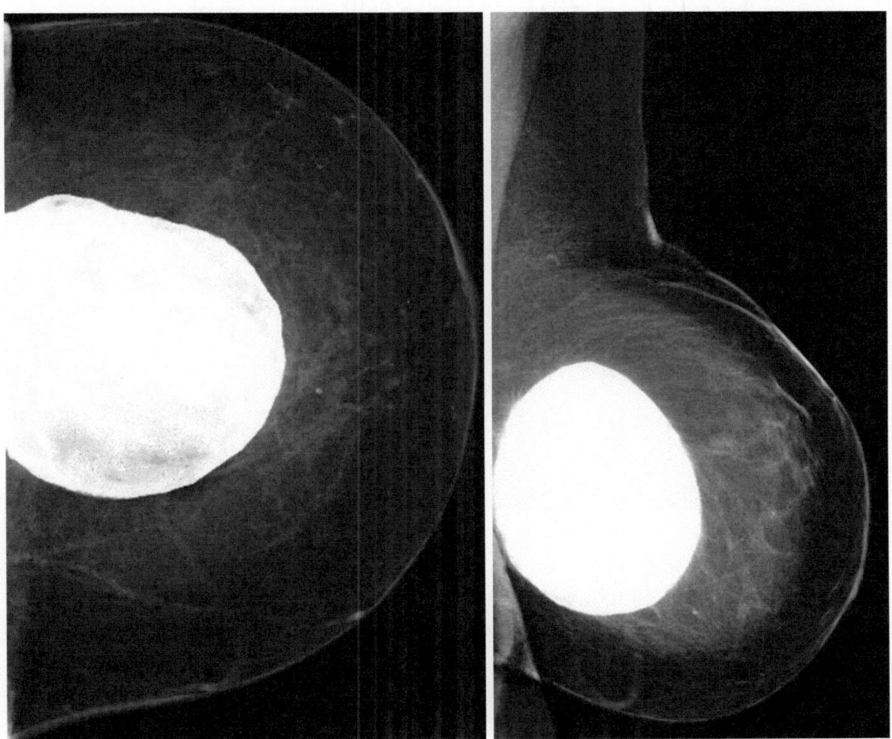

   (a) Extracapsular implant rupture.
   (b) Capsular contracture.
   (c) Free silicone injection.
   (d) Infection.

4b. What is the appropriate management for this condition?
   (a) Nothing.
   (b) Antibiotics.
   (c) Capsulotomy/capsulectomy.
   (d) Mastectomy.

5a. A 54-year-old female from South America presents for screening mammography. She reports no prior history of silicone implants augmentation. CC and MLO views of bilateral breasts are obtained. What would explain the appearance of this patient's breasts on mammography [1]?

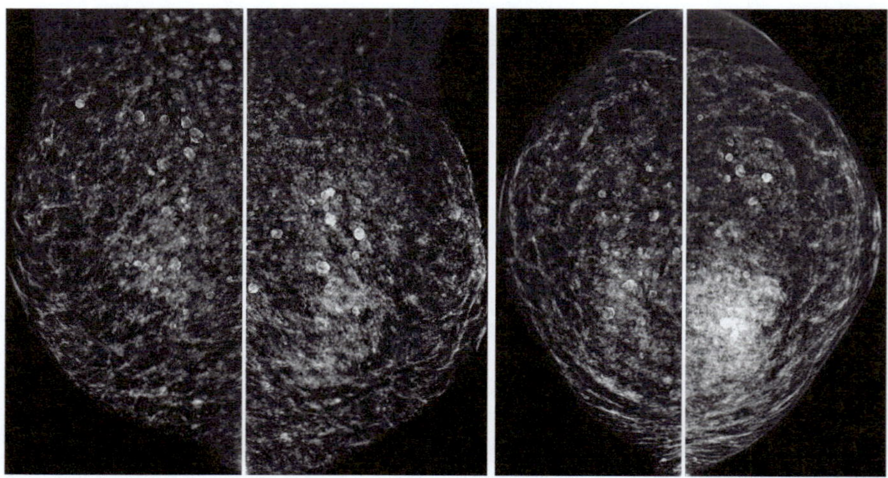

   (a) Fat necrosis.
   (b) Extracapsular silicone implant rupture.
   (c) Free silicone injection granulomas.
   (d) Multiple breast metastases.

5b. Several months later the patient returns with a mass in her left armpit. Ultrasound images are shown. What is the most likely diagnosis?

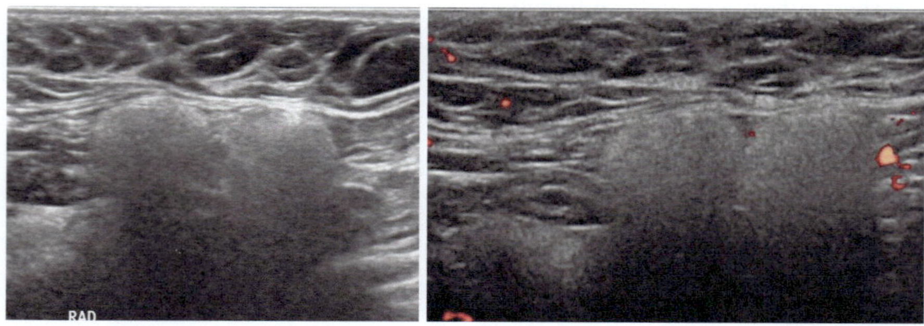

   (a) Silicone-laden lymph nodes.
   (b) Lymphoma.
   (c) Lipoma.
   (d) Reactive lymph nodes.

6. Ultrasound images of a breast with implant are provided. What type of implant is shown and what suggests the implant type?

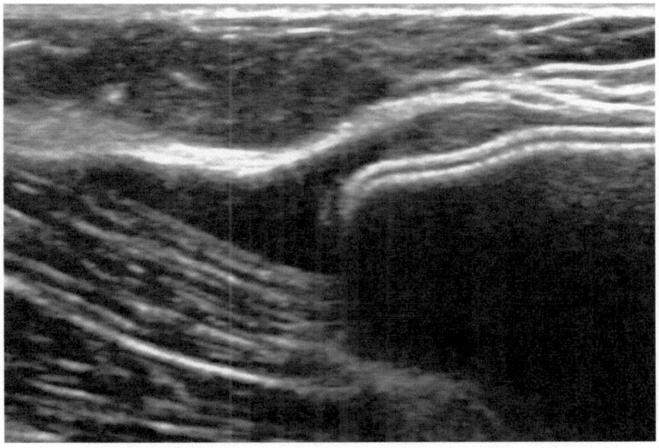

   (a) Silicone; step-off phenomenon.
   (b) Saline; reverberation artifact.
   (c) Silicone; reverberation artifact
   (d) Saline; step-off phenomenon.

7. MRI STIR image of breasts with implants are provided. What type of implant is shown?

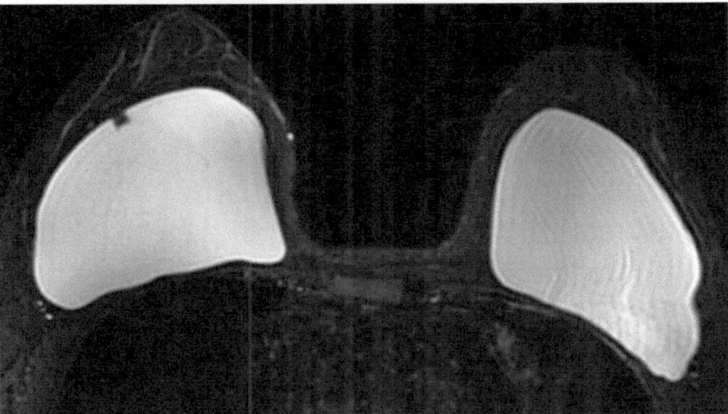

   (a) Silicone.
   (b) Saline.
   (c) Double-lumen.
   (d) Free injection.

8. A 40-year-old female with a history of bilateral breast implants presents complaining of left breast pain and subjective perception of change in left breast shape. Her mammogram was unremarkable. She subsequently received an MRI for her implant concerns. What is seen on MRI? What named sign is observed?

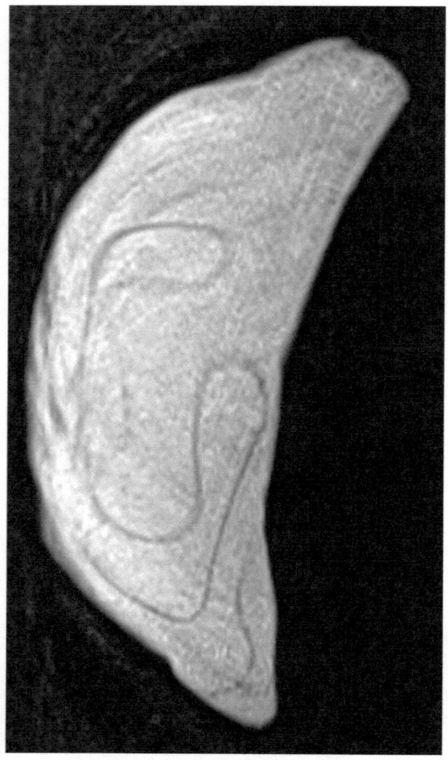

(a) Intracapsular rupture; linguine sign.
(b) Extracapsular rupture; shell sign.
(c) Intracapsular rupture; keyhole sign.
(d) Extracapsular rupture; loop sign.

9. What type of implant is seen on this mammogram?

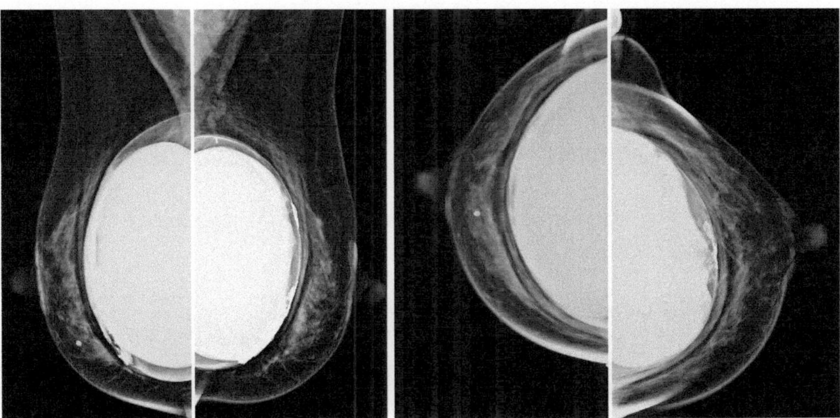

    (a) Single-lumen saline.
    (b) Single-lumen silicone.
    (c) Standard double-lumen.
    (d) Reverse double-lumen.

10. What technique can be employed to improve visualization of breast tissue when implants are present?
    (a) DeBruhl technique.
    (b) Eklund technique.
    (c) Kagetsu and/or Manghisi technique.
    (d) Bassett technique.

11. Ultrasound images are provided of a breast implant. What type of implant is shown?

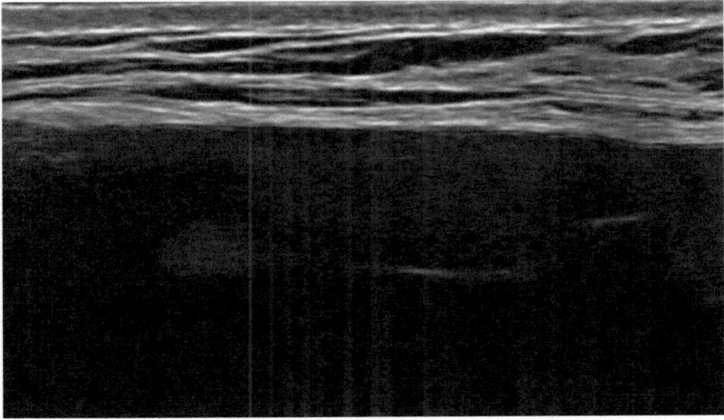

    (a) Silicone.
    (b) Saline.
    (c) Double-lumen.
    (d) Unable to differentiate.

12a. A 55-year-old woman with a remote history of bilateral breast augmentation presents with asymmetric swelling and pain of her right breast. Mammogram was negative. What is the next best step?
 (a) Nothing.
 (b) Ultrasound.
 (c) MRI.
 (d) Surgical consultation.

12b. An ultrasound was performed. What is the differential diagnosis for this peri-implant fluid collection?

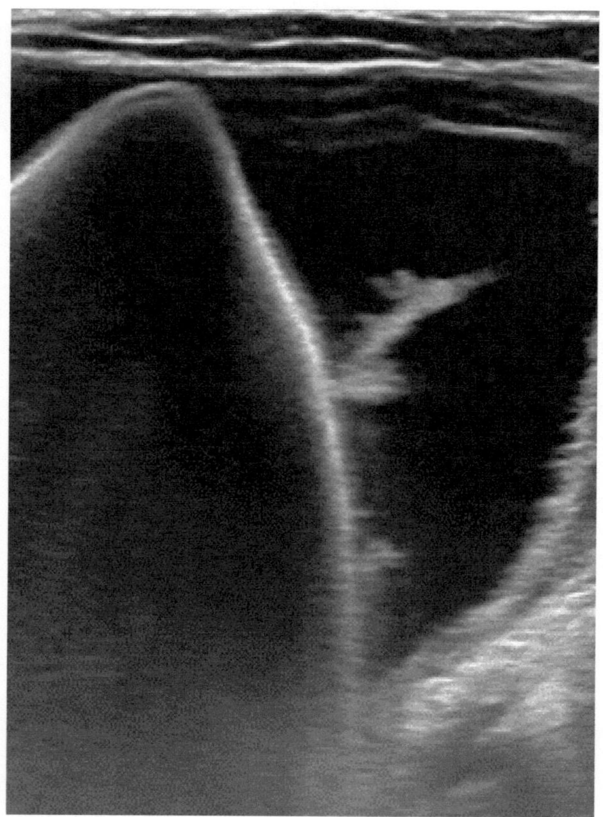

 (a) Infection.
 (b) Implant rupture.
 (c) Late seroma.
 (d) Breast implant-associated anaplastic large cell lymphoma.
 (e) All of the above.

12c. An ultrasound was performed on the patient above, as shown. What is the best next step in the diagnosis and treatment?
    (a) MRI.
    (b) Fluid aspiration.
    (c) Mammography.
    (d) Surgery.
    (e) PET scan.

12d. How common is breast implant-associated lymphoma?
    (a) 0.3–100 in 100,000 women.
    (b) 0.3–100 in 1000 women.
    (c) 1 in 100 women.
    (d) Unknown.

12e. What is a risk factor for breast implant-associated lymphoma?
    (a) Smooth implant.
    (b) Textured implant.
    (c) Saline implant.
    (d) Silicone implant.

12f. What additional imaging can be considered for additional characterization?
    (a) Mammography.
    (b) MRI.
    (c) Nuclear medicine.
    (d) CT.

13. A 50-year-old female seen for diagnostic evaluation of the breast for personal breast cancer history. Ultrasound images are shown. What explains the three echogenic lines seen near the periphery of the implant seen on ultrasound?

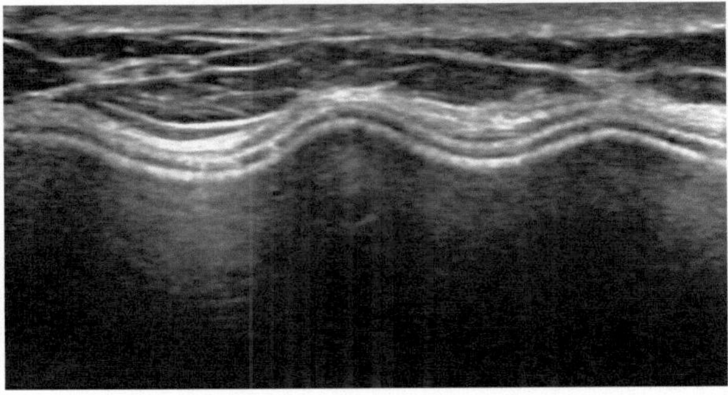

    (a) Intracapsular rupture.
    (b) Extracapsular rupture.
    (c) Normal; trilaminar line.
    (d) Normal; stepladder sign.

14. A 36-year-old female presents for diagnostic evaluation of a lump in the left breast. Ultrasound image is below. What is the most likely diagnosis?

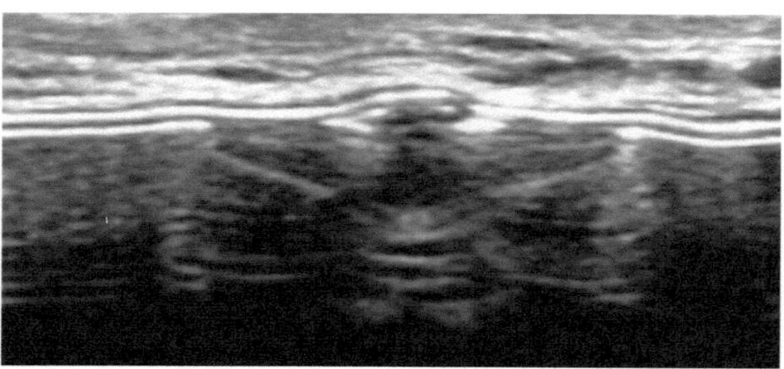

    (a) Saline valve.
    (b) Nipple.
    (c) Intracapsular rupture.
    (d) Lymph node.

15. A 38-year-old female presents for screening. Ultrasound image is shown. What best describes the finding on ultrasound?

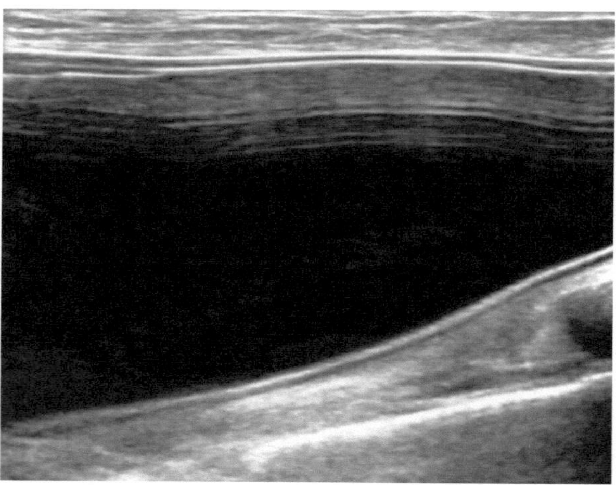

    (a) Reverberation artifact; intact implant.
    (b) Stepladder artifact; extracapsular implant rupture.
    (c) Stepladder artifact; intracapsular implant rupture.
    (d) Shell sign; intact implant.

16. A 70-year-old female is seen for callback from screening. Silicone-sensitive sequence image of the breast is provided. What is the diagnosis?

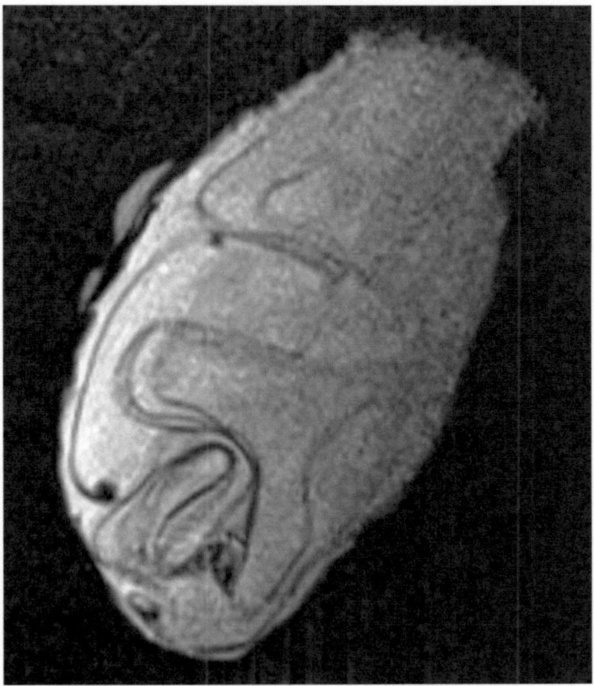

(a) Free silicone injections.
(b) Implant extracapsular rupture.
(c) Normal.
(d) Breast lymphoma.

17. A 50-year-old female with right breast lower inner palpable implant finding, evaluation for implant integrity. A silicone-sensitive sequence of the right breast is provided. What explains the finding?

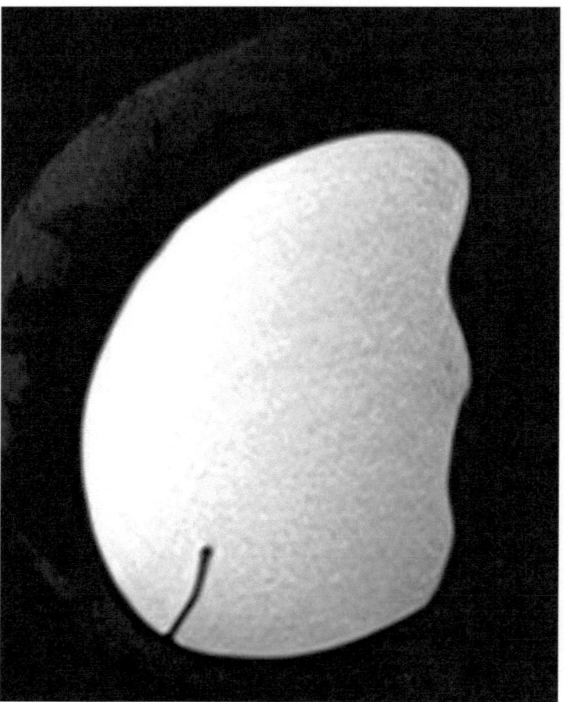

    (a) Radial fold.
    (b) Intracapsular rupture.
    (c) Extracapsular rupture.
    (d) Valve.

Answers

1a. c. Silicone implant; subpectoral.

This patient has a silicone implant as evidenced by the dense contents of the implant on mammography. Single-lumen silicone implants are the most common implant type [2]. Saline implants are typically much less dense in appearance and there is a valve that can be seen in the central part of the implant. The patient's pectoralis major muscle is seen draped over the implant. "Subcutaneous" is not an appropriate term to describe the implant positioning.

1b. c. Ultrasound, followed by a non-contrast MRI if ultrasound is inconclusive.

Given the patient's history, especially change in breast morphology, there is a concern of implant rupture. Although saline implant rupture can be identified on mammography and can be diagnosed clinically, silicone implant rupture—specifically intracapsular rupture—is often challenging to diagnose with mammography alone. Diagnosis of intracapsular rupture can be made by ultrasound. If the ultrasound is inconclusive, a non-contrast MRI can be performed to evaluate the silicone implants and implant integrity.

1c. a. Intracapsular rupture; subcapsular line sign.

No extracapsular silicone content is identified. The fibrous capsule appears intact and the silicone contents are contained entirely within the fibrous capsule. The implant demonstrates intracapsular rupture with the subcapsular line sign (green arrow), teardrop sign (red arrow), and keyhole sign (blue arrow). There is no "shell sign" pertaining to breast implant rupture.

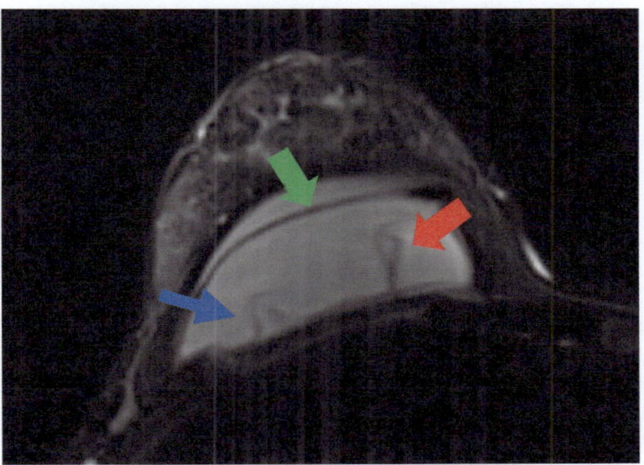

Linguine sign is demonstrated by multiple curvilinear hypointense lines within the silicone gel and describes the collapsed implant shell floating within the silicone. Subcapsular line sign is demonstrated by hypodense wavy lines running parallel and just beneath the fibrous capsule and describes the silicone outside of the implant shell, separating it from the fibrous capsule. Keyhole sign is suggestive of rupture and is depicted by focal invagination of the implant shell, where the two membranes do not touch. Teardrop sign is suggestive of rupture and is depicted by focal invagination of the implant shell containing silicone, where the two membranes touch [3].

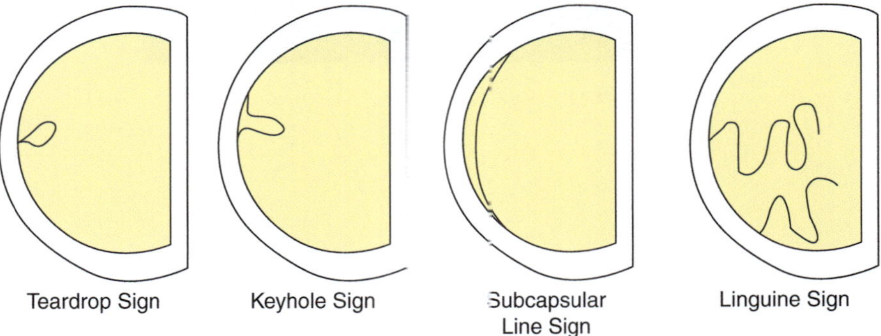

1d. b. Stepladder sign.

On ultrasound, intracapsular rupture may present with the stepladder sign, which is seen as multiple, parallel, discontinuous, hyperechoic lines within the implant lumen. A normal implant should be anechoic. Extracapsular rupture may present with the snowstorm sign. The other two signs do not exist as pertaining to breast implant rupture. Overall, ultrasound is only 59–85% sensitive and 55–79% specific for detecting implant rupture [4].

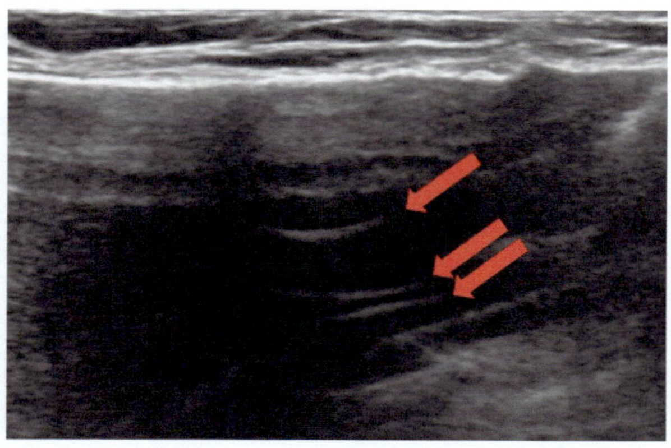

2. b. Snowstorm sign.

Extracapsular rupture presents with the snowstorm sign as demonstrated by a heterogenous echogenic appearance of free silicone droplets mixed with breast tissue. Keyhole sign is suggestive of intracapsular rupture on MRI. There is no donut sign or shadowing sign relating to implant rupture.

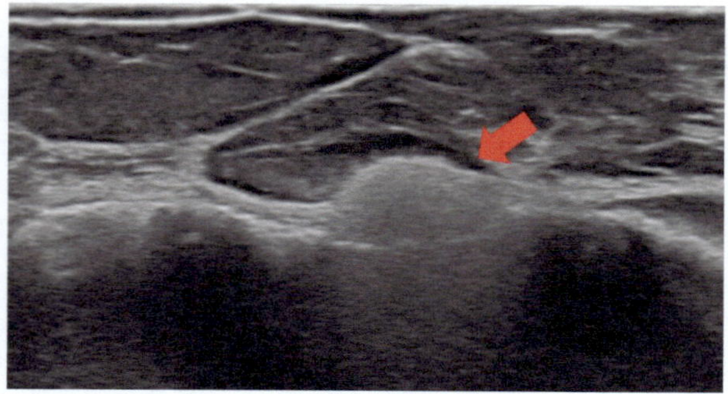

3. a. Left subpectoral saline implant rupture.

The imaging appearance of the left breast on mammography is that of a subpectoral saline implant which has ruptured and collapsed (yellow circle). Saline implants are radiolucent with the presence of a saline implant valve (red arrow). Standard double-lumen implants feature a dense silicone central compartment with the less dense outer saline compartment encircling it. Reverse double-lumen implants feature a central saline compartment with a denser ring of silicone surrounding it.

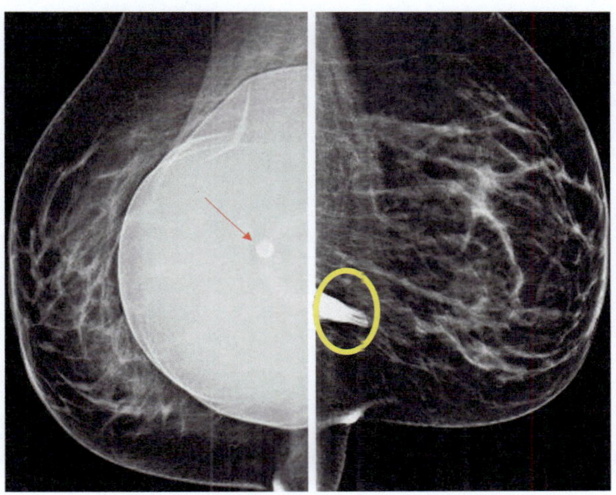

4a. b. Capsular contracture.

The left implant appears rounded and spherical rather than oval in shape, indicating capsular contraction. Another finding include contour irregularity. Capsular contraction is one of the most common complications after breast augmentation. It refers to a tightening of the fibrous capsule surrounding the breast implant, most commonly occurring within months after implantation but can occur at any time [5].

4b. c. Capsulotomy/capsulectomy.

The usual management for capsular contracture is capsulotomy/capsulectomy to relieve pressure on the implant and improve symptoms. This is not an infection, so antibiotics are not warranted. Mastectomy is too radical a solution for this complication. It would not be appropriate to do nothing given the patient's discomfort.

5a. c. Free silicone injection granulomas.

This patient has undergone bilateral breast augmentation with free silicone injections. This practice is still performed in countries throughout Asia and South America, and rarely in the USA. The appearance on mammogram can be difficult to distinguish from extracapsular silicone implant rupture; however, there is no evidence to suggest this patient received silicone breast implants [1].

5b. a. Silicone-laden lymph nodes.

Ultrasound demonstrates two hyperechoic axillary lymph nodes with a well-defined anterior margin and poorly defined posterior margin resulting in a "snowstorm" appearance. These findings coupled with the patient's history of free silicone injections into the breasts are suggestive of silicone-laden lymph nodes. Silicone-laden lymph nodes can be identified on MRI as extracapsular hyperintense signal on silicone-sensitive sequences (red arrows).

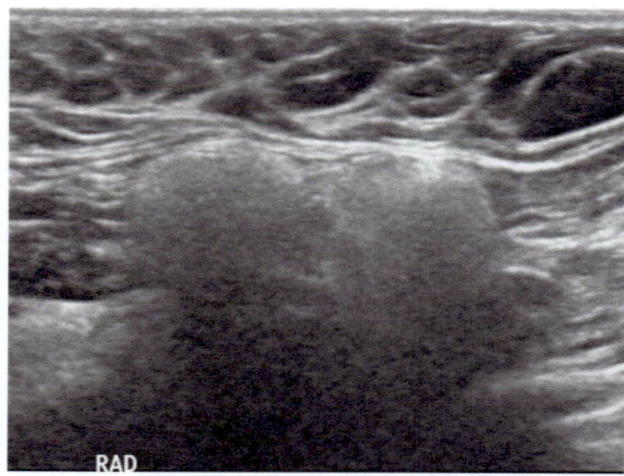
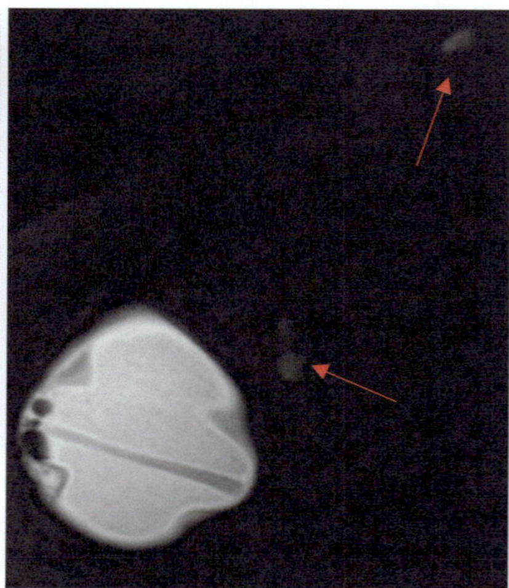

6. a. Silicone; step-off phenomenon.

This patient has silicone implants as evidenced by the step-off phenomenon [2]. Because sound travels more slowly through silicone than saline, soft tissues behind a silicone implant appear farther away and a discontinuity or step-off of the fascia (red bracket) posterior to the silicone implant is seen. The thicker the implant, the more exaggerated the effect [5]. Light compression during scanning can help minimize this effect. Saline implants on ultrasound do not demonstrate step-off effect.

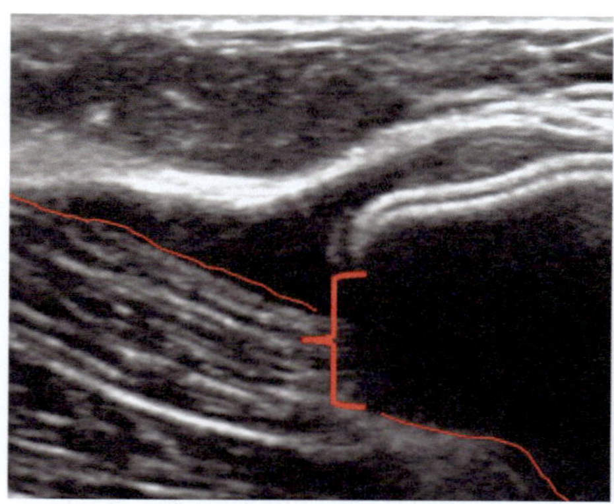
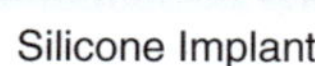

Silicone Implant

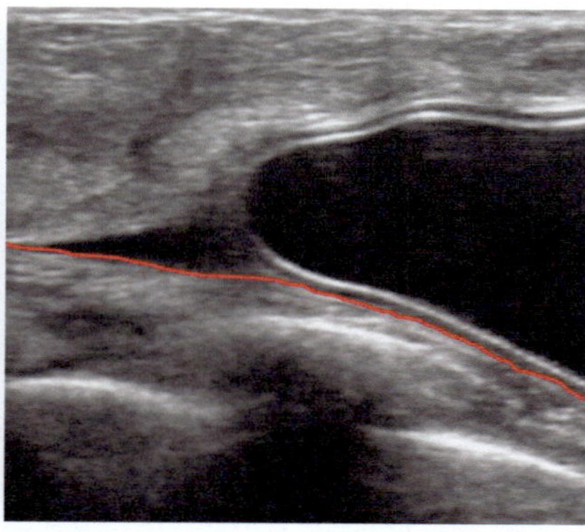

Saline Implant

7. b. Saline.

Based on the images, this patient most likely has saline implants. Distinguishing different implant types on MR can usually be done by examining STIR or T2-weighted images, where saline implants will appear very bright relative to fat and silicone implants will appear intermediate intensity (relative to fat). On T1-weighted images, saline implants are more hypointense compared to silicone implants. An additional finding suggesting saline implant is the presence of a fill valve (also known as injection port), usually seen in a subareolar location at the margin of the implant shell (circle).

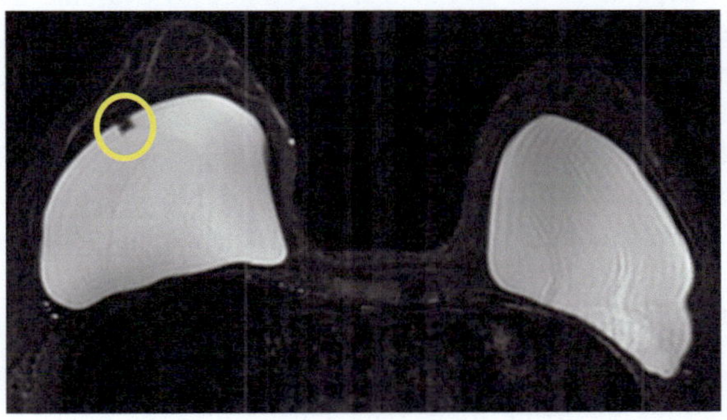

8a. a. Intracapsular rupture; linguine sign.

The fibrous capsule is intact and the silicone contents are contained within it. However, the silicone shell is collapsed and exhibits the linguine sign as demonstrated by multiple curvilinear hypointense lines within the silicone gel.

9. c. Standard double-lumen.

This is the classic imaging appearance of a standard double-lumen implant, comprising approximately 11% of all implants [2], which has a silicone center and inflatable saline outer lumen. Less than 1% of implants are reverse double-lumen, most often used after reconstructive surgery. Additional, even rarer, varieties include triple-lumen and reverse-adjustable double lumen implants.

10. b. Eklund technique.

When implants are present, the Eklund technique is used to improve breast tissue visualization. It involves posterosuperior displacement of the implant (toward the chest wall) with simultaneous anterior traction of the breast tissue forward and around the implant. These implant-displaced images result in maximizing the tissue seen in the mammogram [6].

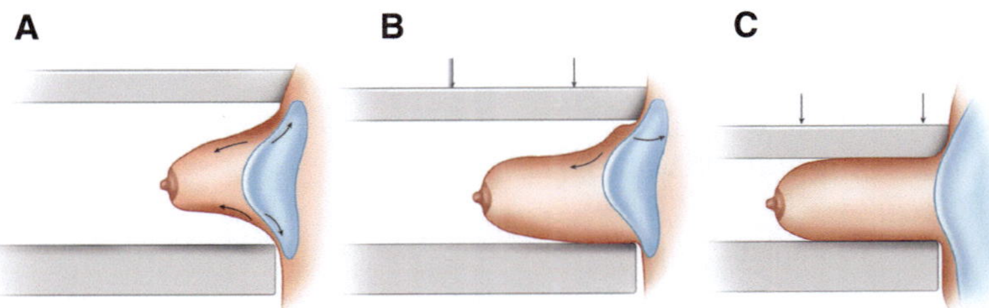

Illustration demonstrating sequential posterior displacement of the implant within the breast during compression for mammography to improve visualization of underlying breast tissue

11. d. Unable to differentiate.

On ultrasound, saline and silicone implants appear similar. They both appear anechoic with a linear echogenic rim capsule. Within the implant, low-level echoes may be seen normally. Additionally, reverberation artifacts can be seen anteriorly and should not be confused with lack of implant integrity.

12a. b. Ultrasound.

Breast ultrasound is the initial test of choice to evaluate swelling or pain related to a breast implant. Ultrasound can assess implant integrity, peri-implant effusion or mass. Mammography does not have the accuracy to detect peri-implant effusion or mass-forming breast implant-associated anaplastic large cell lymphoma. Breast MRI is an imaging test with high accuracy that can be performed after inconclusive ultrasound and can evaluate capsule integrity or contracture, implant rupture, tissue edema, effusion, and mass.

12b. e. All of the above.

A late seroma associated with a breast implant is defined as a periprosthetic fluid collection occurring more than 1 year after the breast augmentation or reconstruction procedure. This complication is rare and usually benign. The symptoms can be indistinguishable from those of Breast Implant-Associated Anaplastic Large Cell Lymphoma (BIA-ALCL). At a median age of 10 years after implant placement, the typical presenting features are sudden onset of breast swelling from peri-implant effusion and less likely a mass [7].

12c. b. Fluid aspiration.

The initial assessment of late onset enlargement of the breast in the setting of breast implants should include a clinical history querying recent trauma or infection. An initial screening with breast ultrasound should be performed to assess for implant integrity, the presence of effusion, the presence of a mass and axillary lymph nodes. If an effusion is present, fluid aspiration is indicated in an attempt to relieve the patient's symptoms and to exclude breast implant-associated anaplastic large cell lymphoma (BIA-ALCL). At least 50 ml of effusion fluid should be analyzed for cytologic analysis and immunopheno-typing, culture, cell count, and protein. In contrast, 5–10 ml of fluid surrounding an implant in an asymptomatic patient is usually normal and generally does not require further investigation. Surgery (en-bloc capsulectomy) followed by chemotherapy and radiation are typically the next steps in management [7]. In this case, cytology revealed a breast implant-associated anaplastic large cell lymphoma.

12d. a. 0.3–100 in 100,000 women [7].

12e. b. Textured implant.

Textured implants are known to increase risk for this type of lymphoma, possibly related to peri-implant inflammation and biofilm formation with chronic subclinical infection, ultimately leading to malignant transformation of T-cells. Smooth implants are not known to increase risk. There is no known association with implant filling [7].

12f. b. MRI.

MRI may demonstrate effusions (arrows) and masses associated with the lymphoma. Additionally, capsular enhancement may be seen in a small number of cases. Neither mammography, nuclear medicine, or PET-CT scans are specific for implant-associated lymphoma [7].

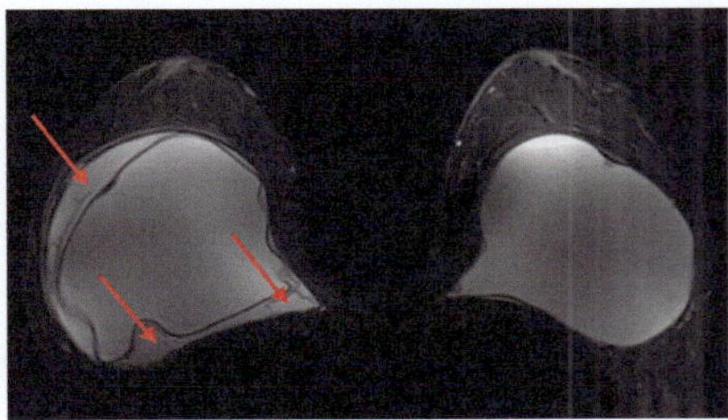
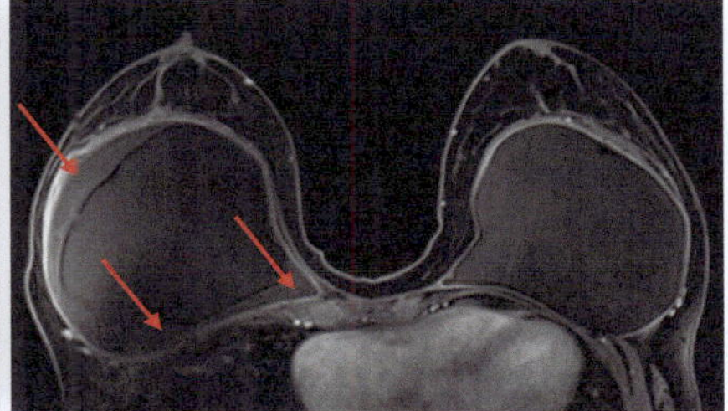

13. c. Normal; trilaminar line.

A fibrous capsule eventually forms around the implant shell and creates a tri-laminar line on ultrasound. The outer echogenic line is the outer surface of the capsule, the middle echogenic line reflects two echogenic lines, which are the inner surface of the capsule and the outer surface of the elastomer shell, and the inner echogenic line corresponds to the inner surface of the elastomer shell. The isoechoic space between the outer and middle echogenic lines represents the fibrous capsule thickness, and the intervening anechoic space between the middle and inner echogenic lines reflects the elastomer shell thickness [5]. The stepladder sign is discussed in question 1.

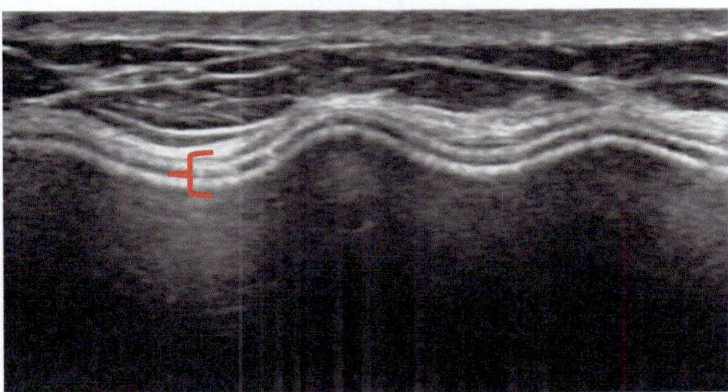

14. a. Saline valve.

This finding in the area of the patient's concern represents a saline valve. The nipple would not be found so deep within the subcutaneous tissues. Intracapsular rupture and lymph node have different ultrasound appearance.

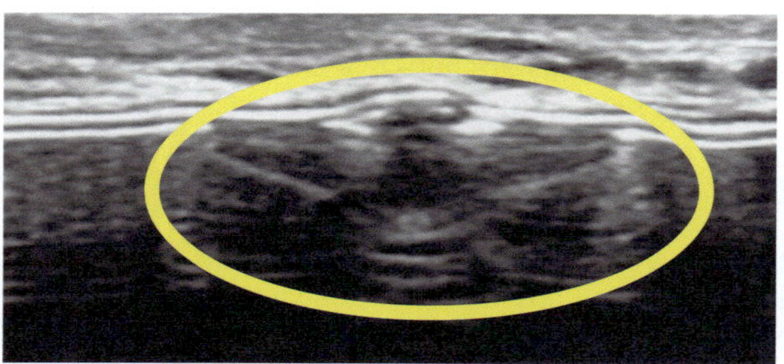

15. a. Reverberation artifact; intact implant.

Ultrasound image shows a band of multiple, closely spaced, echogenic lines (bracket) in the near field parallel to the capsule-shell complex, a finding consistent with reverberation artifact, which can be seen even with an intact implant, as was the case above. There are no imaging findings to suggest implant rupture. Reverberation artifact occurs when the ultrasound beam encounters two strong parallel reflectors, and bounces back and forth between them, resulting in the above artifact. This artifact can be reduced by changing the angle of insonation.

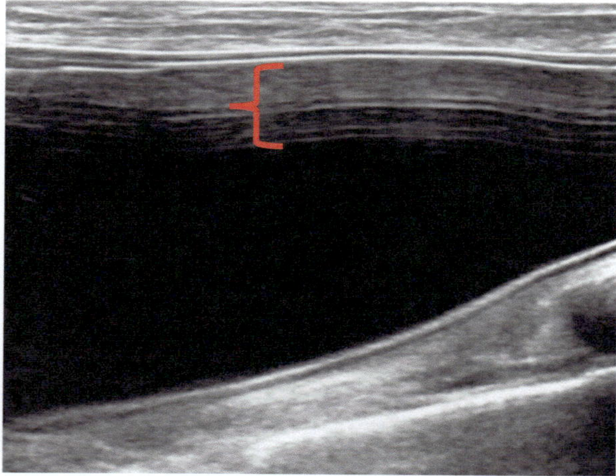

16. b. Implant extracapsular rupture.

The irregular contour of the right breast implant and presence of silicone outside the implant capsule (red arrow) indicate extracapsular silicone rupture of the implant. Free silicone injections and breast lymphoma have an alternate appearance. Linguine sign is also seen which is indicative of intracapsular rupture.

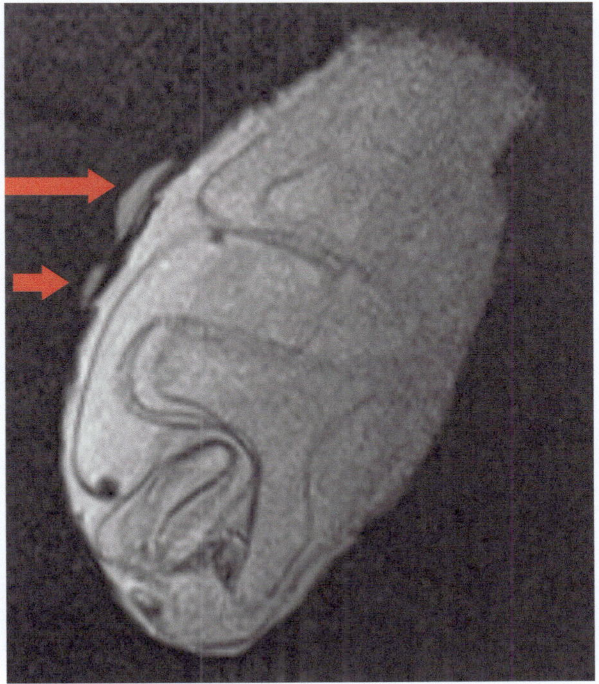

17. a. Radial fold.

The MR image above demonstrates a radial fold, a normal finding of intact breast implants. There is no evidence of intracapsular or extracapsular rupture. Valves appear different, and are seen with saline implants, not silicone.

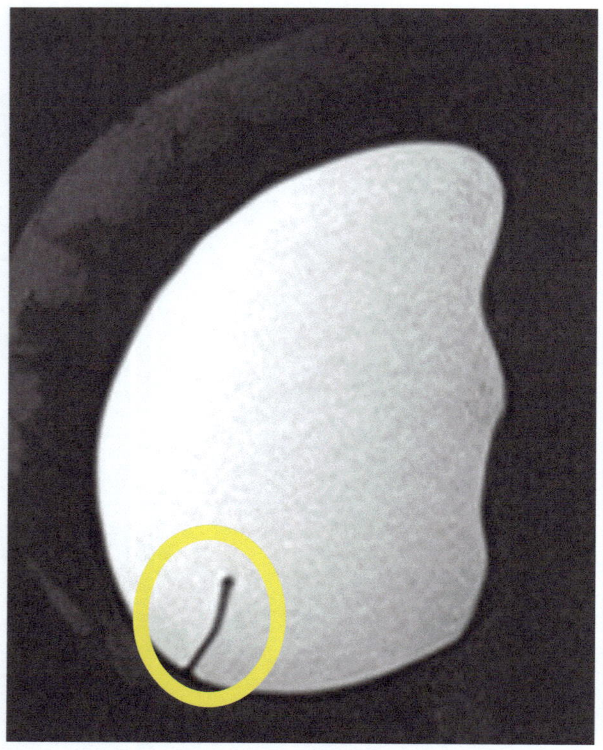

References

1. Leibman AJ, Misra M. Spectrum of imaging findings in the silicone-injected breast. Plast Reconstr Surg. 2011;128(1):28e-9e.
2. Middleton M, McNamara M Jr. Breast implant classification with MR imaging correlation. Radiographics. 2000;20(3):e1-e1.
3. Seiler S, Sharma P, Hayes J, Ganti R, Mootz A, Eads E, Teotia S, Evans WP. Multimodality imaging-based evaluation of single-lumen silicone breast implants for rupture. Radiographics. 2017;37(2):366–82.
4. Paredes ES. Atlas of mammography. Lippincott Williams & Wilkins; 2007.
5. Schaub TA, Ahmad J, Rohrich RJ. Capsular contracture with breast implants in the cosmetic patient: saline versus silicone—a systematic review of the literature. Plast Reconst Surg. 2010;126(6):2140–9.
6. Eklund GW, Busby RC, Miller SH, Job JS. Improved imaging of the augmented breast. AMJ 1988;151(3):469–73.
7. Sharma B, et al. Breast implant-associated anaplastic large cell lymphoma: review and multi-parametric imaging paradigms. Radiographics. 2020;40(3):609–28.

Breast Cancer Workup and Surgical Planning

10

Stephanie Lee-Felker, Natalie Cain, and Mariam Thomas

S. Lee-Felker (✉)
Department of Radiology, West Los Angeles Veterans Affairs Medical Center,
Los Angeles, CA, USA
e-mail: Stephanie.Lee-felker@va.gov

N. Cain
Department of Radiology, David Geffen School of Medicine at UCLA,
Los Angeles, CA, USA
e-mail: ncain@mednet.ucla.edu

M. Thomas
Department of Radiology, David Geffen School of Medicine at UCLA,
Los Angeles, CA, USA

Department of Radiology, Olive View-UCLA Medical Center, Sylmar, CA, USA
e-mail: mathomas@dhs.lacounty.gov

© The Author(s), under exclusive license to Springer Nature
Switzerland AG 2022
L. Chow, B. Li (eds.), *Absolute Breast Imaging Review*,
https://doi.org/10.1007/978-3-031-08274-0_10

1. 57-year-old woman with biopsy-proven invasive ductal carcinoma of the right breast. Ultrasound shows an irregular, hypoechoic mass with angular and indistinct margins. MRI shows an enhancing mass containing biopsy microclip artifact and adjacent enhancing foci. What is the size of the mass for TNM staging?

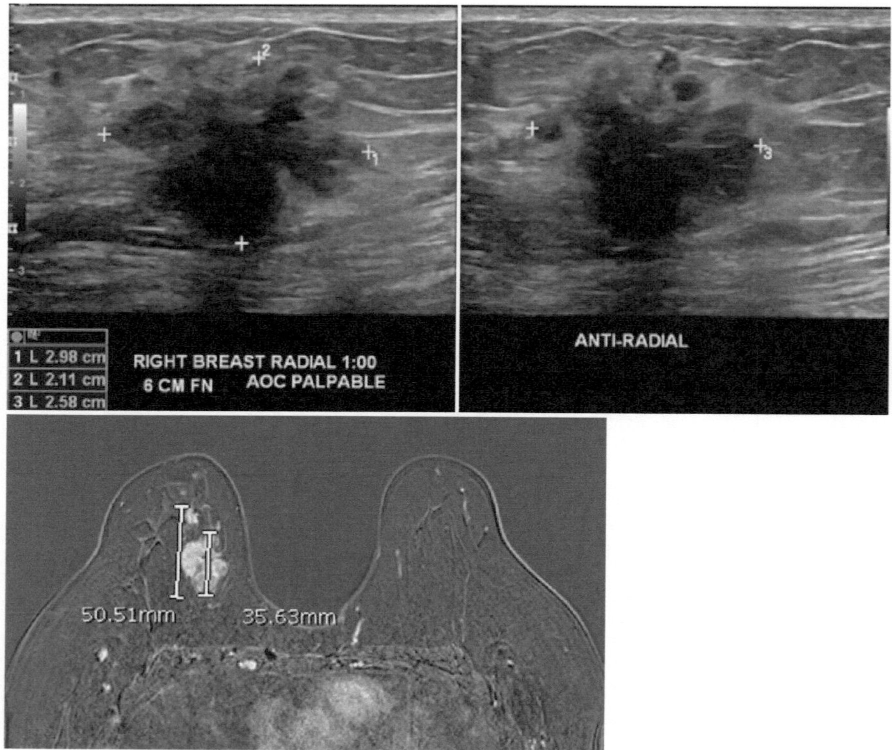

(a) 30 mm.
(b) 36 mm.
(c) 51 mm.
(d) The size of the mass by ultrasound and of the mass by MRI should be averaged.

2. A 49-year-old woman presents with a palpable lump in the right axilla. The ultrasound is shown below. A biopsy of the lymph node was performed, and the biopsy result is metastatic invasive ductal carcinoma from a breast primary. Other than showing abnormal axillary lymph nodes, her mammogram was normal. What is the next step?

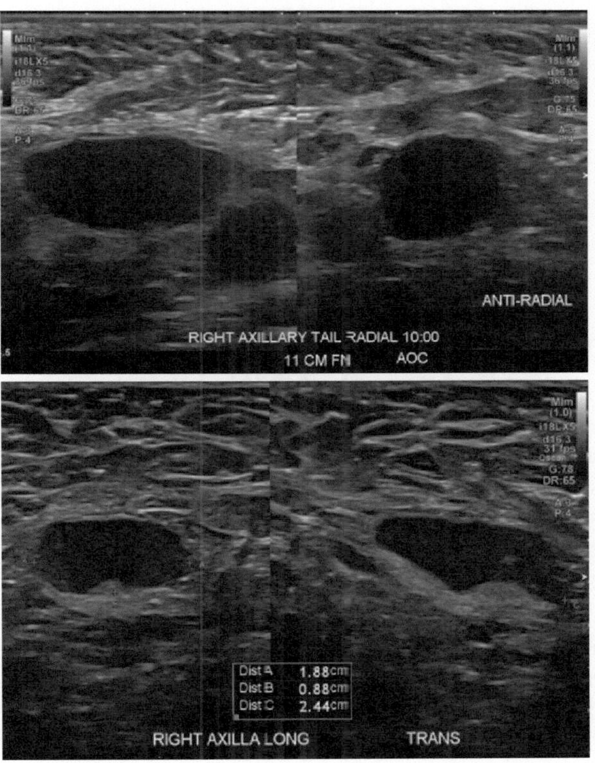

   (a) Contrast-enhanced mammography.
   (b) Breast MRI.
   (c) Molecular breast imaging.
   (d) Surgical excision of the biopsy-proven metastatic axillary lymph node.
   (e) PET examination.

3. Which statement below is incorrect regarding axillary lymph nodes?
   (a) To evaluate axillary lymph nodes, the patient should be positioned supine oblique with the hand above the head, and with the arm abducted and externally rotated.
   (b) Ultrasound is preferred over MRI as the initial exam. Ultrasound is more cost effective and is better at evaluating morphology.
   (c) Sentinel node is usually found at the inferior/lower part of the axilla.
   (d) Tumor infiltration starts at the center of the lymph node.

4. Which axillary lymph node level is marked with the black arrow on the image below?
   (a) I.
   (b) II.
   (c) III.
   (d) The arrow is not in the axillary region.

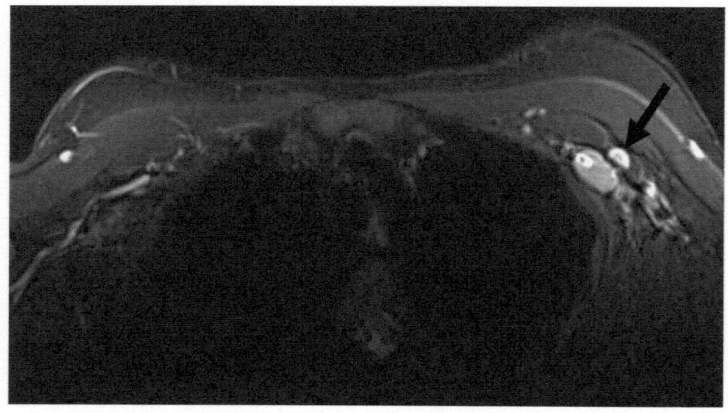

5. Metastases to the cervical, contralateral internal mammary, or contralateral axillary lymph nodes are considered:
   (a) N2 disease.
   (b) N3 disease.
   (c) M0 disease.
   (d) M1 disease.

6. Isolated metastasis to the internal mammary lymph node occurs in what percent of breast cancers?
   (a) Up to 5%.
   (b) Up to 25%.
   (c) Up to 75%.
   (d) Up to 90%.

7a. A 32-year-old woman presents with right nipple erythema and discharge. On physical examination, there is no evidence of skin thickening or ulceration. Her diagnostic mammogram and ultrasound were unrevealing. What is the next best step?
   (a) Contrast-enhanced mammography (CEM).
   (b) MRI.
   (c) PET examination.
   (d) No additional imaging is indicated.

7b. Her MRI is shown below. What is the diagnosis?

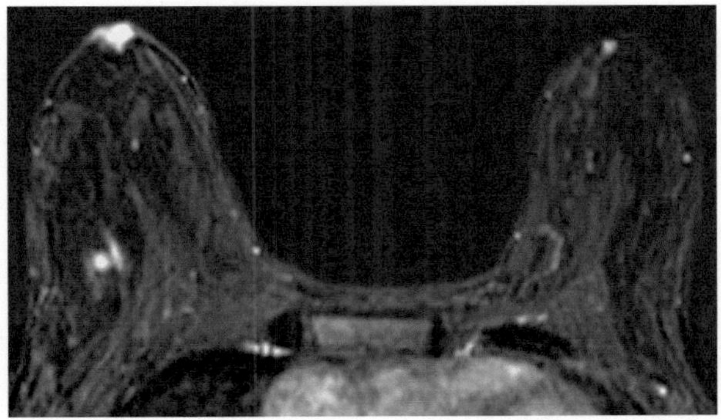

    (a) Paget's disease.
    (b) Eczema.
    (c) Fat necrosis.
    (d) Inflammatory breast cancer.

7c. Her nipple biopsy showed Paget's disease. Her focused ultrasound after the MRI was negative. What is the next step?
    (a) PET.
    (b) Lumpectomy.
    (c) Surgical excision of the nipple.
    (d) MRI-guided biopsy.

8. Paget's disease of the nipple is associated with what other malignancy?
    (a) Phyllodes tumor.
    (b) Lymphoma.
    (c) DCIS.
    (d) Sarcoma.
    (e) Squamous cell carcinoma.

9. 57-year-old woman diagnosed with triple negative invasive ductal carcinoma of the right breast. Fig. A is her breast MRI prior to treatment. Fig. B is her breast MRI after neoadjuvant chemotherapy. What was her response to chemotherapy?

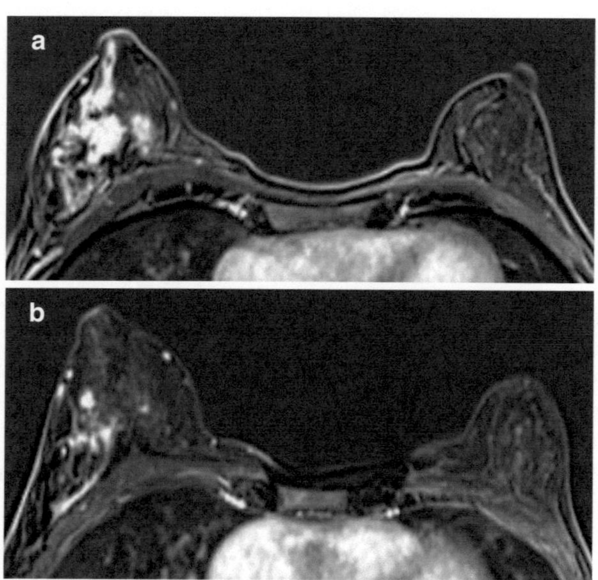

(a) Partial response.
(b) Complete response.
(c) Unable to determine response, need ultrasound images.
(d) Stable disease.

10. Which imaging modality is the most accurate to assess response after neoadjuvant chemotherapy?
(a) Mammogram.
(b) Contrast-enhanced mammogram.
(c) Ultrasound.
(d) MRI.
(e) PET.

11a. A 46-year-old woman presents for screening mammogram. The left screening views are shown. The patient has a history of prior benign surgical excision and core needle biopsy of the left breast. What is the correct BI-RADS assessment for the screening mammogram?

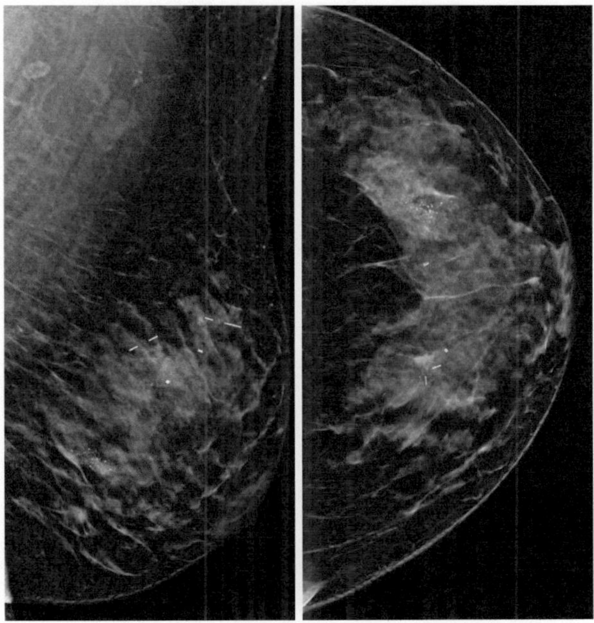

(a) BI-RADS 2. Benign. The surgical scar marker and biopsy clip show that all findings have been evaluated in the past.

(b) BI-RADS 0. Incomplete. Recall the patient.

(c) BI-RADS 4. Suspicious. Recommend stereotactic biopsy.

(d) BI-RADS 1. Negative examination. Return to annual screening.

11b. The patient was recalled, and magnification views of the groups of calcifications were performed. What is the next step?

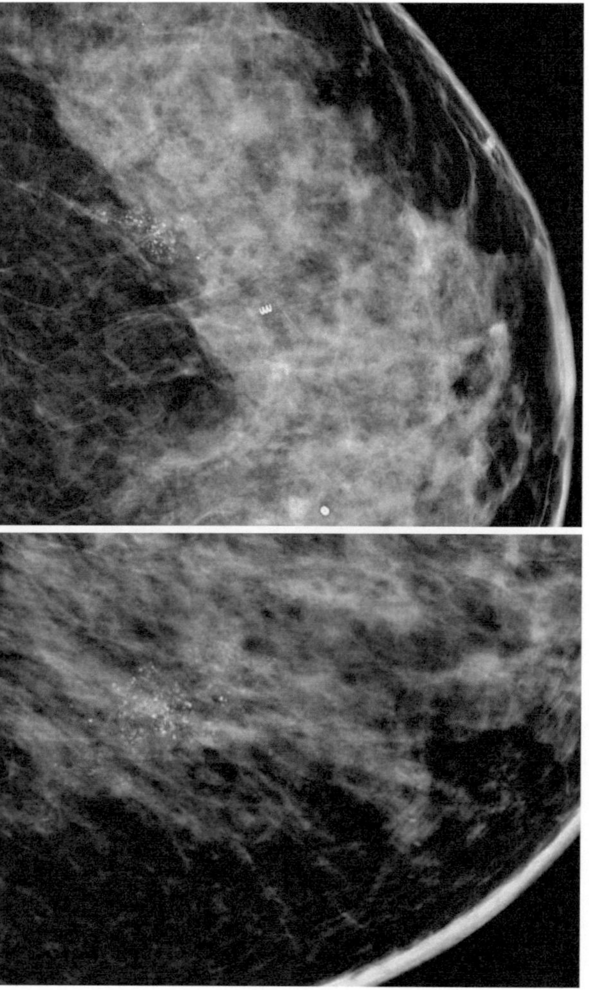

(a) Stereotactic biopsy.
(b) Wait for prior films.
(c) MRI.
(d) Ultrasound.

11c. Subsequent ultrasound was performed. What is the next step?

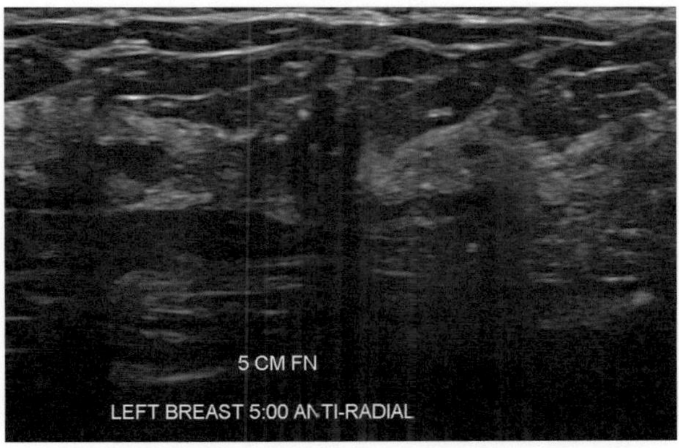

    (a) Stereotactic core biopsy.
    (b) Ultrasound-guided core biopsy.
    (c) MRI to delineate extent of disease.
    (d) Await prior films as the patient had a prior benign biopsy.

11d. There were additional calcifications in the same quadrant and both groups were malignant. What is the correct term for disease?
    (a) Multicentric disease.
    (b) Multiquadrant disease.
    (c) Multifocal disease.
    (d) Multipart disease.

12. An incidentally detected FDG-avid breast lesion greater than 1 cm is identified on FDG PET/CT. What is the likelihood of malignancy?
    (a) 1–5%
    (b) 10–20%
    (c) 30–40%
    (d) 80–90%.

13. 29-year-old BRCA1 positive woman with biopsy-proven invasive ductal carcinoma of the right breast with axillary nodal metastases. Her MRI for initial local staging is shown below. There is non-mass enhancement in the outer right breast. What additional finding on the MRI is important to communicate to the breast surgeon prior to surgery?

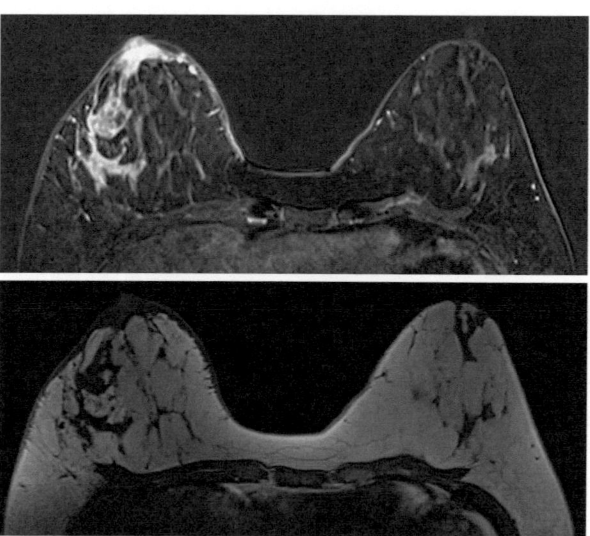

    (a) There is pectoralis muscle involvement.
    (b) There is chest wall involvement.
    (c) There is nipple involvement.
    (d) There are suspicious internal mammary lymph nodes.

14. Which molecular subtype of breast cancer is most likely in a woman with BRCA1 mutation?
    (a) Triple negative.
    (b) Luminal A.
    (c) Luminal B.
    (d) HER2-enriched.

15a. A 38-year-old pregnant woman presents with a palpable breast lump. What is the first-choice imaging modality to work up a palpable breast mass in a pregnant or lactating woman?
    (a) Mammogram.
    (b) MRI.
    (c) Ultrasound.
    (d) The patient should be imaged after she is no longer pregnant or has stopped lactating.

15b. The ultrasound for this woman's palpable lump is shown below. What is the most appropriate next step?

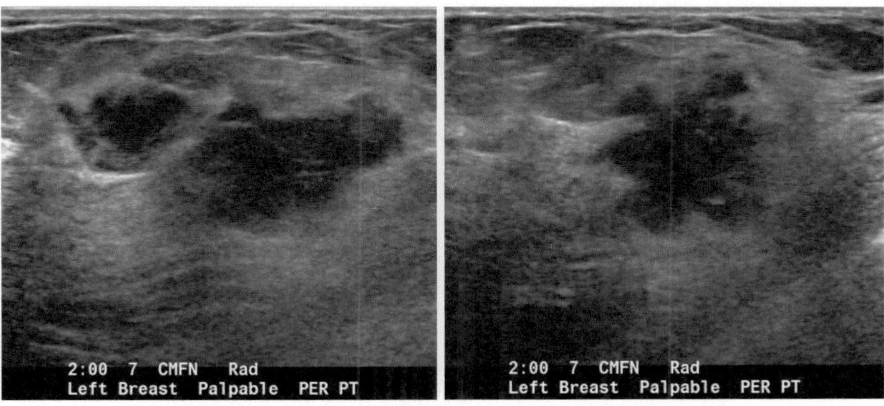

   (a) Close interval ultrasound follow-up in 6 months.
   (b) MRI.
   (c) Biopsy.
   (d) Return after the patient has delivered and stopped breast feeding.

15c. What is the most common presentation of pregnancy-associated breast cancer?
   (a) Nipple discharge.
   (b) Painless breast lump.
   (c) Unilateral breast engorgement.
   (d) Skin thickening and erythema.

16. A type 5 lymph node has what positive predictive value for malignancy?
   (a) 4%
   (b) 29%
   (c) 80%
   (d) 98%.

17. 52-year-old woman with a known invasive ductal carcinoma in the left breast. Ultrasound of the axilla was performed. What is the next step?

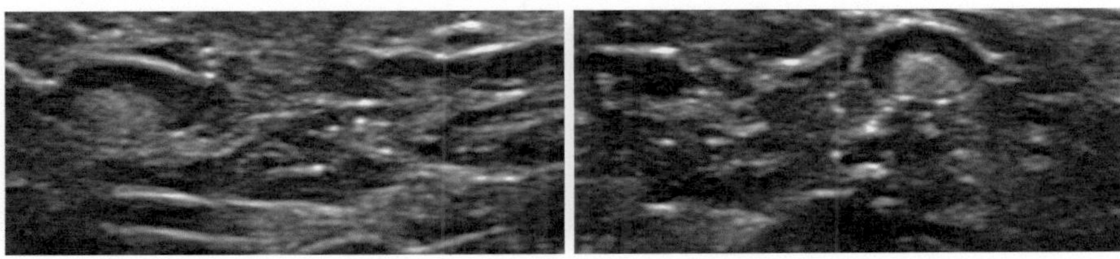

   (a) Ultrasound-guided core needle biopsy of the lymph node.
   (b) Treatment of the primary breast cancer.
   (c) MRI.
   (d) Complete axillary lymph node dissection.

18a. An 88-year-old woman with biopsy-proven DCIS presenting as calcifications underwent surgical resection. The specimen radiograph is shown below. What findings regarding the specimen should be communicated to the surgeon?

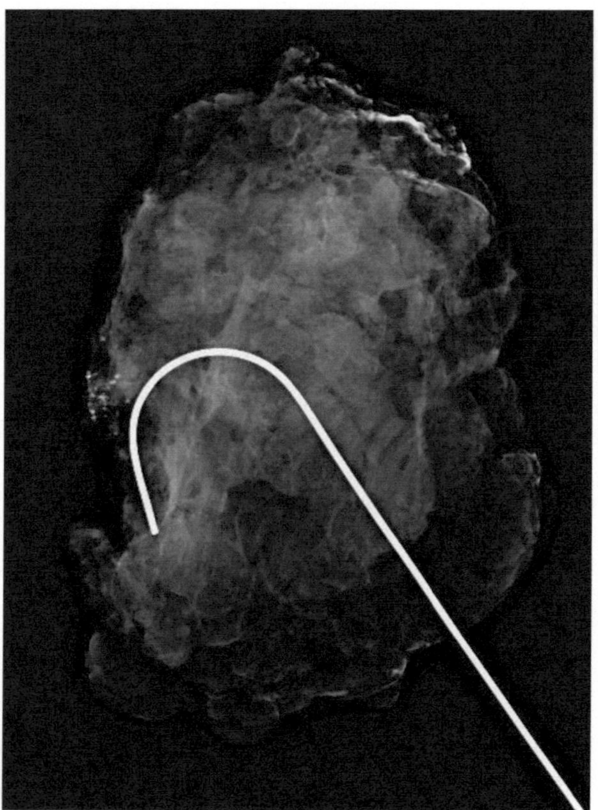

    (a) The specimen is adequate.
    (b) No calcifications are identified in the specimen.
    (c) Measurements of the size of the specimen.
    (d) There are round faint calcifications along the margin.

18b. The surgeon removed additional margins. Due to the presence of extensive calcifications prior to surgery, what is the most appropriate next step prior to starting radiation therapy?
    (a) No additional step is necessary prior to radiation.
    (b) Ultrasound.
    (c) MRI.
    (d) Diagnostic mammogram.

19. The breast radiologist plans to perform mammographically guided seed bracketing in the area of the two biopsy clips that were placed after biopsy of calcifications. What is the optimal distance the seeds should be placed from one another?

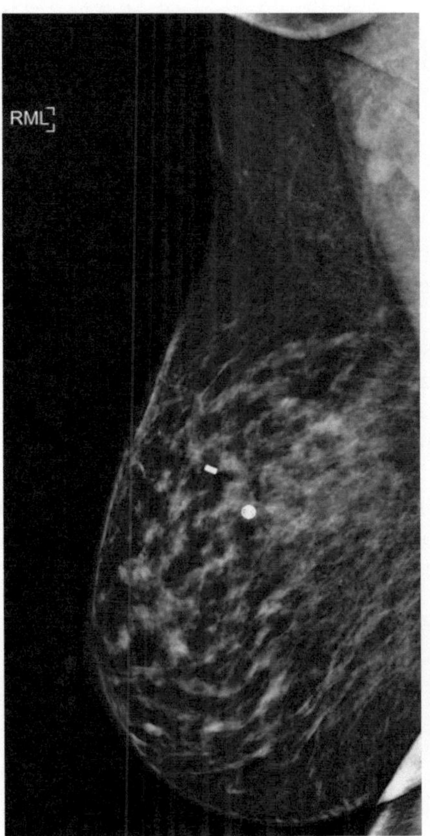

    (a) At most 1 cm.
    (b) 2–3 cm
    (c) The distance between the seeds does not matter; it is important to place the seeds as accurately as possible in every case.
    (d) At least 5 cm.

20. Another patient undergoing radioactive seed placement has a biopsy microclip at the site of microcalcifications that needs to be targeted for surgical removal. What is the optimal placement of the radioactive seed in respect to the microclip?
    (a) Within the prior microclip.
    (b) Adjacent to the site of the prior microclip.
    (c) Do not place the radioactive seed; it is contraindicated in lesions with prior biopsy microclip.
    (d) Anywhere in the lesion of interest; the spatial relationship of the radioactive seed to the biopsy microclip is not important.

21. A 47-year-old woman with infiltrating ductal carcinoma is undergoing right breast lumpectomy with sentinel lymph node biopsy and is referred to you for radioactive seed placement both in the right breast mass and in a suspicious axillary node. What is the best order of seed placement?
    (a) The order of placement does not matter.
    (b) Place a seed in the breast mass first and then the axillary lymph node.
    (c) Place a seed in the axillary lymph node first and then the breast mass.
    (d) Place a seed in the breast mass only; there is no data to support radioactive seed placement in a suspicious axillary lymph node.

22. Another woman is undergoing right breast lumpectomy and sentinel lymph node biopsy for breast cancer. If she is planned for preoperative sentinel node Technetium-99 injection and radioactive seed placement in a suspicious axillary node, which procedure should be done first?
    (a) Radioactive seed placement.
    (b) Sentinel node injection.
    (c) The order does not matter.
    (d) The procedures should be done at the same time.

23a. 58-year-old woman with recently diagnosed invasive ductal carcinoma of the left breast and positive axillary lymph nodes. The image below demonstrates what findings in the left breast?

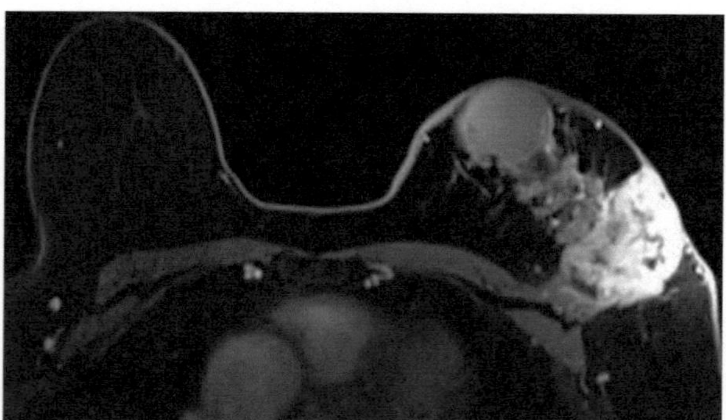

    (a) Irregular masses with a fat plane separating it from the pectoralis muscle.
    (b) Enhancement of the pectoralis muscle, which indicates muscular invasion.
    (c) Irregular masses with involvement of the chest wall.
    (d) Pectoralis muscle involvement, which is considered metastatic disease.

23b. The patient's mammogram is shown below. How would you best characterize her disease?

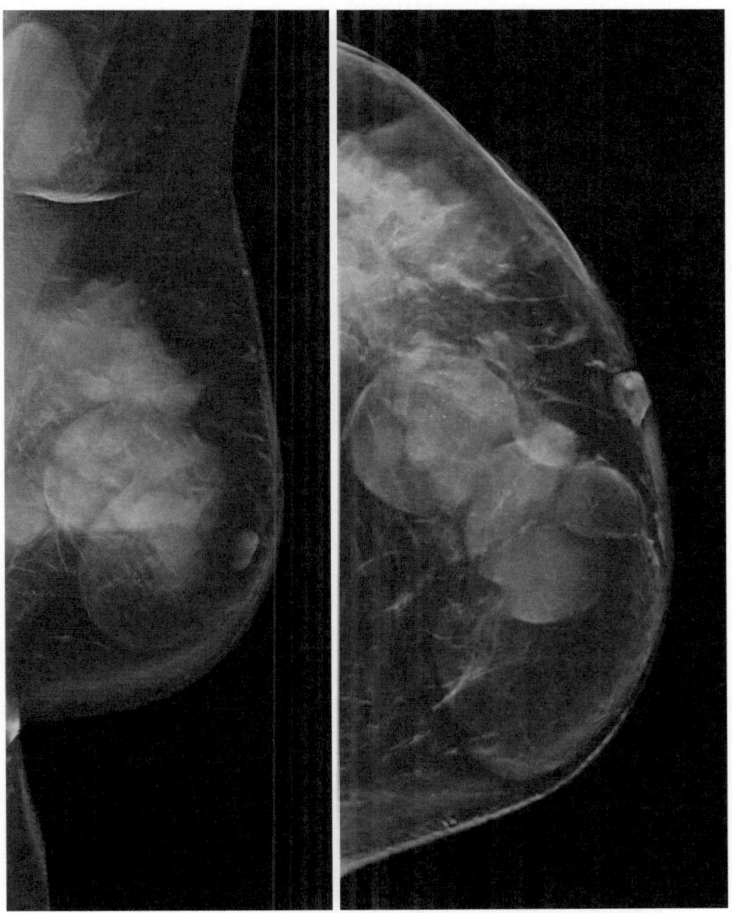

(a) Multilobulated.
(b) Multifocal.
(c) Multicentric.
(d) Multinodular.
(e) Multigeographic.

24. A woman with newly diagnosed left breast cancer underwent FDG PET-CT. The tumor showed avid FDG uptake with high SUV. The tumor most likely has which of the following characteristics?

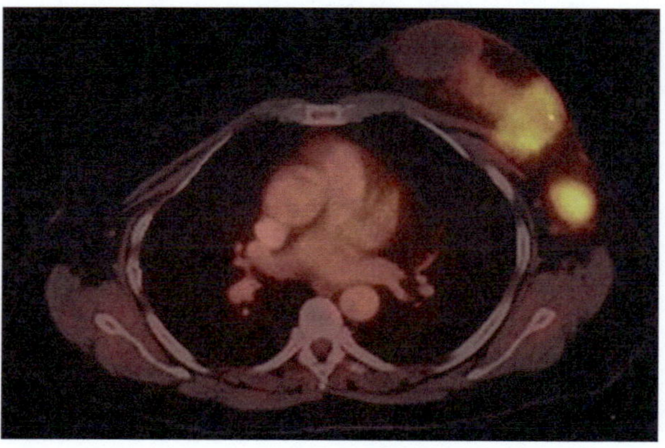

   (a) Triple negative.
   (b) Estrogen receptor positive.
   (c) Lobular cancer.
   (d) Less than 1 cm in size.

25a. A 53-year-old woman with no significant past medical history presents with enlargement and redness of the left breast for the past 2 months, which did not improve after a course of antibiotics. Her MRI is shown below. What is the most likely diagnosis?

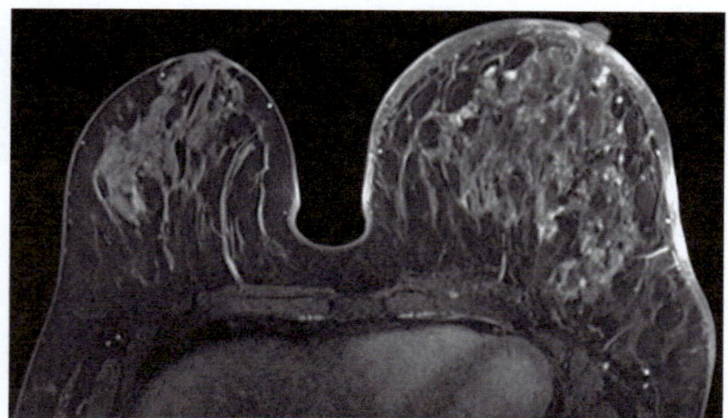

   (a) Infectious mastitis.
   (b) Prior radiation therapy to the region.
   (c) Paget's disease.
   (d) Inflammatory breast cancer.

25b. The patient above had workup and was not found to have any suspicious lymph nodes nor evidence of metastatic disease. What is her TNM stage?
   (a) IIb.
   (b) IIIa.
   (c) IIIb.
   (d) IIIc.

26. For DCIS, what is the TNM stage according to the AJCC staging system eighth edition?
   (a) T1a.
   (b) T1b.
   (c) T1c.
   (d) Tis.

27. Which of the following breast pathologies is included in the current AJCC staging system for breast cancer?
   (a) LCIS.
   (b) Phyllodes tumor.
   (c) Lymphoma.
   (d) Paget's disease of the breast.

28. For which clinical stage of breast cancer should CT chest, abdomen, and pelvis, bone scan, or PET-CT be considered?
   (a) Stage I and above.
   (b) Stage II and above.
   (c) Stage III and above.
   (d) Stage IV and above.

29. A 40-year-old woman presents with a palpable breast lump. Diagnostic mammogram demonstrated a mass. Biopsy was performed and came back as invasive ductal carcinoma. Follow-up mammogram 1 month later was performed (current).

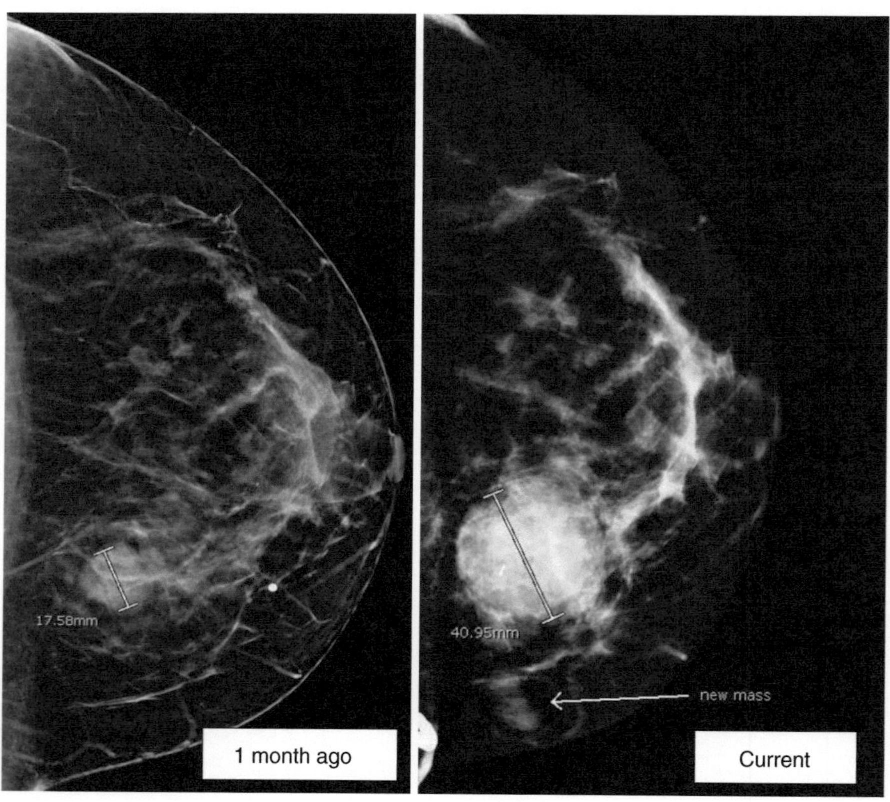

What is the best estimate of the Ki-67 for this patient?
(a) Zero.
(b) Low.
(c) High.
(d) Ki-67 estimation cannot be determined based on these images.

30. For patients with T1 and T2 hormone receptor positive, HER2-negative, and lymph node-negative tumors, what Oncotype DX recurrence score places them in the same AJCC prognostic category as stage I breast cancer?
    (a) Less than 11.
    (b) Less than 21.
    (c) Less than 35.
    (d) Less than 50.

31. Which of the following regarding invasive lobular carcinoma is false?
    (a) It is difficult to determine extent of disease due to its diminished fibrotic reaction.
    (b) It is more often bilateral than invasive ductal carcinoma.
    (c) Preoperative MRI decreases the chances of repeat surgery.
    (d) It accounts for approximately 35% of all breast cancer.

32. Among women with N1 breast cancer receiving neoadjuvant chemotherapy who had two or more sentinel lymph nodes examined in the American College of Surgeons Oncology Group (ACOSOG) Z1071 clinical trial, the false-negative rate of sentinel lymph node biopsy was which of the following?
    (a) 1%
    (b) 4%
    (c) 12.6%
    (d) 74.6%.

33. Which of the following is not an absolute or relative contraindication to whole breast radiation?
    (a) Pregnancy.
    (b) Multicentric disease.
    (c) Prior breast radiation.
    (d) Multifocal disease.

34a. A 33-year-old woman with a history of phyllodes tumor presents with a lump in the right breast. She underwent a diagnostic mammogram and ultrasound.

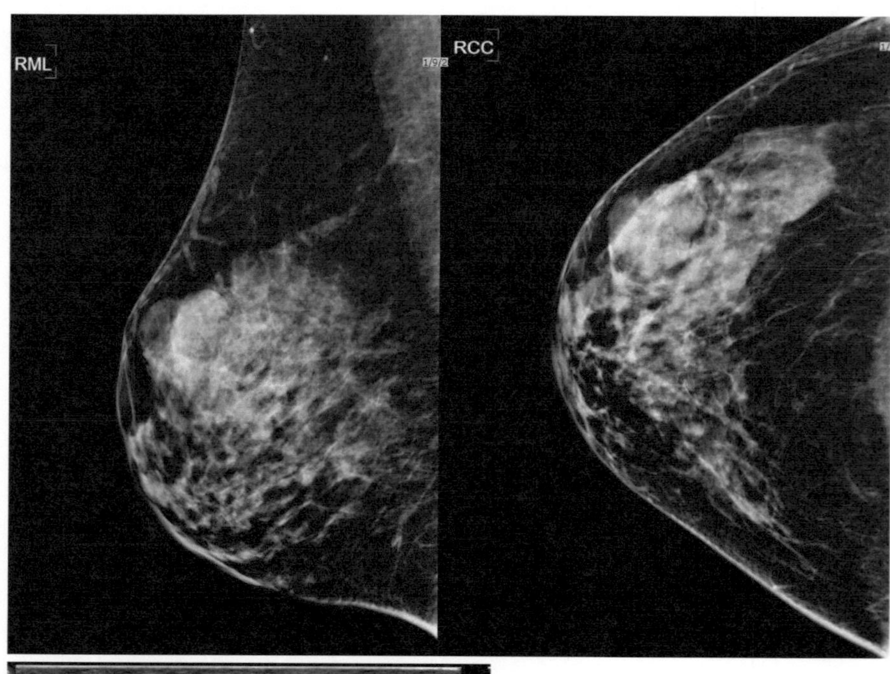

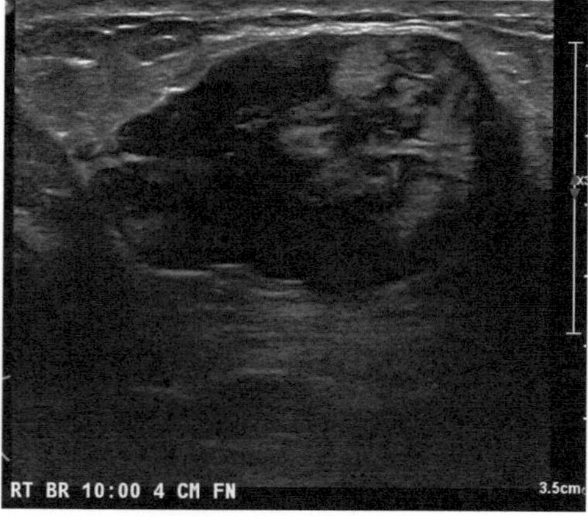

What is the typical treatment for benign phyllodes tumor?
(a) Complete surgical excision with wide margins and chemotherapy.
(b) Complete surgical excision with wide margins.
(c) Complete surgical excision with wide margins, axillary node dissection, chemotherapy, and radiation therapy.
(d) Neoadjuvant chemotherapy followed by wide surgical excision.

34b. What syndrome is associated with the development of phyllodes tumor?
   (a) Li–Fraumeni syndrome.
   (b) Cowdens.
   (c) Von Hippel-Lindau.
   (d) Neurofibromatosis.

35. A 52-year-old woman was recently diagnosed with invasive ductal carcinoma in the left breast. She was found to have an Oncotype DX score of 8. What is the significance of this score?
   (a) The patient has an increased risk of recurrence and should be treated with chemotherapy.
   (b) She has a lower risk of recurrence and may not need chemotherapy.
   (c) She has metastatic disease.
   (d) She has an increased risk of metastatic disease.

36a. A 74-year-old woman was recalled from screening mammogram with tomo-synthesis. Spot compression images were performed at the time of diagnostic imaging and an area of architectural distortion was identified. No ultrasound correlate was identified. What is the next step?

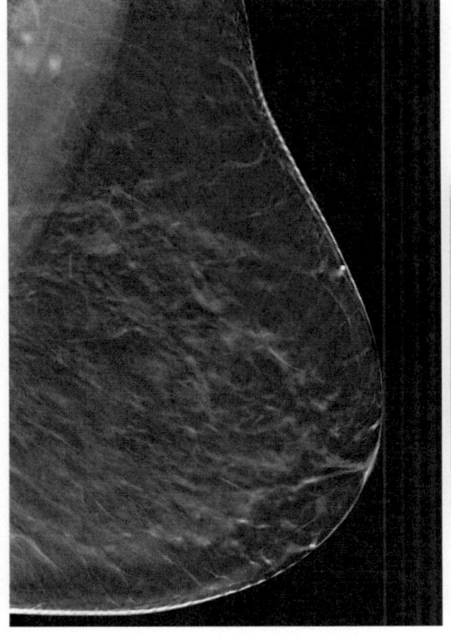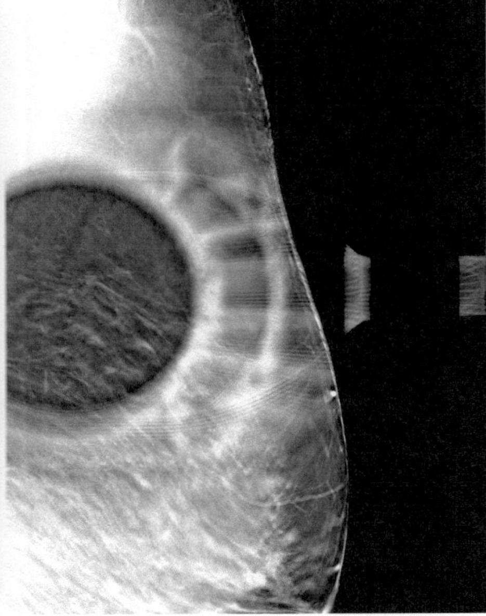

   (a) MRI.
   (b) Contrast-enhanced mammogram.
   (c) Ultrasound-guided biopsy.
   (d) Stereotactic-guided biopsy.
   (e) 6-month follow-up.

36b. What is the malignancy rate of tomosynthesis stereotactic-guided core needle biopsy of architectural distortion without a sonographic correlate?
   (a) 2%
   (b) 19%
   (c) 79%
   (d) 99%.

36c. Surgical excision was performed, and surgical pathology was 2 cm of invasive lobular carcinoma in a background of LCIS. The invasive carcinoma was less than 1 mm from the lateral margin. Which imaging modality would best help evaluate for residual disease prior to re-excision?
   (a) PET-CT.
   (b) Contrast-enhanced mammogram.
   (c) Diagnostic mammogram.
   (d) MRI.
   (e) Ultrasound.

36d. The MRI is shown below. Based on the MRI and the pathology findings, what is the next step?

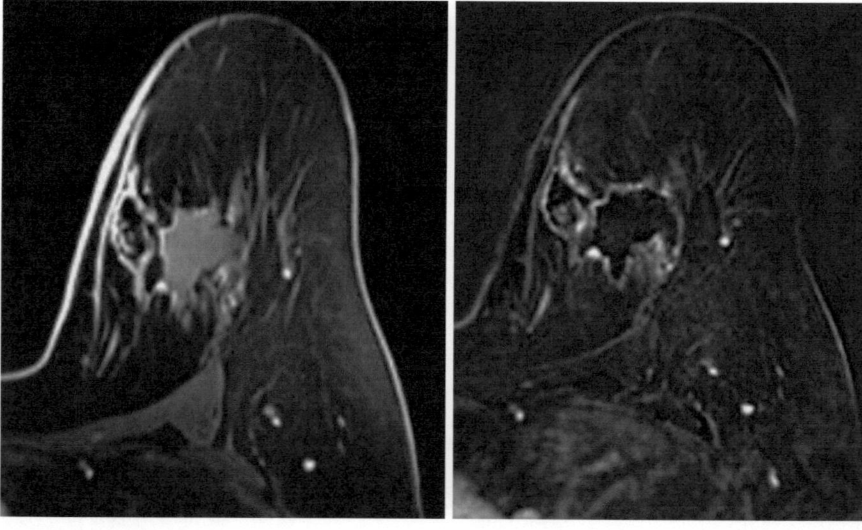

   (a) Re-excision.
   (b) 6-month follow-up MRI
   (c) PET-CT exam.
   (d) Ultrasound.

37. A 66-year-old woman presents with the MRI below. Both lesions were biopsied and showed invasive ductal carcinoma. The primary tumor measures 18 mm, and the satellite lesion measures 7 mm. What is the T of the TNM staging of this patient's breast cancer?

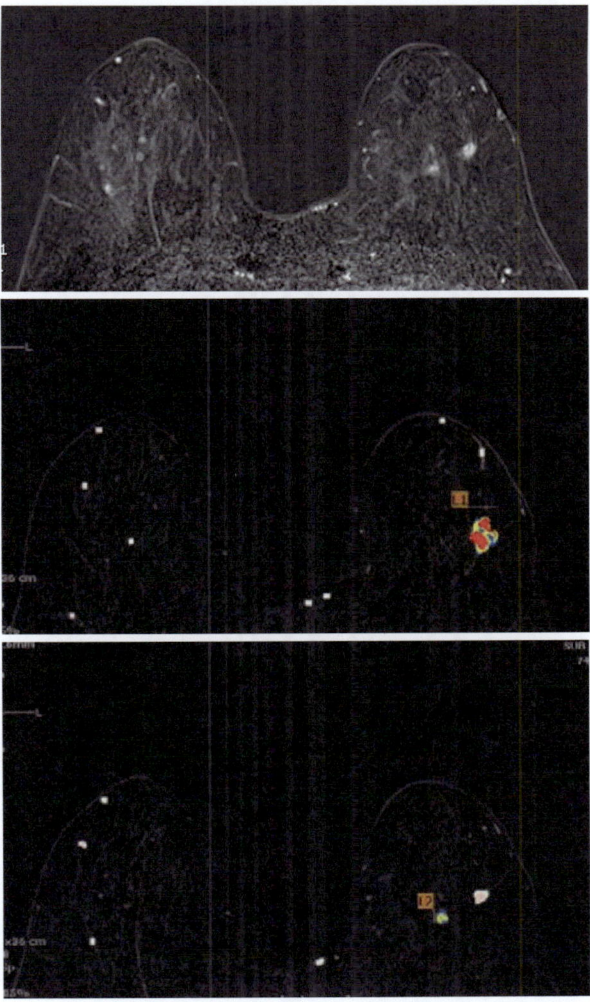

    (a) T1.
    (b) T2.
    (c) T3.
    (d) T4.

38. A mass measures 15 mm on ultrasound but 21 mm on MRI. What is the correct measurement of the mass for TNM staging?
    (a) MRI measurement.
    (b) Ultrasound measurement.
    (c) Both measurements should be averaged.
    (d) The patient should be recalled, and a repeat ultrasound should be performed to obtain a new measurement.

39. Excellent tumor response to neoadjuvant chemotherapy is best seen in which molecular subtypes of breast cancer?
    (a) Triple negative and HER2 positive breast cancer.
    (b) Hormone receptor positive and HER2 negative breast cancer.
    (c) Hormone receptor positive and HER2 positive breast cancer.
    (d) There is no difference among the molecular subtypes of breast cancer for response to neoadjuvant chemotherapy.

40. A 53-year-old woman underwent surgery for DCIS and subsequent MRI images are shown following surgery. What is the most appropriate next step?

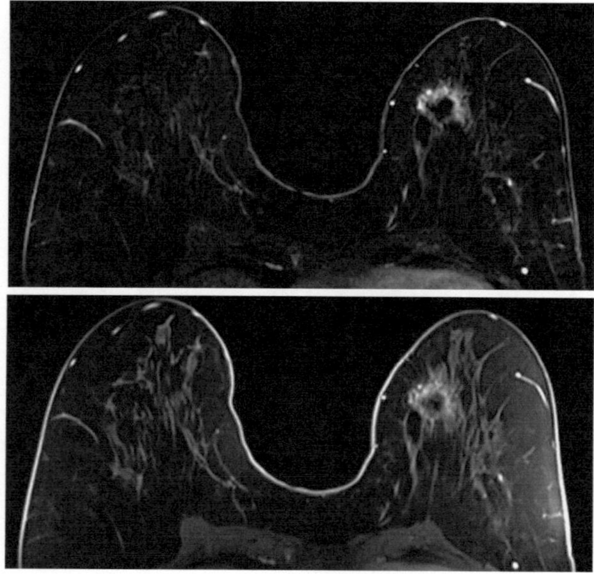

    (a) Radiation.
    (b) Re-excision.
    (c) Routine follow-up.
    (d) PET/CT scan.

41a. 61-year-old woman with a history of right breast cancer. Screening mammogram is shown with comparison images from 2 years prior. What is the most appropriate BI-RADS assessment?

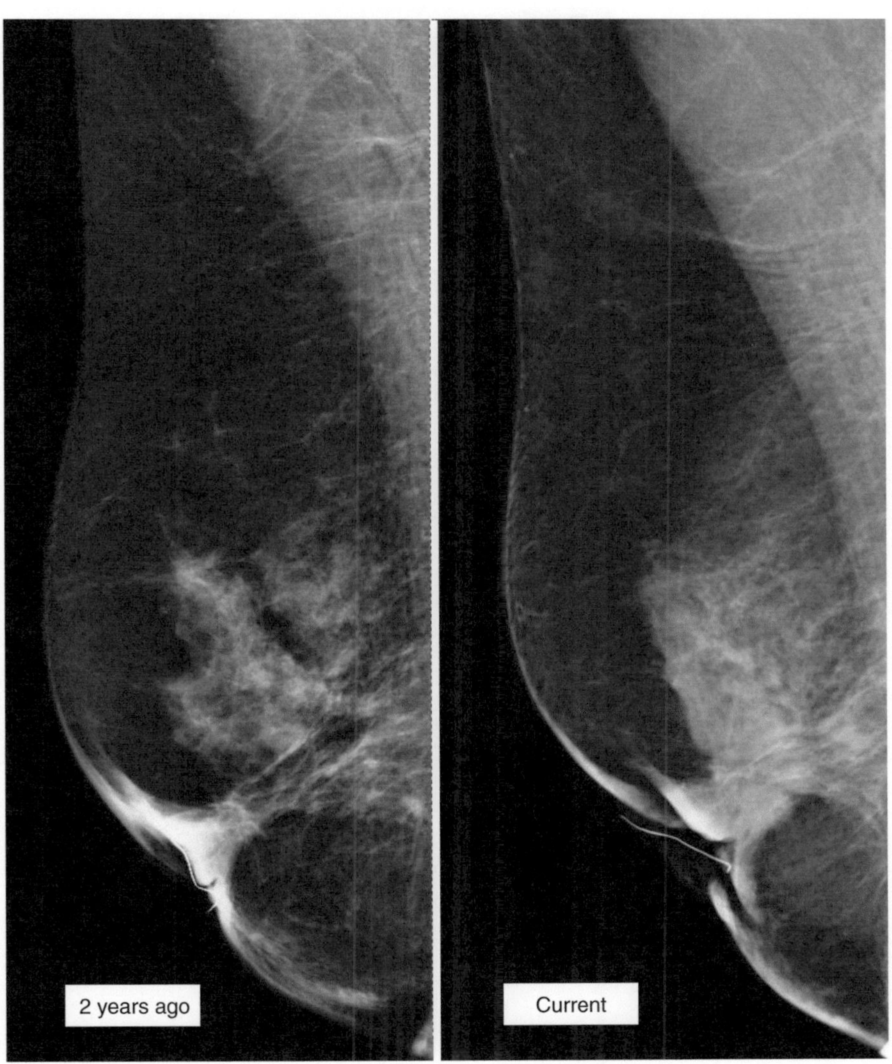

   (a) BI-RADS 0 additional imaging.
   (b) BI-RADS 3 probably benign post-surgical changes.
   (c) BI-RADS 2 benign post-surgical changes.
   (d) BI-RADS 4 suspicious.

41b. The patient was recalled, and additional imaging was performed. What is the most appropriate assessment and management plan?

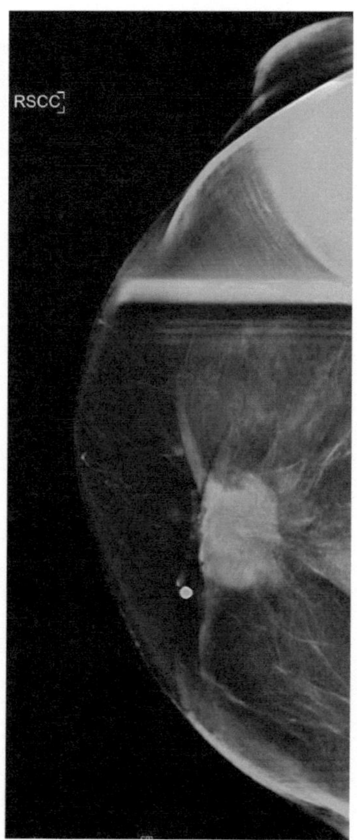

(a) The finding represents benign post-surgical changes; return in 1 year.
(b) The finding represents benign post-surgical changes; return in 6 months.
(c) Ultrasound.
(d) MRI.

41c. An ultrasound was performed, and biopsy showed invasive ductal carcinoma. The patient has already undergone radiation in the past as part of initial breast conserving treatment. What is the traditional treatment for the recurrent cancer at the lumpectomy site?

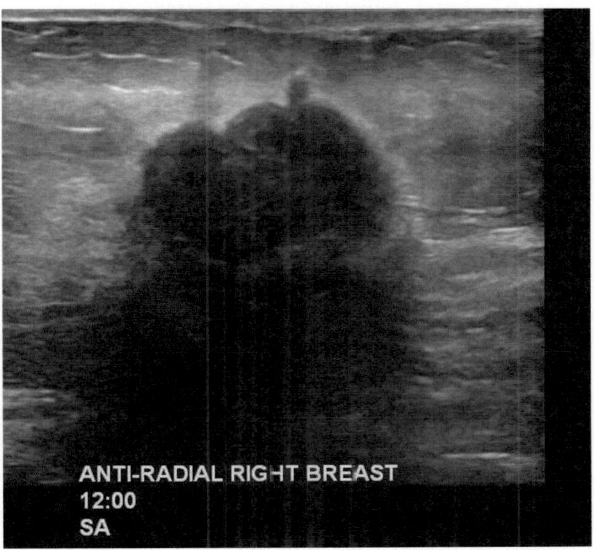

  (a) Radiation therapy.
  (b) Re-excision with radiation.
  (c) Mastectomy.
  (d) No surgical management.

Answers

1. b. 36 mm.

By ultrasound, the index cancer measures 30 mm. By MR, the index cancer measures 36 mm. Including adjacent enhancing foci, the span of suspicious enhancements measures 51 mm in conglomerate.

For TNM staging, the maximum dimension of the dominant mass measured to the nearest millimeter is used. Associated satellites of non-contiguous tumor should not be included in the T measurement but should be reported for surgical planning [1, 2].

Although size measurements vary between ultrasound and MRI, that by MRI is considered more accurate and should therefore be used [1, 2]. In this case, the answer is 36 mm. If a substantial discrepancy between measurements on different imaging modalities exists such that T staging is affected, additional imaging workup and/or biopsy should be performed to better delineate the extent of disease [1, 2].

2. b. Breast MRI.

Breast MRI should be performed for unilateral metastatic axillary adenopathy to assess for underlying breast disease. MRI has been shown to identify the occult primary breast malignancy in 62–86% of women presenting with axillary lymph node metastasis [3]. Better delineation of the extent of disease is important for treatment planning.

3. d. Tumor infiltration begins at the periphery, not the center, of the axillary lymph node.

All other answer choices are true [4].

4. a. I.

The three major sites of lymphatic drainage of the breast are the axillary, interpectoral, and internal mammary lymph nodes. The regional lymph nodes in the breast for staging breast cancer include the axillary, interpectoral, internal mammary, and supraclavicular lymph nodes. Although intramammary lymph nodes are located within the breast, they are considered axillary lymph nodes for staging purposes [2] Please see question 14 in Chap. 5 for additional anatomic details.

The axillary lymph nodes can be classified as level I (low axilla) nodes, which are located lateral to the lateral border of the pectoralis minor muscle. Level II (mid-axilla) nodes are located between the medial and lateral borders of the pectoralis minor muscle and include interpectoral nodes (Rotter's nodes). Level III (apical axilla or infraclavicular) nodes are located medial to the medial margin of the pectoralis minor muscle and inferior to the clavicle. The level III nodes designate a worse prognosis. The internal mammary lymph nodes are located in the intercostal spaces along the edge of the sternum. The supraclavicular lymph nodes are located in the supraclavicular fossa, which is bounded laterally and superiorly by the omohyoid muscle and tendon, medially by the internal jugular vein, and inferiorly by the clavicle and subclavian vein [1, 2]. Please see question 14 in chapter 5 for additional anatomic details.

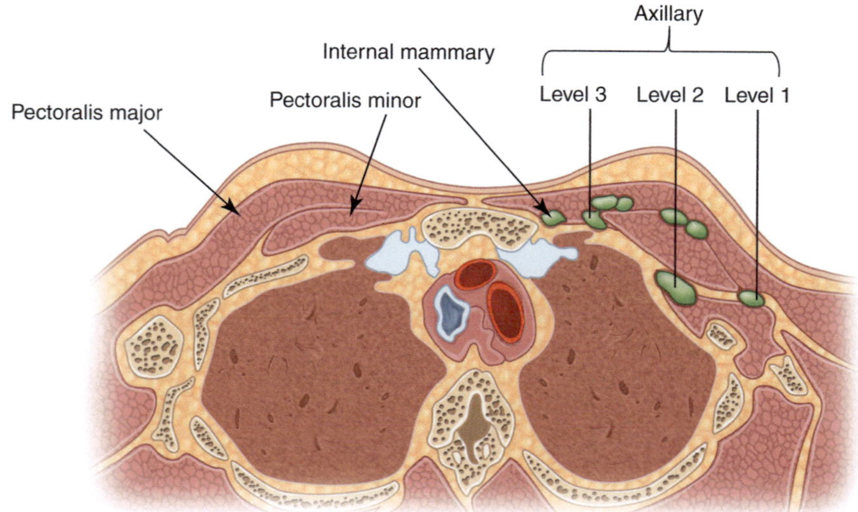

5. d. M1.

Metastasis to cervical lymph nodes, contralateral internal mammary lymph nodes, or contralateral axillary lymph nodes are considered distant metastases, classified as M1 disease [1, 2]. The clinical anatomic nodal staging and the pathological anatomical nodal staging are different, designated as c for clinical and p for pathological. The clinical anatomical nodal staging is more relevant for the radiologist as this is based on imaging findings [1, 2]. Refer to the tables below for an overview of the clinical anatomical nodal and metastasis criteria.

Clinical Regional Lymph nodes (cN)

cN Category	cN Criteria
cNX	Regional lymph nodes cannot be assessed
cN0	No regional lymph node metastasis by clinical exam or imaging
cN1	Metastasis to movable ipsilateral level I or II axillary
cN2	Fixed or matted ipsilateral level I or II axillary nodes (cN2a) or ipsilateral internal mammary nodes in the absence of axillary node metastasis (cN2b)
cN3	Metastases in ipsilateral level III (cN3a) or ipsilateral internal mammary nodes with level I, II axillary nodes (cN3b) or metastases in ipsilateral supraclavicular nodes (cN3c)

Metastasis

M category	M criteria
M0	No clinical or imaging evidence of metastases
cM1	Clinical or imaging evidence of metastases

6. a. Up to 5%.

Normal internal mammary nodes are less than 6 mm in short-axis dimension [2, 4]. Isolated metastases to the internal mammary nodes occur in 1–5% of breast cancers [4]. The metastases usually come from medial or deep lesions. Usually, metastases to the internal mammary nodes occur after a tumor has metastasized to the axilla, which is considered N3b disease [2, 4]. When there are isolated metastases to the internal mammary nodes, it is considered N2b disease [2, 4].

Surgical dissection is not performed for internal mammary nodal metastases because there is no survival benefit and there is increased morbidity [4]. In such cases, radiation treatment planning is tailored to include the internal mammary nodes. Standard tangential external beam radiation therapy of the breast does not typically include these nodes [4].

7a. b. MRI.

Paget's disease of the breast is a rare malignancy of the breast and accounts for approximately 1–3% of all breast cancers [5]. The clinical presentation of Paget's disease of the nipple includes itching, eczema, and erythema of the nipple and areola, nipple erosion, ulceration, or retraction, scaly or flaky skin, or isolated bloody discharge from the nipple. Mammography may be unrevealing in 50% of cases [5]. If the mammogram and ultrasound are negative, MRI is recommended as a next step because 90% of cases of Paget's disease of the nipple are associated with an additional underlying breast malignancy [5].

7b. a. Paget's disease.

The MRI image shows asymmetric enhancement of the right nipple and an enhancing mass in the outer right breast. The MR findings of the right nipple in conjunction with the history are consistent with Paget's disease. If the mammogram and ultrasound are negative, MRI is recommended as a next step [5].

7c. d. MRI-guided biopsy.

In addition to the asymmetric enhancement of the right nipple, there is an enhancing mass in the outer right breast on MRI. This finding is suspicious and should undergo biopsy. Over 90% of Paget's disease cases are associated with either ductal carcinoma in situ (DCIS) or invasive carcinoma [5]. This woman underwent mastectomy with surgical pathology showing both Paget's disease and invasive ductal carcinoma.

8. c. DCIS.

Ninety percent of cases of Paget's disease of the nipple are associated with an additional underlying breast malignancy, most frequently DCIS in the lactiferous ducts of the nipple-areolar complex [5]. Paget's disease can also be associated with DCIS or invasive cancer elsewhere in the breast [5].

9. a. Partial response.

Based on Response Evaluation Criteria in Solid Tumors (RECIST), the resolution of all lesions indicates complete response [6]. A decrease in the maximum diameter of target lesions by greater than or equal to 30% compared with baseline indicates partial response. An increase in diameter of greater than or equal to 20% is consistent with progression of disease. When the criteria for neither partial response nor progression of disease is met, it is considered stable disease [6]. On the initial MRI (Fig. A), there is extensive non-mass enhancement throughout the right breast. On her subsequent MRI (Fig. B), the non-mass enhancement has decreased by greater than 30%, consistent with partial response.

10. d. MRI.

MRI is the most accurate imaging modality for assessing tumor response to neoadjuvant therapy after treatment [7–9]. A meta-analysis that compared MRI and FDG PET/CT for evaluation of pathologic response to neoadjuvant chemotherapy in patients with breast cancer found that when performed after completion of neoadjuvant therapy, MRI outperformed FDG PET/CT through its higher sensitivity (0.88 vs 0.57) [7].

11a. b. BI-RADS 0. Incomplete. Recall the patient.

Although the patient has undergone prior benign surgical excision and prior benign biopsy, there are calcifications that require further evaluation. The patient should be recalled for magnification views of the calcifications.

11b. d. Ultrasound.

There are suspicious grouped fine pleomorphic calcifications in the lower outer left breast. There is an additional smaller group of suspicious calcifications seen in the medial left breast (magnification views not shown). Although the suspicious calcifications can be biopsied by stereotactic guidance, an ultrasound should first be performed to evaluate for an underlying sonographic mass representing a potential invasive component, which can be targeted by ultrasound for biopsy.

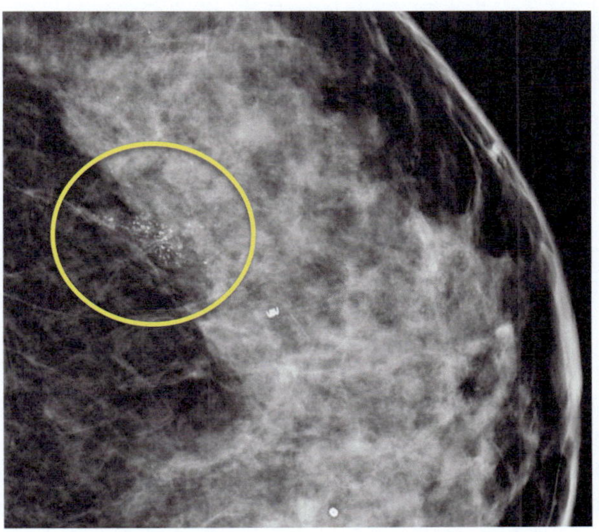

11c. b. Ultrasound-guided core biopsy.

The ultrasound shows an irregular hypoechoic mass with calcifications within and adjacent to the mass. The constellation of findings is worrisome for malignancy, and an ultrasound-guided core needle biopsy should be performed. Although the calcifications can be targeted by stereotactic guidance, the mass seen on ultrasound is worrisome for an invasive component and should be targeted by ultrasound guidance. Specimen radiograph of the tissue obtained from ultrasound-guided biopsy can be obtained to confirm sampling of calcifications.

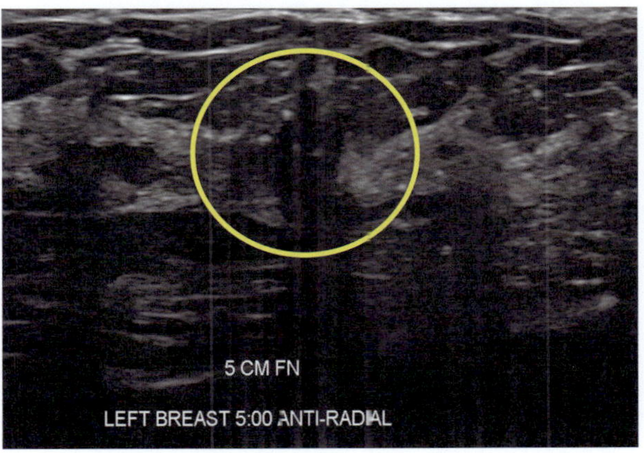

11d. c. Multifocal disease.

Multifocal disease involves one quadrant of the breast, while multicentric disease involves two or more quadrants of the breast or lesions that are greater than 5 cm apart [10]. Multicentric breast cancer typically is not amenable to breast conservation therapy due to distance of lesions and resultant distortion of the breast; mastectomy is the standard of care in these cases [10]. MRI is more sensitive than mammography for the detection of multifocal or multicentric disease in dense breasts [11]. If the patient desires breast conservation therapy, an additional area in another quadrant should be biopsied to document extent of disease [11].

12. c. 30–40%.

Incidentally detected FDG-avid breast soft tissue lesions have a 30–40% chance of malignancy, including unsuspected primary breast cancer, metastases to the breast, and breast lymphoma [12]. These lesions should be further evaluated with dedicated mammography and/or ultrasound. Lesions with suspicious characteristics on subsequent workup warrant targeted biopsy [12].

13. c. There is nipple involvement.

The MRI shows extensive non-mass enhancement in the outer right breast, which extends to the nipple. There is suspicious enhancement of the nipple itself. Breast cancer invasion of the nipple-areolar complex is considered skin involvement, T4 disease, and precludes nipple-sparing mastectomy [13]. The MRI does not show pectoralis muscle, chest wall, or internal mammary lymph node involvement.

14. a. Triple negative.

Breast cancers in BRCA1 positive women are associated with the triple negative molecular subtype, whereas those in BRCA2 positive women are associated with the luminal B molecular subtype [14–16]. BRCA1 carriers are more likely to present with breast cancer at a younger age, have higher nuclear grade, worse histologic grade, earlier development of metastasis, and decreased survival compared to BRCA2 carriers [14].

Molecular subtype	ER/PR	HER2	Associations
Luminal A	ER (+) and/or PR (+)	(−)	Favorable prognosis, low Ki-67 (<14%), responds to endocrine therapy
Luminal B	ER (+) and/or PR (+)	(−) or (+)	BRCA2, high Ki-67 (>14%), endocrine therapy not reliable
HER2-enriched	(−)	(+)	Responds to trastuzumab (Herceptin) and responds to anthracycline-based chemotherapy
Basal like	(−)	(−)	Most often triple negative, often seen in BRCA1, common in African American women, sensitive to platinum-based chemotherapy and PARP inhibitors

15a. c. Ultrasound.

Ultrasound is the first-choice imaging modality in a pregnant or lactating woman with a palpable breast mass [17]. Ultrasound does not utilize ionizing radiation and has a high sensitivity for detecting breast cancer [17]. Ultrasound has a reported sensitivity and negative predictive value of 100% in these women [17].

If suspicious findings are seen on ultrasound, a full workup with mammography is warranted to help identify calcifications and to delineate extent of disease [17].

15b. c. Biopsy.

The ultrasound shows suspicious irregular hypoechoic masses with angular, microlobulated, and indistinct margins. Ultrasound-guided biopsy is the most appropriate next step. In this case, the biopsy result was triple negative invasive ductal carcinoma with DCIS.

Pregnancy-associated breast cancer is the most common malignancy in pregnancy and is the most common cause of cancer-related death in pregnant and lactating women [17]. The imaging features have been reported to be similar to those of non-gestational breast cancers [17]. Biopsy of any new solid mass detected on ultrasound during pregnancy should be considered to avoid a delay in diagnosis [17].

15c. b. Painless breast lump.

The most common presentation of pregnancy-associated breast cancer is a painless, palpable breast lump [17]. Other less common clinical presentations include unilateral breast enlargement with skin thickening, focal pain, and nipple discharge associated with a mass. The "milk rejection" sign has been described, in which the infant refuses to nurse from the affected breast [17].

16. b. 29%.

Axillary lymph nodes can be classified according to cortical morphologic features. Usually types 1–3 can be considered benign. Type 1 lymph nodes are hyperechoic with almost no discernible cortex. Type 2 lymph nodes have a uniformly thin hypoechoic cortex of <3 mm, while type 3 lymph nodes have a uniformly thick cortex of >3 mm and may have minor surface lobulations. Type 4 lymph nodes are hypoechoic with generalized cortical lobulation [18]. Type 5 lymph nodes demonstrate asymmetric focal hypoechoic cortical lobulation and have a positive predictive value of 29% [18]. Type 6 are completely hypoechoic with no hilum, and its positive predictive value for malignancy is 58% [18].

17. b. Treatment of the primary breast cancer.

The images show an axillary lymph node with normal morphology, including reniform shape and central echogenic hilum. Although normal-appearing lymph nodes can still harbor micrometastases, there are no suspicious imaging findings to warrant biopsy or dissection.

Evaluation of axillary lymph node involvement in breast cancer is an integral part of determining extent of disease for treatment planning [19]. Based on the American College of Surgeons Oncology Group (ACSOG) Z0011 trial, current recommendations are to offer sentinel lymph node biopsy in lieu of complete axillary lymph node dissection to select women with stage T1 or T2 tumors without palpable lymphadenopathy [19]. In this trial, complete axillary lymph node dissection did not improve survival and resulted in increased morbidity [19].

18a. d. There are round faint calcifications along the margin.

Prior to localization, all prior breast imaging should be reviewed carefully [20]. This patient had biopsy-proven DCIS presenting as extensive calcifications. At the time of specimen review, the radiologist should inform the surgeon whether the targeted lesion and/or biopsy microclip(s) are seen in the specimen and whether the specimen margins appear adequate by imaging [20]. The faint calcifications along the margin of the specimen should be communicated to the surgeon, as these appear suspicious and warrant wider excision. The final pathology on this specimen did have positive surgical margins.

18b. d. Diagnostic mammogram.

Due to the large extent of calcifications that were biopsy-proven as DCIS, the treatment team should obtain a post-surgical, pre-radiation diagnostic mammogram with magnification views to assess for any residual calcifications. Although MRI can be performed to assess for residual disease, the area of calcifications may not enhance on MRI.

19. b. 2–3 cm.

A separation of at least 2–3 cm between radioactive seeds enables the surgeon to better detect each site and to remove both seeds in one specimen [21]. Close proximity of seeds can limit intraoperative detection of separate radioactive sites, leading to an unrecovered seed [21].

20. b. Adjacent to the site of the prior microclip.

A preoperative radioactive seed should be placed adjacent to a prior biopsy microclip. Placing a seed at the site of the prior microclip can result in it residing in the gelatinous substance of the microclip, making intraoperative recovery of the seed more difficult due to the slippery nature of the bioabsorbable polymer surrounding the metallic microclip [21]. Intraoperatively, the microclip, seed, or both can be expelled from the surgical bed or suctioned out without the surgeon's knowledge [21].

21. c. Place a seed in the axillary lymph node first and then the breast mass,

A radioactive seed should be placed first in the axillary lymph node, with confirmation of placement using a Geiger counter, before any additional seeds are placed in the breast, since its location in the axilla may be beyond the field of view of the post-procedure mammogram [21].

22. a. Radioactive seed placement.

A radioactive seed should be placed in the suspicious axillary lymph node before sentinel node injection of Technetium-99 [21]. Since the seed may be beyond the field of view of the post-procedure mammogram, its placement can be confirmed with a Geiger counter [21]. However, if the seed is placed after Technetium-99 injection, the Geiger counter cannot distinguish between radioactivity from the seed and radioactivity from the Technitium-99 injection [21].

23a. b. Enhancement of the pectoralis muscle, which indicates muscular invasion.

The MRI shows invasion of the pectoralis muscle, which is not considered chest wall and does not affect TNM staging [2]. Pectoralis muscle involvement may be seen as direct muscle enhancement with loss of the fat plane between tumor and muscle [2, 22]. Obliteration of the fat plane without associated muscle enhancement does not necessarily indicate pectoralis muscle involvement [2, 22]. Pectoralis muscle involvement is important to describe because it may affect surgical approach [2, 22]. In contrast, chest wall invasion is involvement of ribs, intercostal muscles, and/or serratus anterior muscle, and upgrades the stage to T4 [2].

23b. c. Multicentric disease.

Multicentric disease involves two or more quadrants of the breast or consists of lesions that are more than 5 cm apart, as seen in this case [10, 11]. Multifocal disease involves multiple masses involving one quadrant of the breast [10, 11]. MRI is more sensitive than mammography for the detection of multifocal or multicentric disease in dense breasts [11]. Multilobulated, multinodular, and multigeographic are not standardized descriptors for breast cancer tumor distribution.

24. a. Triple negative.

Higher FDG uptake and SUV can be seen in more aggressive disease, including high grade and estrogen receptor negative cancer such as triple negative cancer [23]. False-negative PET-CT results can be seen in tumors that are less than 1 cm due to small size and in lobular cancers [23]. False-positive uptake can be seen in infectious and inflammatory processes, post-surgical changes, radiation necrosis, and proliferative changes such as gynecomastia and lactation, and uncommonly fibroadenomas [23].

25a. d. Inflammatory breast cancer.

The main differential diagnosis for inflammatory breast cancer (IBC) is mastitis with or without associated abscess [24]. If the patient fails appropriate antibiotic treatment or has an incomplete response to antibiotics, then IBC should be considered [24]. Both clinical evidence of inflammatory disease and tissue diagnosis of malignancy are required to confirm the diagnosis of IBC [1, 24]. On this MRI, there is marked diffuse skin thickening of the enlarged left breast with diffuse asymmetric enhancement.

25b. c. IIIb.

The AJCC defines inflammatory breast cancer (IBC) as a clinical-pathologic entity with diffuse skin erythema and edema (peau d'orange) involving at least one-third of the skin of the breast with symptoms occurring for less than 6 months [1, 22]. IBC typically progresses rapidly over weeks to months due to tumor emboli obstructing flow in the dermal lymphatic vessels [22]. T4d staging is reserved for disease that meets criteria for IBC regardless of tumor size [1, 22].

The staging system for breast cancer is shown in the chart below.

Anatomic staging is utilized when biomarker tests are not available [1, 2]. If favorable, biomarker tests can decrease the staging by one level [1].

Tumor Stage by TNM Grade

Stage	TNM
0	Tis, N0, M0
IA	T1, N0, M0
IB	T0, N1mi, M0
	T1, N1mi, M0
IIA	T0, N1, M0
	T1, N1, M0
	T2, N0, M0
IIB	T2, N1, M0
	T3, N0, M0
IIIA	T0, N2, M0
	T1, N2, M0
	T2, N2, M0
	T3, N1, M0
	T3, N2, M0
IIIB	T4, N0, M0
	T4, N1, M0
	T4, N2, M0
IIIC	Any T, N3, M0
IV	Any T, any N with M1

Definition of Primary Tumor (T) for Clinical and Pathological Staging. All measurements should be taken of the greatest dimension of the tumor.

T category	T criteria
TX	Primary tumor unable to be assessed
T0	No evidence of primary tumor
Tis	DCIS
	Paget disease of the nipple (not associated with invasive carcinoma or DCIS in the ipsilateral breast)
T1	Tumor less than or equal to 20 mm
T1mi	Tumor less than or equal to 1 mm

T category	T criteria
T1a	Tumor greater than 1 mm but less than or equal to 5 mm (please note that any measurement greater than 1–1.9 mm should be rounded up to 2 mm)
T1b	Tumor greater than 5 mm but less than or equal to 10 mm
T1c	Tumor greater than 10 mm but less than or equal to 20 mm
T2	Tumor greater than 20 mm but less than or equal to 50 mm
T3	Tumor greater than 50 mm
T4	Tumor extension to the chest wall
T4a	Extension to the chest wall only
T4b	Ulceration and/or ipsilateral macroscopic satellite nodules and/or edema of the skin that does not meet the criteria for inflammatory cancer
T4c	Both T4a and T4b
T4d	Inflammatory breast cancer

Clinical Regional Lymph nodes (cN)

cN Category	cN Criteria
cNX	Regional lymph nodes cannot be assessed
cN0	No regional lymph node metastasis by clinical exam or imaging
cN1	Metastasis to movable ipsilateral level I or II axillary
cN2	Fixed or matted ipsilateral level I or II axillary nodes (cN2a) or ipsilateral internal mammary nodes in the absence of axillary node metastasis (cN2b)
cN3	Metastases in ipsilateral level III (cN3a) or ipsilateral internal mammary nodes with level I, II axillary nodes (cN3b) or metastases in ipsilateral supraclavicular nodes (cN3c)

Metastasis

M category	M criteria
M0	No clinical or imaging evidence of metastases
cM1	Clinical or imaging evidence of metastases

26. d. Tis.

DCIS and Paget's disease (without associated invasive carcinoma or DCIS) are categorized as Tis [1, 2]. T1 disease is invasive carcinomas subcategorized as T1mi (tumor size ≤1 mm), T1a (tumor size >1 mm but ≤5 mm), T1b (tumor size >5 mm but ≤10 mm), and T1c (tumor size >10 mm but ≤20 mm) [1, 2]. Previous editions included LCIS in the Tis category, but in the AJCC eighth edition update, LCIS is excluded [1, 2].

27. d. Paget's disease of the breast.

Paget's disease without associated invasive carcinoma or DCIS is classified as Tis in the current AJCC staging system for breast cancer [1, 2]. LCIS is no longer included in the Tis category but rather is considered a benign entity that confers a higher lifetime risk of future breast cancer [1, 2]. Phyllodes tumor and lymphoma are not included in the AJCC staging system for breast cancer [1, 2].

28. c. Stage III and above.

According to the guidelines of the National Comprehensive Cancer Network, for patients with clinical stage I to stage IIB disease, imaging studies should be directed by signs or symptoms (i.e., bone scan should be performed if the patient reports bone pain or has an elevated serum alkaline phosphatase) [2]. For patients with clinical stage IIIA disease, CT or MRI chest, abdomen, and pelvis, bone scan, or PET-CT using fluorine 18 fluorodeoxyglucose or radioactive sodium fluoride should be considered [2].

29. c. High.

The rapid progression of disease over 1 month manifesting as increase in size of the index cancer and development of an adjacent new mass is consistent with a high Ki-67 level. The Ki-67 corresponds to the tumor proliferation status [25]. A higher Ki-67 is associated with a worse clinical outcome and changes in Ki-67 during neoadjuvant chemotherapy are used to assess treatment response [25].

Ki-67 plays a role in differentiating luminal A and luminal B molecular subtypes of breast cancer [25]. Both luminal types are hormone receptor positive, but type A has a lower Ki-67 less than 14, and type B has a higher Ki-67 greater than or equal to 14 [25]. Luminal A tends to be less responsive to chemotherapy but is responsive to endocrine therapy [25]. Luminal B treatment may involve both endocrine therapy and chemotherapy, as well as molecular targeted drugs [25].

30. a. Less than 11.

The Oncotype DX recurrence score is a validated multigene panel used for hormone-positive, node-negative tumors to evaluate the benefit of implementing adjuvant chemotherapy in addition to endocrine therapy [2]. It evaluates 16 genes and 5 reference genes to predict the likelihood of recurrence in patients undergoing endocrine therapy alone, categorizing each patient into low, intermediate, or high-risk categories for recurrence [2]. An Oncotype DX recurrence score of less than 18 denotes a patient with a low risk of recurrence, predicting no additional benefit of chemotherapy. In the eighth edition of the AJCC staging system for breast cancer, the incorporation of the Oncotype DX recurrence score can potentially downstage tumors, as in this case [2].

31. d.

Invasive lobular carcinoma accounts for approximately 5-15% of all breast cancer [26].

32. c. 12.6%.

Sentinel lymph node surgery provides reliable nodal staging information with less morbidity than axillary lymph node dissection for patients with clinically node-negative breast cancer (N0) [27]. However, the ACOSOG Z1071 clinical trial demonstrated a false-negative rate of 12.6% in those initially presenting with biopsy-proven N1 breast cancer receiving neoadjuvant chemotherapy [28]. The increased false-negative threshold greater than 10% in this patient population shows that sentinel lymph node surgery alone is not appropriate in N1 breast cancer receiving neoadjuvant chemotherapy [28]. For these patients, preoperative localization of the biopsy-proven metastatic axillary lymph node with targeted axillary dissection is an option [28].

33. d. Multifocal disease.

Relative contraindications for breast radiation include pregnancy, extensive multicentric disease, collagen vascular disease, prior breast radiation, or anticipated poor cosmetic result [29].

34a. b. Complete surgical excision with wide margins.

Phyllodes tumors account for approximately 1% of all breast neoplasms [30]. Classically, they occur in women in their fifth decade and can be quite large, up to 5 cm, when first detected. Phyllodes tumors usually present as a dense round or oval, non-calcified mass and can mimic a fibroadenoma. Occasionally, they can contain cystic spaces [31]. Phyllodes tumors are fibroepithelial neoplasms with both stromal and epithelial elements. They have a characteristic leaf-like architecture with abundant cellular stroma [30, 31].
Phyllodes tumors are subclassified as benign, borderline, or malignant. Approximately 25% of phyllodes tumors are malignant, and approximately 13–40% of the malignant subtype can metastasize [32]. Metastasis is usually via hematogenous spread for the borderline and malignant types [30].

All phyllodes tumors should be completely excised, with negative surgical margins greater than or equal to 1 cm [30]. Axillary lymph node dissection is not necessary. Local recurrence ranges from 5% to 30% in benign phyllodes and up to 65% in borderline and malignant phyllodes if there is incomplete excision [30].

Adjuvant radiation therapy may treat borderline or malignant tumors, but not usually used in cases of benign phyllodes tumors. Chemotherapy is used for certain patients with large, high-risk, or recurrent malignant phyllodes tumors [32].

34b. a. Li–Fraumeni Syndrome [32].

35. b. She has a lower risk of recurrence and may not need chemotherapy.

The Oncotype DX recurrence score is a validated multigene panel used for hormone-positive, node-negative tumors to evaluate the benefit of adjuvant chemotherapy in addition to endocrine therapy [2, 23]. The large randomized prospective trials showed recurrence of less than 10% at 10 years in patients with a score of 18 or less [23]. Data suggest that patients with a score of 10 or less, as in this patient's case, have an overall survival of 98%, with 99.3% metastasis-free disease at 5 years [23].

36a. d. Stereotactic-guided biopsy.

On the provided mammograms, an area of architectural distortion is identified in the upper left breast. Although a sonographic correlate was not identified, this persisted on the spot compression images and therefore is still suspicious and should be categorized as BI-RADS 4. The lack of sonographic correlate should not preclude biopsy of a suspicious mammographic finding [33]. Since the distortion is identified mammographically, this can be biopsied by stereotactic guidance.

36b. b. 19%.

In a study of tomosynthesis-guided biopsy of architectural distortion without a sonographic correlate, the cancer yield was 19% [32]. This study suggests that a high index of suspicion should be maintained for distortions, and biopsy is warranted [33].

36c. d. MRI.

Breast MRI is a sensitive tool in the detection of residual disease in a patient with positive or close surgical margins [34]. The other imaging modalities listed are not as sensitive.

36d. a. Re-excision.

There is suspicious nodular enhancement along the periphery of the lumpectomy bed (curved red arrow). The patient should undergo re-excision, especially in the context of close surgical margin on the surgical specimen. Re-excision was performed, and atypical lobular carcinoma and lobular carcinoma in situ were seen. No residual invasive carcinoma was identified on re-excision in this case.

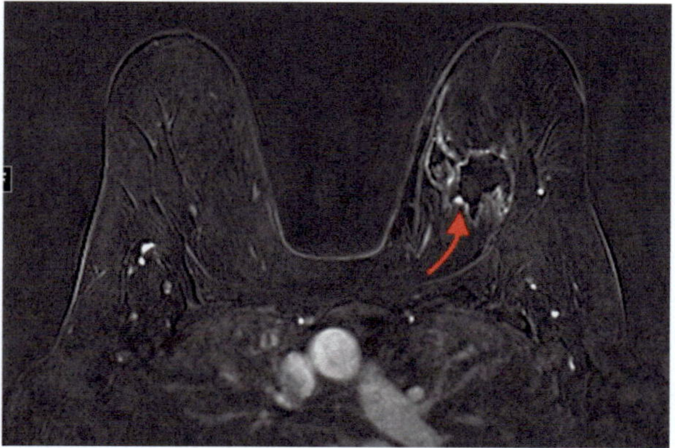

37. a. T1.

The index tumor defines the T in TNM staging [1, 2]. The satellite lesion is not included in the measurement [1, 2]. A T1 tumor measures less than or equal to

20 mm. A T2 lesion is greater than 20 mm but less than 50 mm. A T3 tumor is greater than 50 mm. A T4 tumor has direct extension to the chest wall and/or the skin with macroscopic changes [1, 2].

38. a. MRI measurement.

The largest tumor dimension should be measured on all imaging modalities [1]. If there is a discrepancy between the ultrasound and the MRI measurements, the MRI measurement should be used as it is considered more accurate [1]. If there is a large variation in measurements, such as due to additional disease revealed by one imaging modality, additional biopsies should be considered to document the true extent of disease [1].

39. a. Triple negative and HER2 positive breast cancer.

Tumor response to neoadjuvant chemotherapy can provide prognostic information as pathologic complete response after neoadjuvant chemotherapy and surgical resection is associated with improved disease-free survival [9]. This correlation is strongest for patients with triple negative and HER2 positive breast cancers [9].

40. b. Re-excision.

The MRI shows suspicious nodular enhancement at the periphery of the lumpectomy site and is suspicious for residual disease. Mass like enhancement, nodularity greater than 5 mm around a seroma cavity or segmental or clumped non-mass enhancement around a seroma cavity is suspicious [34]. However, minimal or focal area of enhancement or thin non-mass enhancement may be seen up to 18 months post-surgery [34]. If it is not associated with a mass or nodularity, it can be considered probably benign and a 6 month follow-up can be performed [34]. In this case, re-excision showed dense fibrosis and signs of prior surgical site without evidence of recurrence.

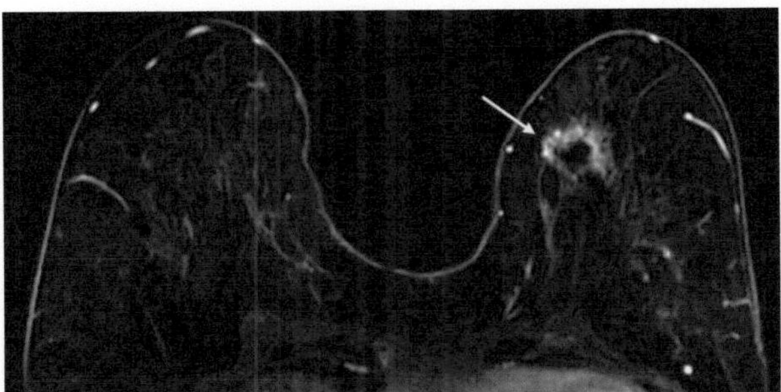

41a. a. BI-RADS 0 additional imaging.

A radiopaque scar marker is present denoting the area of prior surgery and there are post-surgical changes consistent with the history of lumpectomy. However, there is a new asymmetry in the retroareolar right breast with distortion. Although distortion can be seen in the setting of surgery, the distortion and asymmetry are new and associated with nipple retraction. The constellation of findings is highly worrisome, and the patient should be called back (BI-RADS 0) for further workup.

41b. c. Ultrasound.

The finding is a new mass in the subareolar region with associated nipple retraction. Ultrasound is the most appropriate next step for further evaluation.

41c. c. Mastectomy.

Imaging of patients previously treated for breast cancer can be challenging. Any new areas of asymmetry, breast edema, distortion, or suspicious calcifications should be viewed with a high level of suspicion and warrants further evaluation to assess for the presence of tumor recurrence [35]. This was subsequently biopsied and was invasive ductal carcinoma. Mastectomy is the traditional treatment of a breast cancer in a previously irradiated breast; although in some cases, breast radiation after a second breast conserving surgery is a viable option to mastectomy [36].

References

1. Hortobagyi GN, Connolly JL, D'Orsi CJ, et al. Breast. In: Amin MB, Edge S, Greene F, et al., editors. AJCC cancer staging manual. 8th ed. New York: Springer; 2017. p. 589–633.
2. Kalli S, et al. American joint committee on Cancer's staging system for breast cancer, eighth edition: what the radiologist needs to know. Radiographics. 2018;38(7):1921–33.
3. Argus A, Mahoney MC. Indications for breast MRI: *case-based review*. Am J Roentgenol. 2011;196:WS1–WS14.
4. Ecanow JS, et al. Axillary staging of breast cancer: what the radiologist should know. Radiographics. 2013;33(6):1589–612.
5. Lim HS, et al. Paget disease of the breast: mammographic, US, and MR imaging findings with pathologic correlation. Radiographics. 2011;31:1973–87.
6. Eisenhauer, et al. New response evaluation criteria in solid tumours: revised RECIST guideline (version1.1). Eur J Cancer. 2009;45:228–47.
7. Sheikhbahaei S, et al. FDG-PET/CT and MRI for evaluation of pathologic response to neoadjuvant chemotherapy in patients with breast cancer: a meta-analysis of diagnostic accuracy studies. Oncologist. 2016;21(8):931–9.
8. Kaufmann M, et al. Recommendations from an international consensus conference on the current status and future of neoadjuvant systemic therapy in primary breast cancer. Ann Surg Oncol. 2012;19(5):1508–16.
9. Fowler AM, Mankoff DA, Joe BN. Imaging adjuvant therapy response in breast cancer. Radiology. 2017;285(2):359–75.
10. Zhou M, et al. Clinical and pathologic features of multifocal and multicentric breast cancer in Chinese women: a retrospective cohort study. J Breast Cancer. 2013;16(1):77–83.
11. Sardanelli F, et al. Sensitivity of MRI versus mammography for detecting foci of multifocal, multicentric breast cancer in fatty and dense breasts using the whole-breast pathologic examination as a gold standard. Am J Roentgenol. 2004;183:1149–57.
12. Ulaner GA. PET/CT for patients with breast cancer: where is the clinical impact? Am J Roentgenol. 2019;213:254–65.

13. Gao Y, Brachtel EF, Hernandez O, Heller SL. An analysis of nipple enhancement at breast MRI with radiologic-pathologic correlation. Radiographics. 2019;39(1):10–27.
14. Ha SM, et al. Association of BRCA mutation types, imaging features, and pathologic findings in patients with breast cancer with BRCA1 and BRCA2 mutations. Am J Roentgenol. 2017;209(4):920–8.
15. Schnitt SJ. Classification and prognosis of invasive breast cancer: from morphology to molecular taxonomy. Mod Pathol. 2010;23(2):S60–4.
16. Tran B, Bedard PL. Luminal-B breast cancer and novel therapeutic targets. Breast Cancer Res. 2011;13(6):221.
17. Vashi R, et al. Breast imaging of the pregnant and lactating patient: imaging modalities and pregnancy-associated breast cancer. Am J Roentgenol. 2013;200(2):321–8.
18. Bedi DG, et al. Cortical morphologic features of axillary lymph nodes as a predictor of metastasis in breast cancer: in vitro sonographic study. Am J Roentgenol. 2008;191(3):646–52.
19. Humphrey KL, et al. To do or not to do: axillary nodal evaluation after ACOSOG Z0011 trial. Radiographics. 2014;34:1807–16.
20. Homer MJ, Berlin L. Radiography of the surgical breast biopsy specimen. Am J Roentgenol. 1998;171(5):1197–9.
21. Goudreau SH, Joseph JP, Seiler SJ. Preoperative radioactive seed localization for nonpalpable breast lesions: technique, pitfalls, and solutions. Radiographics. 2015;35:1319–34.
22. Lee SC, et al. Radiologist's role in breast cancer staging: providing key information for clinicians. Radiographics. 2014;34:330–42.
23. Lee CI, Lehman CD, Bassett LW. Breast imaging (rotations in radiology). 1st ed. Oxford University Press; 2018.
24. Yeh ED, et al. What radiologists need to know about diagnosis and treatment of inflammatory breast cancer: a multidisciplinary approach. Radiographics. 2013;33:2003–17.
25. Mori N, et al. Luminal-type breast cancer: correlation of apparent diffusion coefficients with the Ki-67 Labeling index. Radiology. 2015;274:66–73.
26. Ha SM, et al. Breast MR imaging before surgery: outcomes in patients with invasive lobular carcinoma by using propensity score matching. Radiology. 2018;287(3):771–7.
27. Boughey JC, et al. Sentinel lymph node surgery after neoadjuvant chemotherapy in patients with node-positive breast cancer: the ACOSOG Z1071 (Alliance) clinical trial. JAMA. 2013;310(14):1455–61.
28. Shin K, et al. Radiologic mapping for targeted axillary dissection: needle biopsy to excision. Am J Roentgenol. 2016;207:1372–9.
29. Ikeda DM. Breast imaging: the requisites. 2nd ed. ELSEVIER MOSBY; 2004. p. 233.
30. Kalambo M, et al. Phyllodes tumor of the breast: ultrasound-pathology correlation. Am J Roentgenol. 2018;210(4):W173–9.
31. Ikeda DM. Breast imaging: the requisites. 2nd ed. ELSEVIER MOSBY; 2004. p. 110–3.
32. Grau A, et al. Phyllodes tumors of the breast UpToDate. Wolters Kuwer Health; 2021. https://www.uptodate.com/contents/phyllodes-tumors-of-the-breast. Accessed December 19, 2021
33. Ambinder EB, et al. Tomosynthesis-guided vacuum-assisted breast biopsy of architectural distortion without a sonographic correlate: a retrospective review. Am J Roentgenol. 2021;2017:845–54.
34. Drukteinis JS, et al. MR imaging assessment of the breast after breast conservation therapy: distinguishing benign from malignant lesions. Radiographics. 2012;32(1):219–34.
35. Chansakul T, Lai KC, Slanetz PJ. The postconservation breast: part 2, imaging findings of tumor recurrence and other long-term sequelae. Am J Roentgenol. 2012;198(2):331–43.
36. Harms W, et al. Current treatment of isolated locoregional breast cancer recurrences. Breast Care. 2015;10:265–71.

Postsurgical Breast

11

Jennifer Choi, Lucy Chow, Bill Zhou, and Bo Li

J. Choi (✉)
Department of Radiology, LAC+USC (GH), Los Angeles, CA, USA

L. Chow · B. Zhou · B. Li
Department of Radiology, David Geffen School of Medicine at UCLA, Los Angeles, CA, USA

© The Author(s), under exclusive license to Springer Nature Switzerland AG 2022

L. Chow, B. Li (eds.), *Absolute Breast Imaging Review*, https://doi.org/10.1007/978-3-031-08274-0_11

1. A 47-year-old woman presents for her annual screening mammogram. What is the most likely clinical history to explain the interval changes seen on the current screening mammogram?

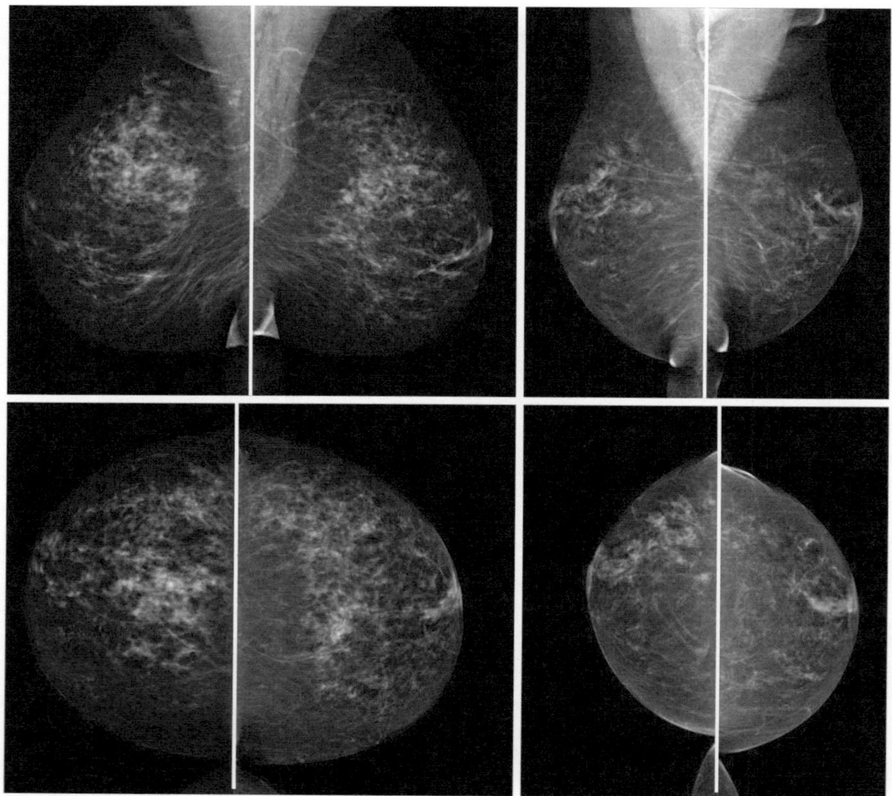

Screening mammogram from 1 year   Current screening mammogram

(a) Weight loss.
(b) Discontinued use of hormone replacement therapy.
(c) Shrinking breast due to invasive lobular carcinoma.
(d) Reduction mammoplasty.

2a. What type of calcifications are seen on this mammogram?

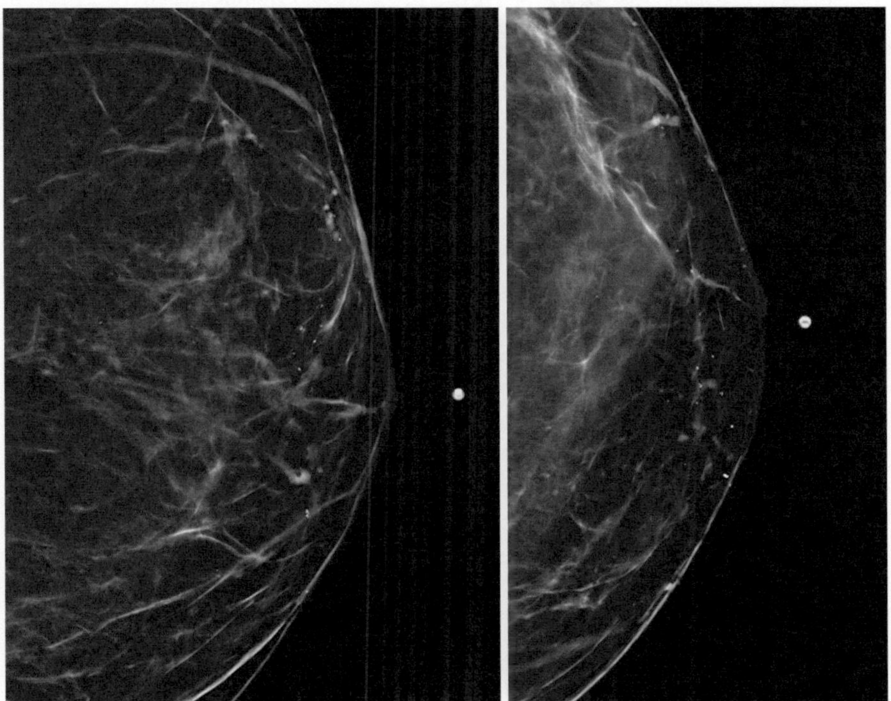

   (a) Secretory.
   (b) Dystrophic.
   (c) Dermal.
   (d) Vascular.
   (e) Milk of calcium.

2b. What is the appropriate BI-RADS category assessment for the mammogram?
    Patient reports history of breast reduction.
    (a) BI-RADS Category 0: Incomplete—Need additional imaging evaluation.
    (b) BI-RADS Category 2: Benign.
    (c) BI-RADS Category 3: Probably Benign.
    (d) BI-RADS Category 4: Suspicious.

3a. A 65-year-old woman with history of left lumpectomy followed by radiation therapy 7 months ago for a small invasive ductal carcinoma presents for her first mammogram following treatment. She has a palpable lump in the area of her lumpectomy scar. A radiopaque BB marker has been placed in the area of lump. What is the most appropriate next step?

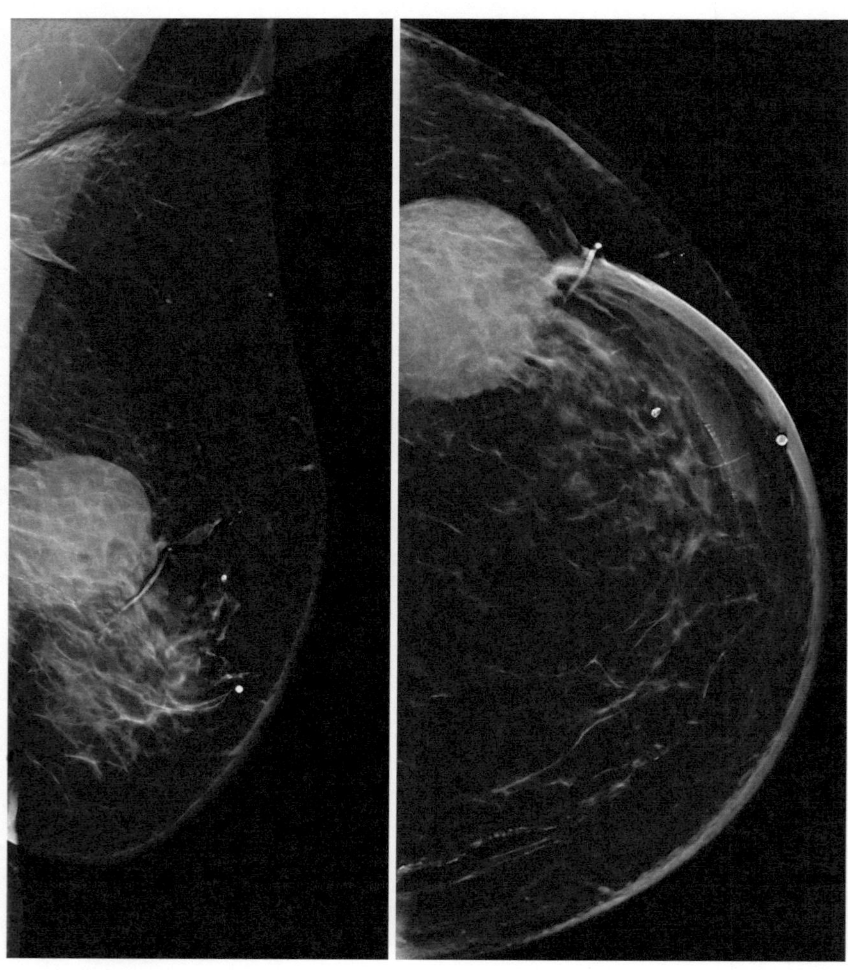

(a) Biopsy.
(b) Ultrasound.
(c) Return to annual screening mammogram.
(d) Short-term follow-up.

3b. What is the most likely etiology for the palpable finding seen on mammogram and ultrasound in the setting of negative surgical margins and compliance with treatment?

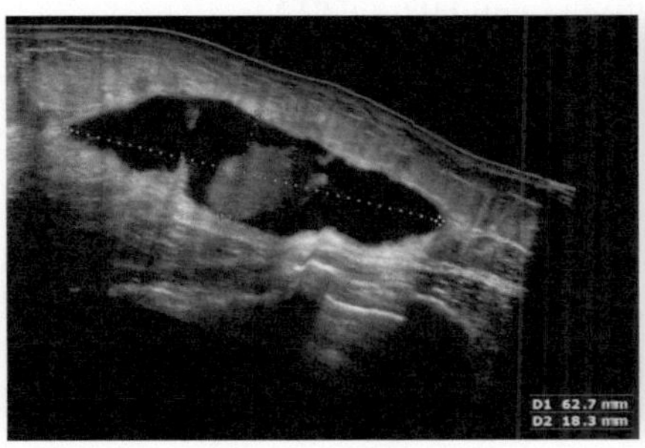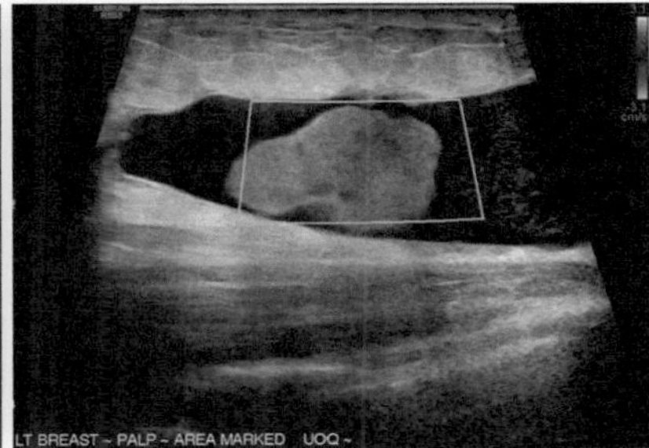

(a) Seroma.
(b) Abscess.
(c) Metachronous cancer.
(d) Recurrence.

4. What are the expected signal and enhancing characteristics of a seroma on a breast MRI?
   (a) T1 hypointense, STIR hyperintense, smooth, thin rim enhancement.
   (b) T1 hyperintense, STIR hyperintense, smooth, thin rim enhancement.
   (c) T1 hypointense, STIR hypointense, smooth, thin rim enhancement.
   (d) T1 hyperintense, STIR hypointense, smooth, thin rim enhancement.

5. A 58-year-old woman who had breast conservation therapy for left breast cancer presents for a routine annual mammogram. The left MLO views from current exam and an exam from 2 years ago are shown. What is the appropriate BI-RADS category assessment for the current mammogram exam?

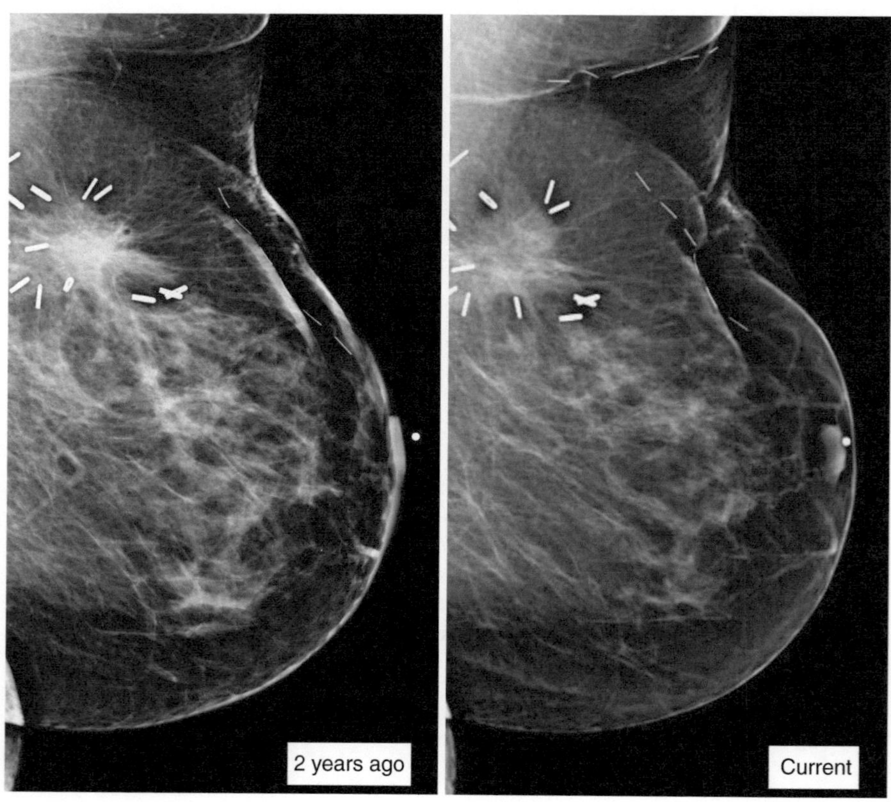

(a) BI-RADS Category 6: Known biopsy-proven malignancy.
(b) BI-RADS Category 2: Benign.
(c) BI-RADS Category 3: Probably benign.
(d) BI-RADS Category 4: Suspicious.

6a. A PET/CT of a 49-year-old woman with history of bilateral mastectomies for left breast cancer is shown. What is the most appropriate next step?

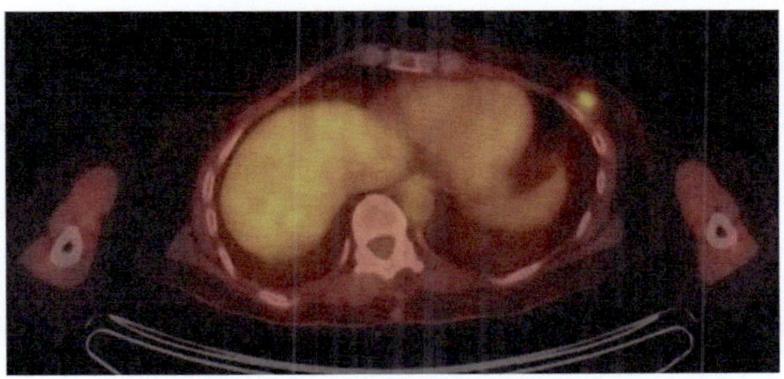

(a) Biopsy.
(b) Ultrasound.
(c) Mammogram.
(d) Surgical excision.
(e) Breast MRI.

6b. The patient subsequently had a targeted left breast ultrasound. What is the most appropriate BI-RADS category assessment for the ultrasound finding?

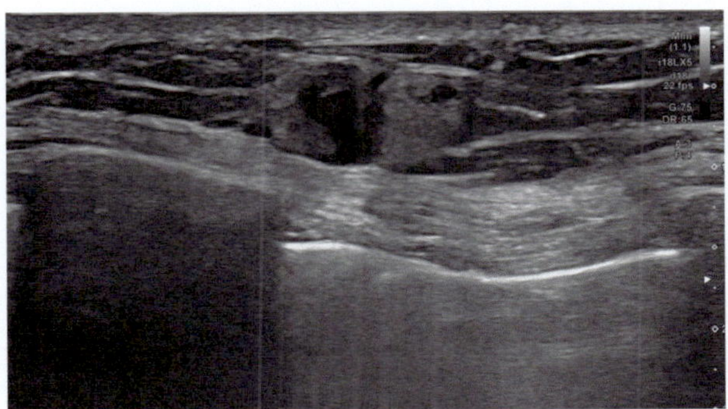

(a) BI-RADS Category 2: Benign.
(b) BI-RADS Category 3: Probably benign.
(c) BI-RADS Category 6: Known biopsy-proven malignancy.
(d) BI-RADS Category 4: Suspicious.

7. What is the best description of a modified radical mastectomy?
   (a) Modified radical mastectomy removes breast tissue, skin envelope, nipple areolar complex.
   (b) Modified radical mastectomy removes breast tissue, skin envelope, level I-II axillary lymph nodes.
   (c) Modified radical mastectomy removes breast tissue, skin envelope, nipple areolar complex, level I-II axillary lymph nodes.
   (d) Modified radical mastectomy removes breast tissue, skin envelope, nipple areolar complex, pectoralis muscles.

8. What components are surgically removed in a nipple-sparing mastectomy (also known as a total-skin-sparing mastectomy or subcutaneous mastectomy)?
   i. Skin envelope.
   ii. Nipple areolar complex.
   iii. Breast tissue.
   iv. Axillary lymph nodes.
   v. Pectoralis muscles.

   (a) iii.
   (b) ii, iii.
   (c) i, ii, iii.
   (d) i, ii, iii, v.
   (e) ii, iii, iv.

9. What is the most likely explanation for the appearance of this woman's mammogram?

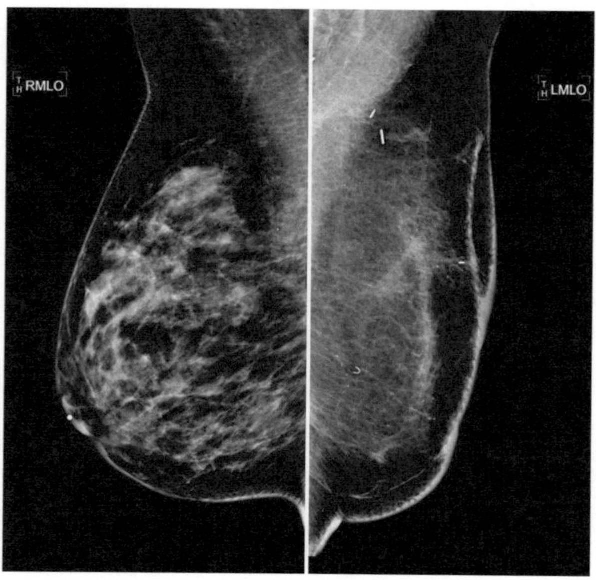

(a) Poland syndrome.
(b) Left mastectomy and autologous reconstruction.
(c) Mastectomy.
(d) Asymmetric breast tissue composition.

10. A sagittal contrast enhanced fat-suppressed T1-weighted MR subtraction image of a 43-year-old woman with history of bilateral skin-sparing mastectomies with TRAM flap reconstruction for left breast cancer is shown. Where is the most likely location of a possible recurrence of her breast cancer?

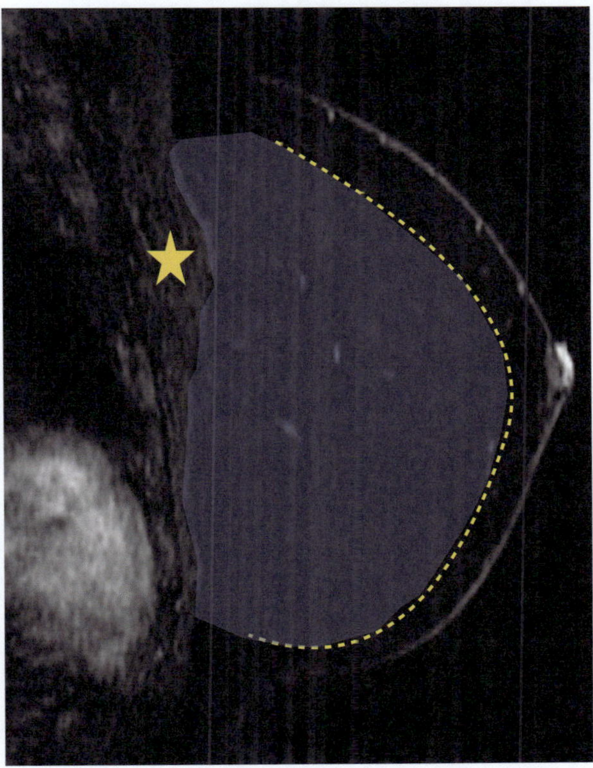

(a) Chest wall—Star.
(b) TRAM flap—Blue area.
(c) Contact zone—Dashed line.

11a. What is the best description for the calcifications located between the arrows
      on this patient's mamm©ogram?

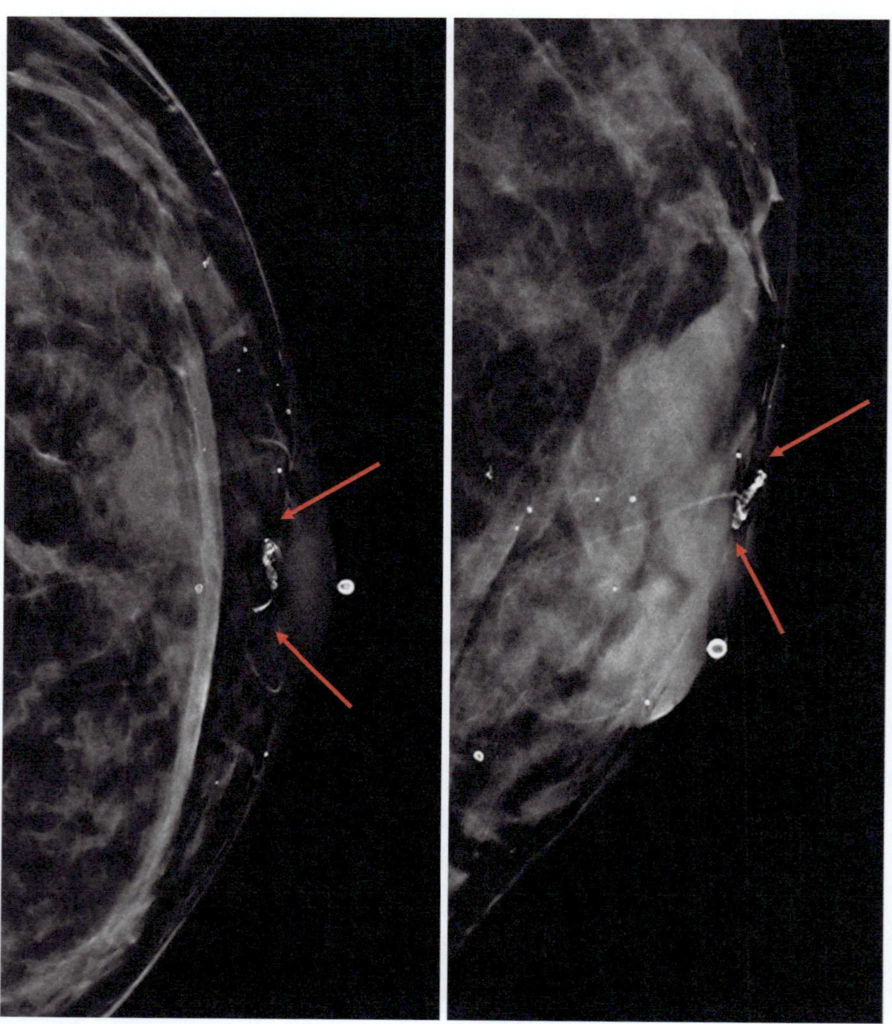

    (a) Fine pleomorphic.
    (b) Fine linear branching.
    (c) Vascular.
    (d) Suture.

11b. What is the most appropriate next step?
    (a) Recall from screening mammogram.
    (b) Annual screening mammogram.
    (c) Biopsy.
    (d) Six-month follow-up.

12a. A 52-year-old woman with history of right excisional biopsy for atypical ductal hyperplasia presents for routine screening mammogram. Final surgical pathology on excision showed atypical ductal hyperplasia, no evidence of carcinoma. The excisional biopsy occurred a few years ago. What is the most likely etiology of the finding indicated by the arrows?

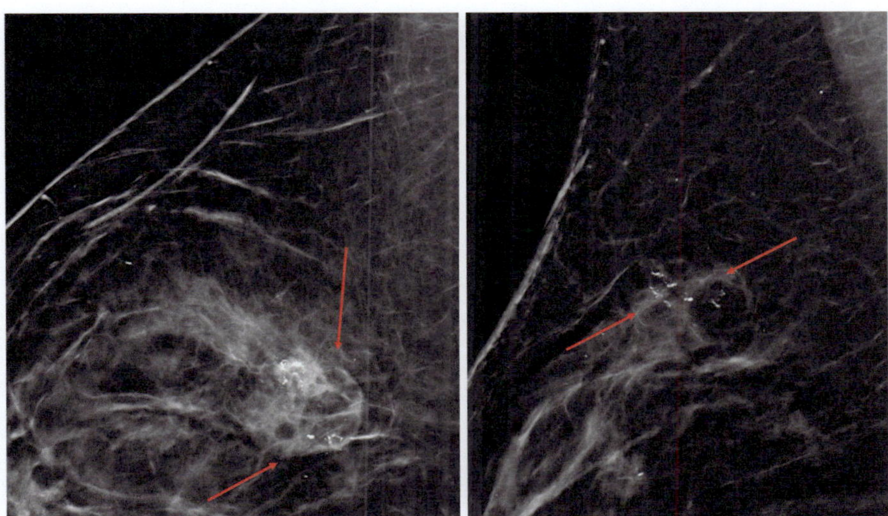

    (a) Hamartoma.
    (b) Lipoma.
    (c) Fat necrosis.
    (d) Seroma.
    (e) DCIS.

12b. If the same patient presented with a palpable lump at the area indicated by the arrows, what would be the most appropriate next step?
    (a) Ultrasound.
    (b) Biopsy.
    (c) Six-month follow-up.
    (d) Reassurance and return to screening mammogram.

13a. A 44-year-old woman with history of breast conservation therapy for a medial left breast cancer 3 years ago presents for annual high risk screening MRI. Axial (B) and sagittal (A) T1-weighted postcontrast images with (C) subtraction are shown. Kinetic enhancement curve (D) is also shown. What is the most appropriate description of the pertinent finding?

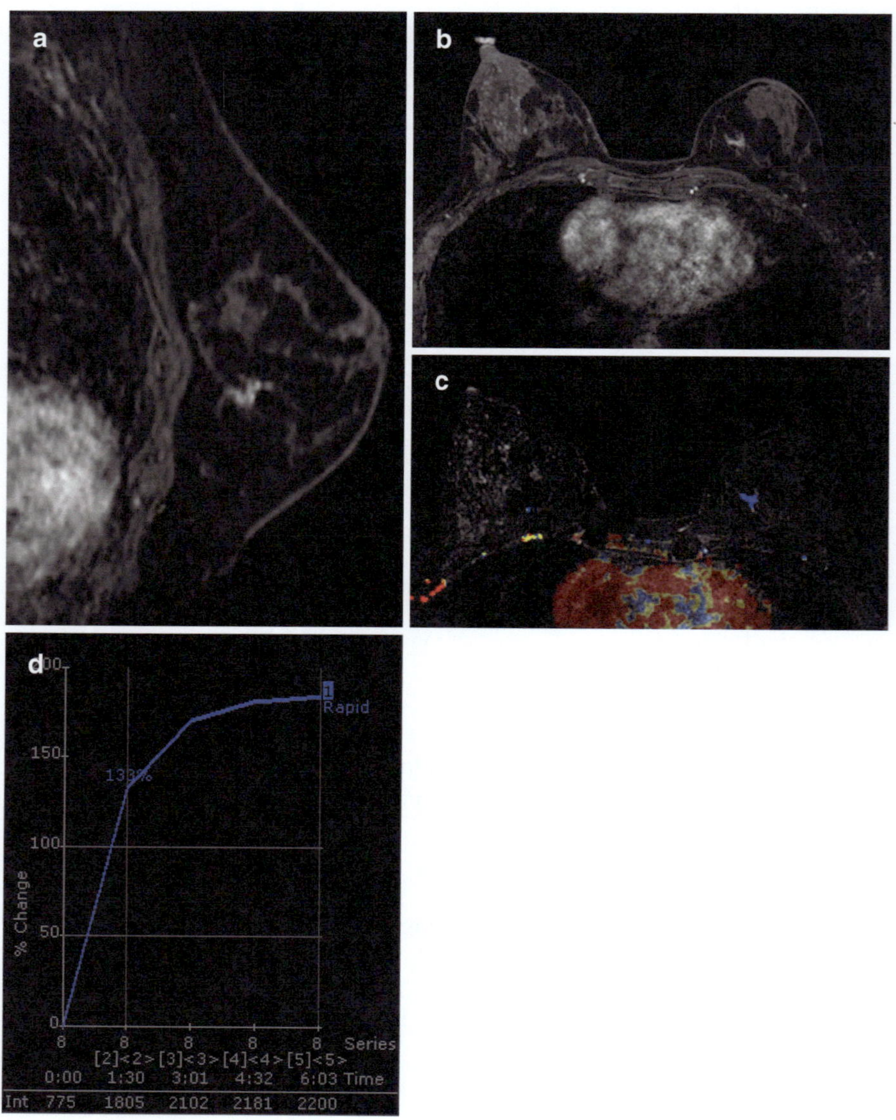

(a) Enhancing focus with persistent kinetics.
(b) Focal non-mass enhancement with washout kinetics.
(c) Enhancing focus with plateau kinetics.
(d) Focal non-mass enhancement with persistent kinetics.

13b. Prior images have been retrieved for this patient. Axial T1-weighted fat-suppressed subtraction images from this year's MRI are shown along with her MRI from last year. What is the most concerning feature of the pertinent finding?

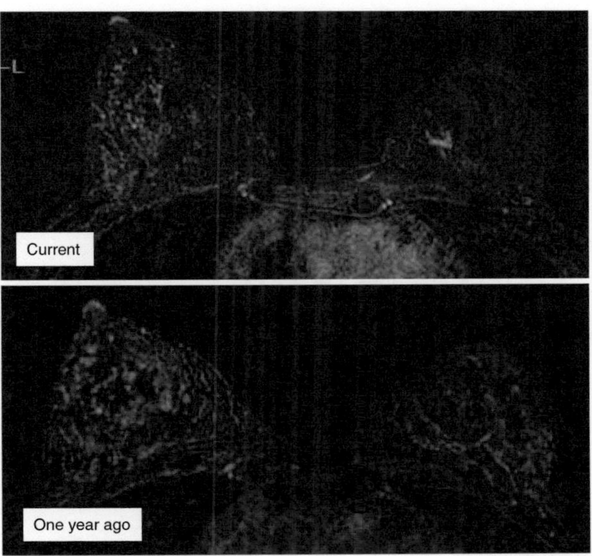

(a) Kinetics.
(b) Size.
(c) Location at the lumpectomy site.
(d) New/increasing enhancement.

14. A 50-year-old female status post right sided mastectomy without reconstruction presents with a palpable lump. What is the best initial imaging exam?
(a) Ultrasound.
(b) Mammogram.
(c) MRI.
(d) Defer to surgical consultation.

15a. 43-year-old female with history of biopsy-proven right breast cancer status post recent lumpectomy. Recent surgery reported positive margins and surgical specimen did not show the biopsy microclip. What is the best descriptor for the microcalcifications seen in the right inner breast?

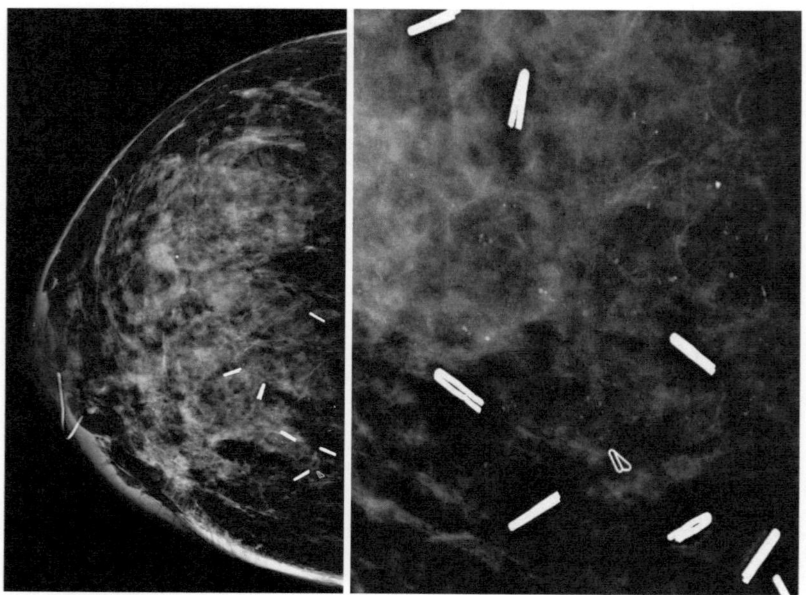

    (a) Round.
    (b) Coarse heterogenous.
    (c) Fine pleomorphic.
    (d) Layering.

15b. What is the appropriate next step for the patient?
    (a) Ultrasound.
    (b) Close surveillance.
    (c) Surgical excision.
    (d) Radiation therapy.

16. Which of the following statement about microcalcifications following breast-conserving therapy with radiation therapy is FALSE?
    (a) Majority of recurrent tumors appear mammographically similar to primary tumor.
    (b) Majority of recurrent tumors recur in the same quadrant as the primary tumor.
    (c) Majority of recurrent tumors have similar histopathology as primary tumor.
    (d) New calcifications that arise in the lumpectomy bed 6–18 months after therapy are usually malignant.
    (e) New microcalcifications that arise in the lumpectomy bed with benign appearing morphology are frequently benign.

17. Which of the following about dermal calcifications is FALSE?
    (a) They can be artifactual from deodorant.
    (b) Their spatial relationship may change on different projections.
    (c) Tangential views can be obtained to confirm position.
    (d) They have lucent centers.
    (e) They are round or oval.

18a. A 70-year-old female with history of multifocal left breast invasive ductal carcinoma status post lumpectomy presents for screening. What is the appropriate next step for the increasing calcifications in her breast?

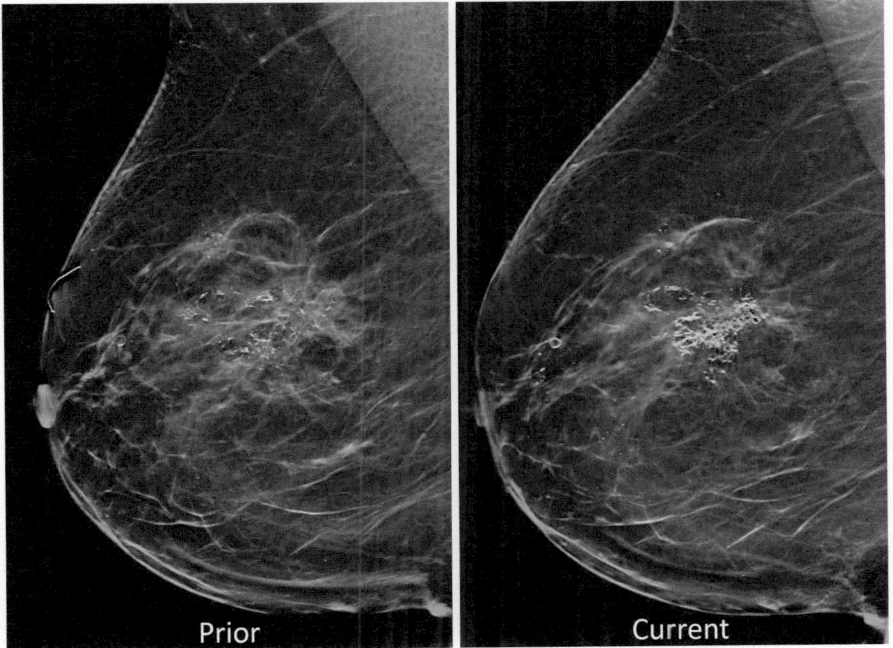

    (a) Ultrasound.
    (b) Biopsy.
    (c) Close surveillance.
    (d) Return to screening.

18b. Patient incidentally had a recent MR breast. What is the most appropriate BI-RADS assessment?

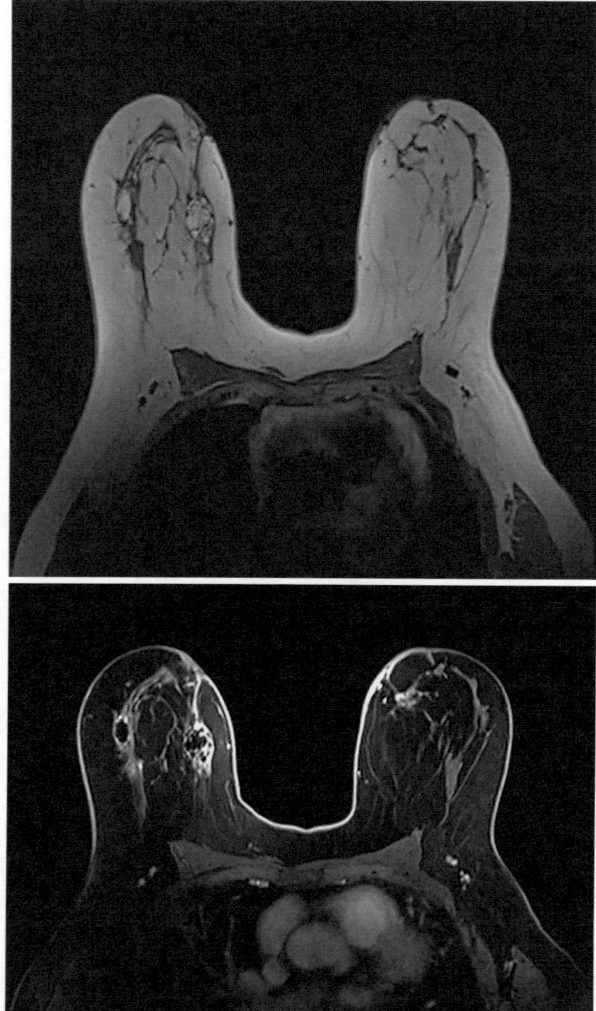

    (a) BI-RADS Category 1: Negative.
    (b) BI-RADS Category 2: Benign.
    (c) BI-RADS Category 3: Probably Benign.
    (d) BI-RADS Category 4: Suspicious.

18c. Given the MRI findings, what is the appropriate next step for the right breast?
    (a) Second-look ultrasound.
    (b) Biopsy.
    (c) Follow-up MRI in 6 months.
    (d) Return to screening.

19. Which of the following statement about fat necrosis is FALSE?
    (a) Fat necrosis can be differentiated from malignancy with PET-FDG.
    (b) Fat necrosis can have rapid enhancement with washout kinetics.
    (c) Fat necrosis can have internal septations with heterogenous enhancement.
    (d) Fat necrosis is commonly seen in inferior, central breast after reduction mammoplasty.
    (e) Fat necrosis is commonly seen in periphery of flap after breast reconstruction.

20. Which of the following is NOT usually associated with breast fat necrosis?
    (a) Recent breast surgery.
    (b) Trauma.
    (c) Radiation therapy.
    (d) Scleroderma.

21. What is the most common appearance of fat necrosis on mammogram?
    (a) Smooth-bordered lucent mass.
    (b) Pleomorphic calcifications.
    (c) Irregular hyperdense mass.
    (d) Architectural distortion.

22. 75-year-old female with history of multicentric right breast cancer presenting for imaging. Which of the following complication is most commonly associated with the patient's bilateral surgery?

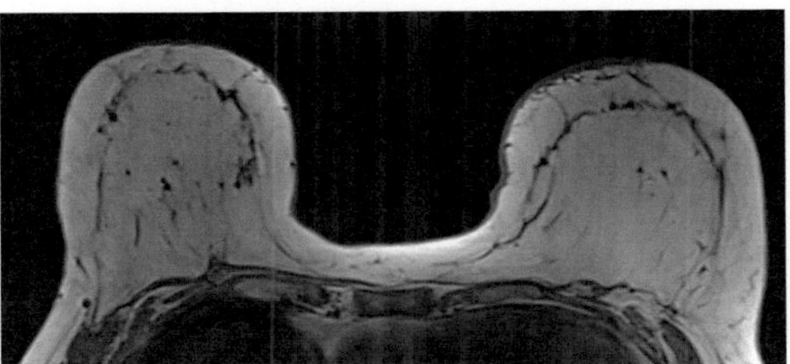

    (a) Implant rupture.
    (b) Capsular contracture of the implant after radiation therapy.
    (c) Anaplastic large cell lymphoma.
    (d) Fat necrosis.

23. Following mastectomy, post-reconstruction seromas are expected to resolve by what time?
    (a) 2 months.
    (b) 6 months.
    (c) 1 year.
    (d) 3 years.

24. Patient had a left mastectomy and flap reconstruction. A coronal T2 HASTE image was obtained. What type of reconstruction has the patient received?

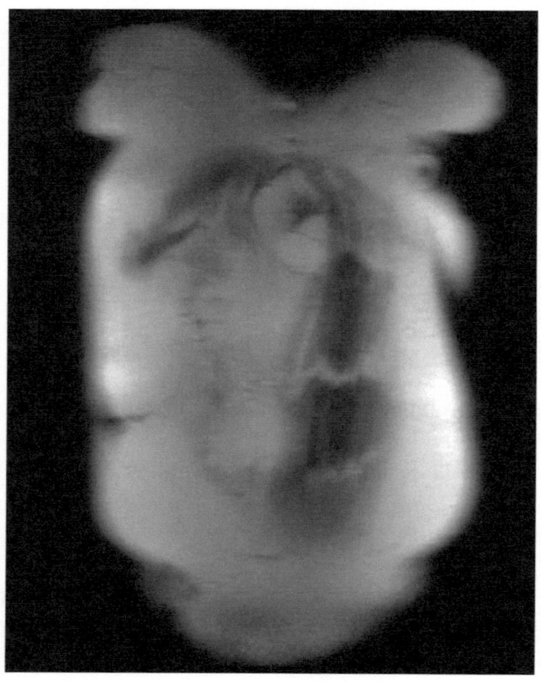

(a) Latissimus dorsi flap.
(b) TRAM (transverse rectus abdominis myocutaneous) flap.
(c) DIEP (deep inferior epigastric perforator) flap.
(d) SIEA (superficial inferior epigastric artery) flap.

Answers

1. d. Reduction Mammoplasty.

   The patient had a reduction mammoplasty since her prior mammogram. Reduction mammoplasty or breast reduction is typically performed for cosmetic reasons or to relieve shoulder/back pain symptoms related to large breast size. With reduction mammoplasty, excess breast tissue and skin are surgically removed and the nipples are surgically relocated superiorly to achieve the patient's desired breast size and appearance. The current screening mammogram demonstrates characteristic mammographic changes that can be seen after a reduction mammoplasty, most notably the reduction in the size of the breasts, redistribution of the remaining fibroglandular tissue (circles), and elevation of the nipples (arrows). Additional imaging findings which can be seen after reduction mammoplasty include dermal calcifications, postsurgical architectural distortion, islands of fibroglandular tissue, fat necrosis, and skin thickening [1, 2].

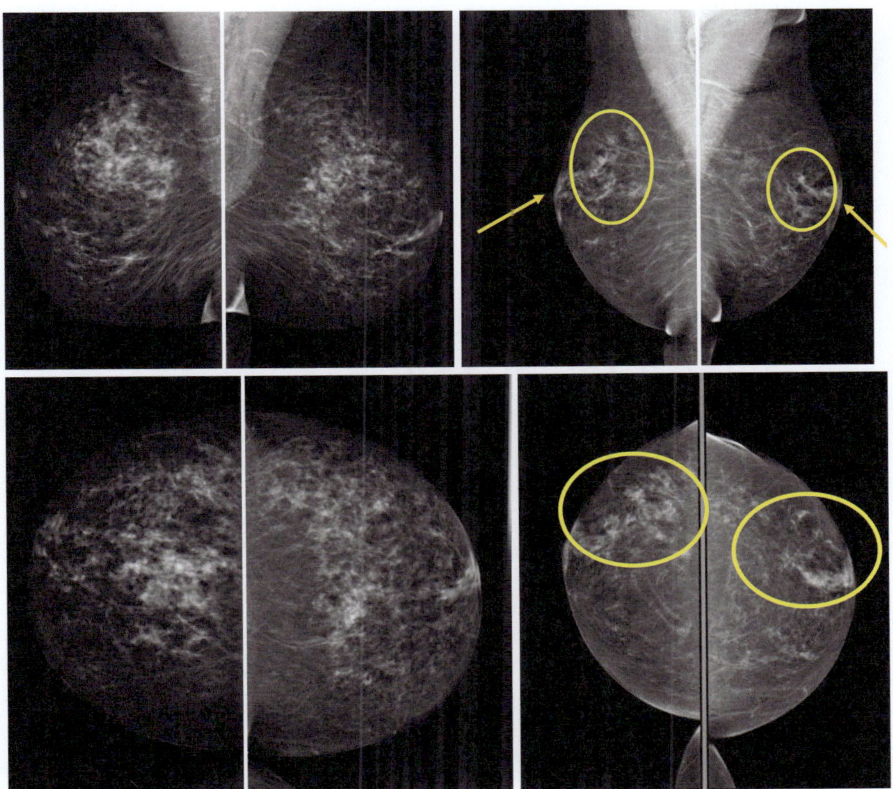

Screening mammogram from 1 year ago   Current screening mammogram

2a. c. Dermal calcifications.

The mammogram demonstrates dermal calcifications along the nipple areolar region in a circumferential pattern. In patients who have undergone reduction mammoplasty or breast augmentation, dermal calcifications are commonly seen along the scars and skin incision sites, typically around the areolas and the inferior breasts [1, 2].

2b. b. BI-RADS Category 2: Benign Findings.

With the appropriate clinical history, characteristic post-reduction mammo-plasty changes are benign findings and, in most cases, can be distinguished from screening mammography and do not require additional workup. It is not appropriate to assign BI-RADS 3 and 4 category assessments on screening mammogram.

3a. b. Ultrasound.

Ultrasound is the most appropriate next step in the evaluation of a palpable lump unless a clearly benign etiology is identified on mammogram, such as a lipoma, hamartoma, or calcified involuting fibroadenoma. Mammogram dem-onstrates a partially obscured, iso- to hyperdense round mass at the lumpec-tomy site.

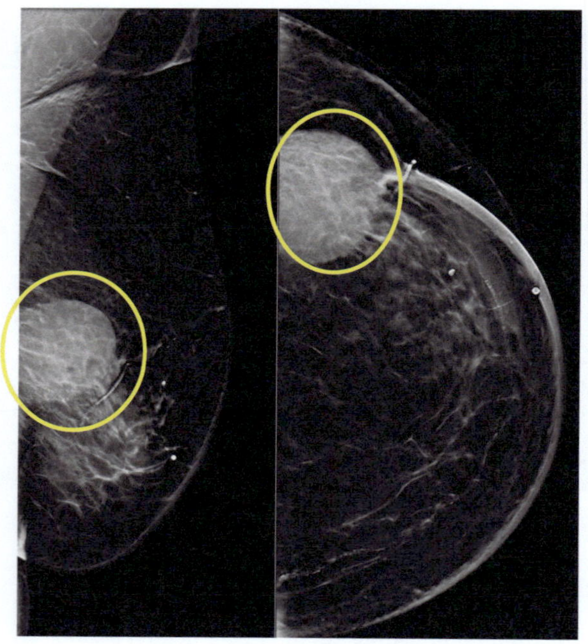

3b. a. Seroma.

Seromas are common postsurgical fluid collections. Seromas typically decrease in size over time and can even resolve (see below example). Mammography findings can show an oval or round, iso- or hyperdense mass with circumscribed or obscured margins [3, 4]. There can be adjacent postsurgical architectural distortion. Ultrasound findings show a fluid collection with varying degrees of complexity due to debris, wall thickening, or septations, which should demonstrate no vascularity on color Doppler interrogation.

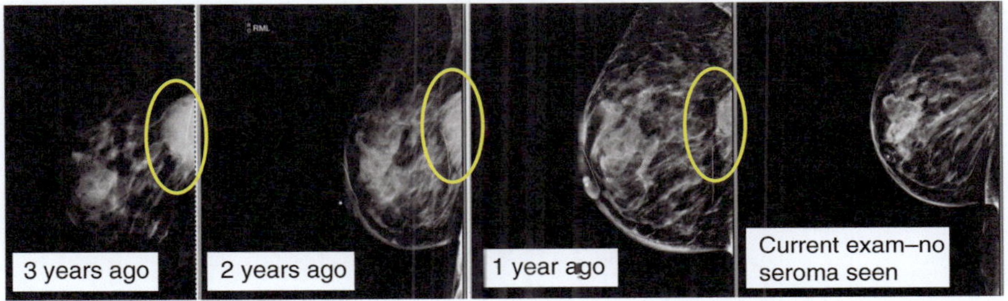

4. a. T1 hypointense, STIR hyperintense, smooth, thin rim enhancement,

Axial T1-weighted (A), STIR (B) and postcontrast subtraction images (C) show a benign T1-hypointense, STIR hyperintense mass within the surgical bed. There is thin peripheral rim enhancement. These findings are consistent with seroma [5, 6].

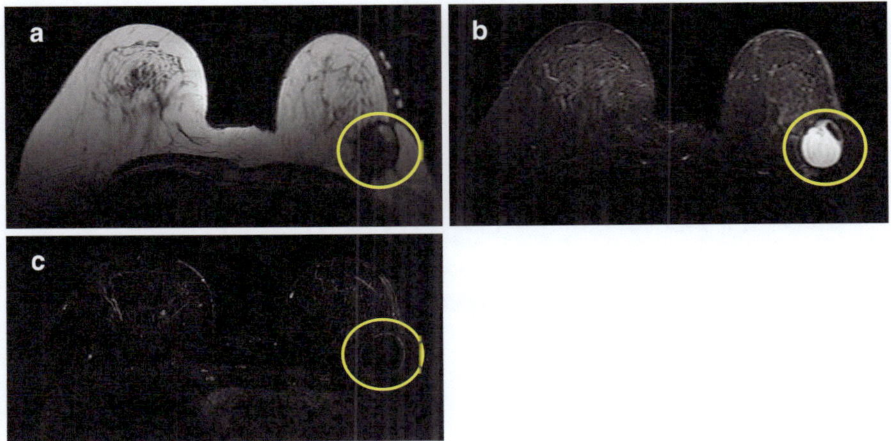

5. b. BI-RADS Category 2—Benign Findings.

The current MLO view demonstrates the lumpectomy changes in the posterior superior left breast. Compared to the MLO view from 2 years ago, the scar is decreased in density, which is expected for a healing scar. Lumpectomy changes that increase in size and density over time are suspicious and should be further evaluated with ultrasound and biopsied as indicated. If present, postsurgical distortion should also decrease in prominence over time [2].

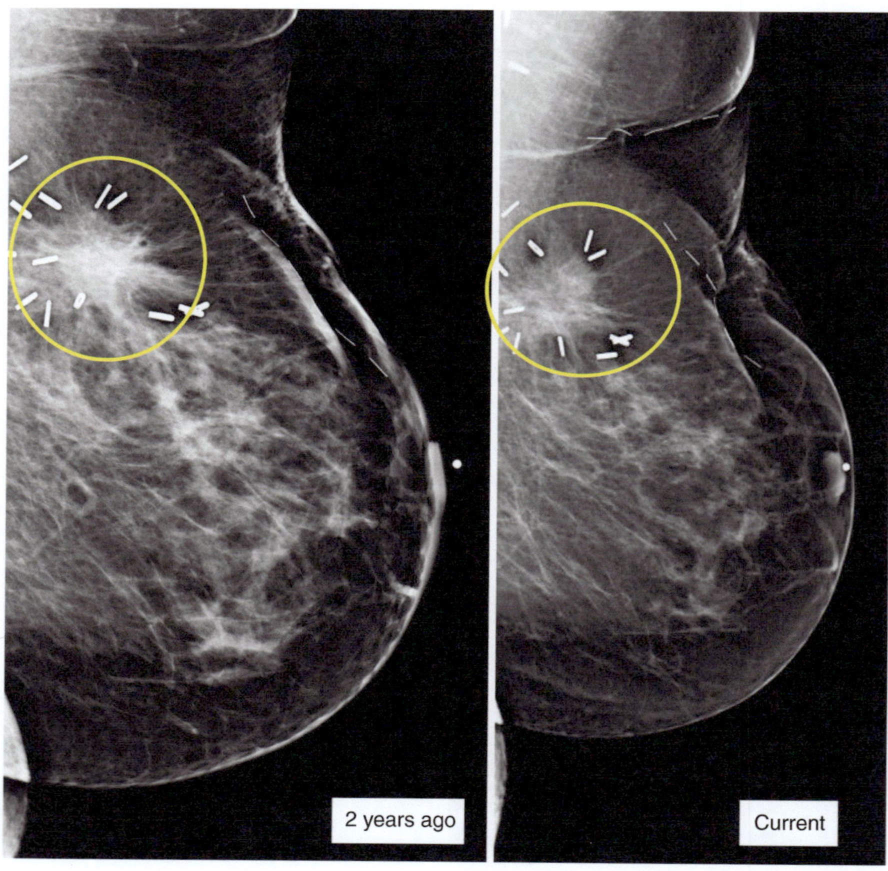

6a. b. Ultrasound.

There is a hypermetabolic mass in the left mastectomy site (circle). Ultrasound is the most appropriate next step in the evaluation of this mass.

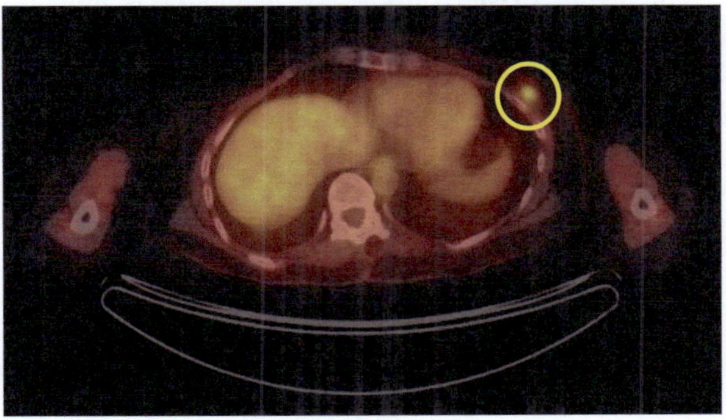

6b. d. BI-RADS Category 4: Suspicious.

Ultrasound demonstrates a complex cystic and solid oval mass with indistinct margins that correlates with the hypermetabolic mass seen on the PET/CT. This suspicious mass is worrisome for recurrence given the history of left breast cancer. Biopsy is indicated and BI-RADS 4 is the appropriate assessment. Ultrasound guided core biopsy demonstrated invasive ductal carcinoma.

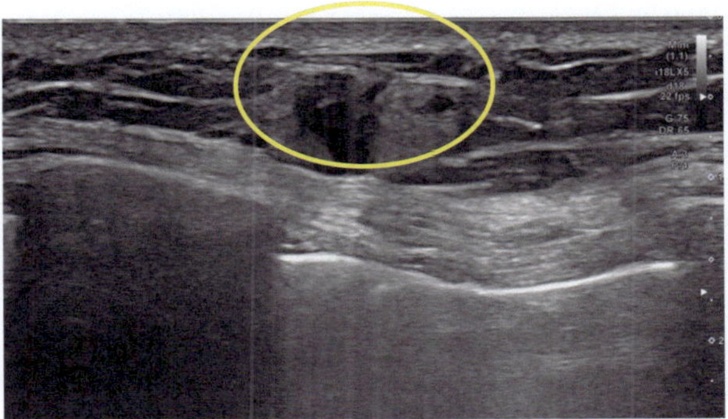

7. c. Modified radical mastectomy entails the complete removal of the breast parenchymal tissue, skin envelope, nipple areolar complex, and level I and II axillary lymph nodes [1]. The pectoralis muscles are not removed in a modified radical mastectomy. The muscles are removed in a radical mastectomy, which is an older surgical technique that is still sometimes utilized for advanced cases of breast cancer.

8. a. iii—Breast tissue.

The nipple-sparing mastectomy (NSM) preserves both the skin envelope and the nipple areolar complex. NSM is also known as total-skin-sparing mastectomy or subcutaneous mastectomy. NSM technique is most often performed for women undergoing prophylactic mastectomies. A skin-sparing mastectomy (SSM) is a different mastectomy technique that preserves just the skin envelope. It involves the complete removal of the breast parenchymal tissue and the nipple areolar complex. Both NSM and SSM are considered conservative mastectomies and are associated with promising aesthetic outcomes and improved patient satisfaction [1, 7].

9. b. Left mastectomy and autologous reconstruction.

The patient has had a left mastectomy with autologous TRAM (transverse rectus abdomens myocutaneous) reconstruction. The left mammogram demonstrates fatty tissue from the flap which originated from the abdomen. In some patients, the muscular pedicle can be seen posteriorly on mammogram [8].

10. c. Contact Zone—Dashed Lines.

The dashed line delineates the junction or contact zone between the native residual subcutaneous fat and the TRAM flap. Most recurrences occur at this contact zone and within the skin envelope, reported to be up to 72% [1, 9, 10]. Recurrences in the chest wall are less common but can occur and tend to have a poorer prognosis [9].

11a. d. Suture.

Sutural calcifications can have a variable imaging appearance but classically they demonstrate a curvilinear appearance following the shape of a knotted suture. Sutural calcifications can often be seen in patients with history of breast cancer following treatment; however, they can also be seen after benign breast surgery and augmentation [11, 12].

11b. b. Annual screening mammogram.

Sutural calcifications are considered benign and do not warrant further workup.

12a. c. Fat necrosis.

The mammogram demonstrates coarse and rim calcifications associated with fat-containing masses in the area of postsurgical scar (as denoted by the skin scar marker). This is most consistent with fat necrosis related to the excisional biopsy. Fat necrosis can have a widely variable appearance on mammogram, sometimes manifesting as asymmetries, suspicious calcifications, or spiculated masses [13, 14].

12b. d. Reassurance and return to screening mammogram.

With the typical mammographic appearance for fat necrosis and the absence of suspicious mammographic findings as in this case, the patient can be reassured of the benign etiology of her palpable lump and return to annual screening mammography. Mammogram is more specific than ultrasound when evaluating for fat necrosis. If there are no worrisome features on mammogram, then ultrasound may not be needed to make the diagnosis. For any mammogram where the findings are equivocal or worrisome, ultrasound can be helpful. The ultrasound appearance of fat necrosis varies and depends on the amount of fibrosis. While no vascularity within the sonographic finding does not exclude malignancy entirely, it is a reassuring finding that helps support the diagnosis of fat necrosis [13, 14]. The following three examples show the varying sonographic appearances of biopsy-proven fat necrosis. As shown, fat necrosis can have a cystic or solid appearance on ultrasound.

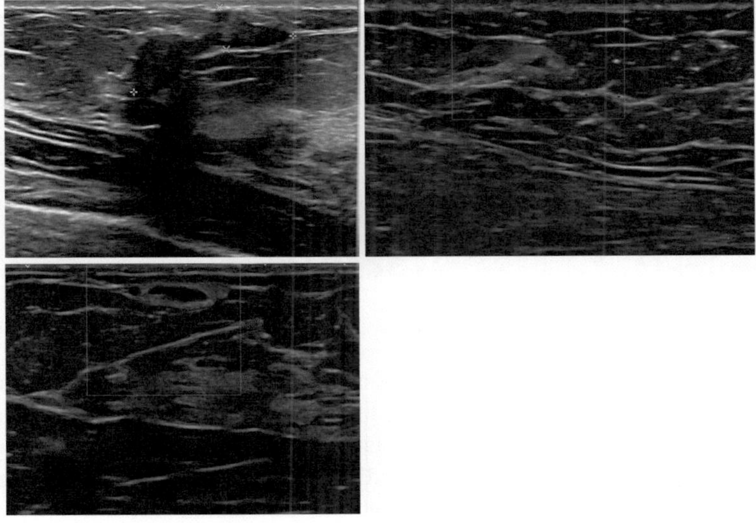

13a. d. Focal non-mass enhancement with persistent kinetics.

The pertinent finding on the breast MRI is within the medial left breast where there is a focal area of non-mass enhancement demonstrating persistent kinetics, as indicated by the kinetics curve and blue color on the color overlay map.

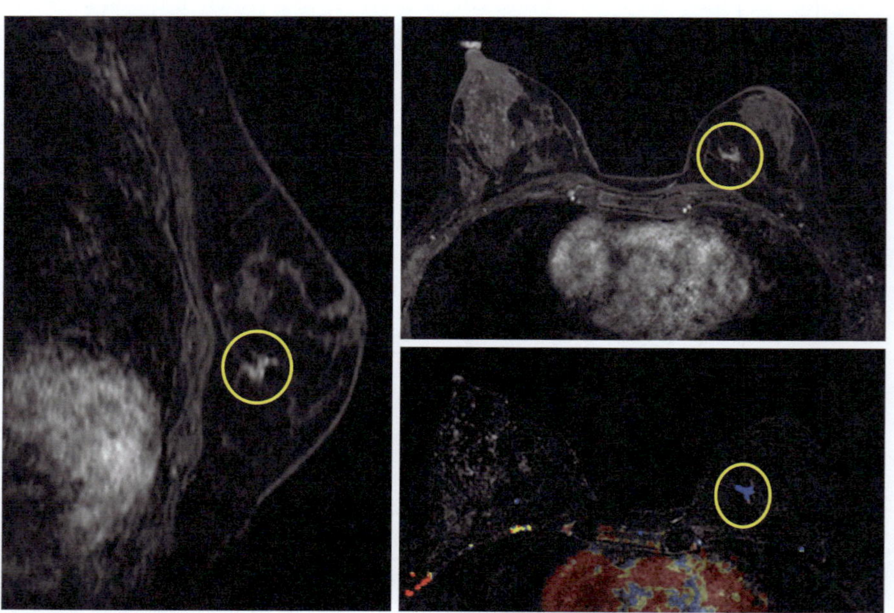

13b. d. New/increasing enhancement.

The most suspicious feature of the non-mass enhancement seen at the left lumpectomy site on the current breast MRI is that it is new/increasing from the prior exam. It is common to see enhancement at a lumpectomy scar during the immediate post-operative period. Radiation can also cause increased enhancement in the surgical bed, up to 3 months after radiation [15].

Lumpectomy scars can continue to demonstrate enhancement years after treatment but should demonstrate stability or decrease in prominence on subsequent exams. An increase in size or prominence of enhancement should be viewed as suspicious and warrants further evaluation to exclude recurrence. In patients with breast conservation treatment, enhancement may be present in the surgical bed up to 5 years after surgery [16]. Enhancement after 5 years was uncommon [16].

14. a. Ultrasound.

Per ACR Appropriateness criteria [17], ultrasound of the breast is given the appropriateness category of "usually appropriate". Mammogram "may be appropriate", but there is insufficient evidence for use of mammogram as the initial imaging test. Mammograms can also be technically challenging or not possible if very little tissue remains. Dashevsky et al. evaluated 118 palpable cases with a history of mastectomy and demonstrated that targeted ultrasound had a high negative predictive value of 97% [18]. Of note, mammography did not show any additional cancers but did help to confirm benign findings such as fat necrosis [18].

15a. c. Fine pleomorphic.

CC (left) and magnified (right) views of the right breast demonstrate pleomorphic calcifications (red circle) adjacent to surgical clips. A heart-shaped biopsy microclip is seen (blue circle).

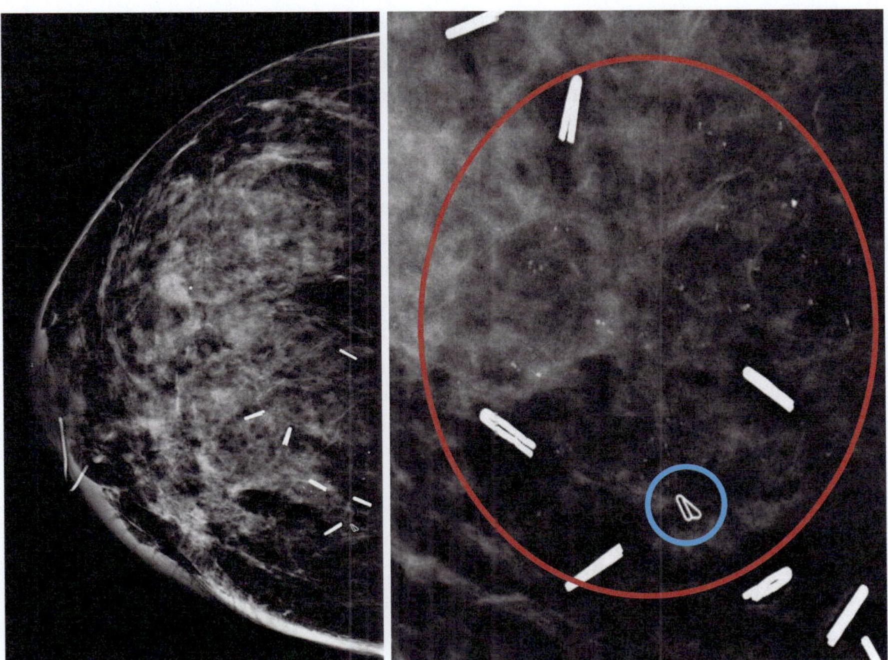

15b. c. Surgical excision.

Breast-conserving therapy includes breast-conserving surgery followed by radiation therapy to eradicate residual microscopic disease. Positive margins are associated with twofold increase of local recurrence. Given the history of positive margins, residual calcifications in the lumpectomy bed are suspicious for residual disease. In this case, patient's mammogram demonstrates fine pleomorphic calcifications within the lumpectomy bed. In addition, the previously placed biopsy microclip was not excised. Patient will need repeat surgical resection of the remaining calcifications prior to receiving radiation therapy to reduce the chance for recurrence. Breast-conserving surgery has a reoperation rate of 21.6% in the United States.

16. d. New calcifications that arise in the lumpectomy bed 6–18 months after therapy are usually malignant.

New microcalcifications that arise in the lumpectomy bed after breast-conserving therapy are common. Though microcalcifications are frequently seen with recurrent tumor (positive predictive value ranging from 33% to 100% in various studies), most microcalcifications are benign (studies range from 50–91%) [19]. This poses a conundrum for radiologists. Higher suspicion should be given to calcifications with the same appearance and occur in the same quadrant as the primary tumor. Furthermore, microcalcifications that occur early (6–18 months) tend to be benign while those that occur later tend to be malignant (median 52 months) [19]. Nevertheless, morphology and distribution should always be the most important factors in determining the need for biopsy.

17. b. Their spatial relationship may change on different projections.

Dermal calcifications have fixed relationships to each other on different mammographic views in what is known as the tattoo sign.

18a. d. Return to screening.

Serial MLO images of the right breast demonstrate increasing regional rim and dystrophic calcifications, consistent with evolution of fat necrosis. Mammographic appearances of fat necrosis is highly varied with the most common findings being dystrophic or coarse calcifications and radiolucent oil cysts. Other findings include calcifications with indeterminate morphology, ill-defined spiculated mass, asymmetry, and deformity of skin and subcutaneous tissue, emphasizing the difficulty of distinguishing fat necrosis from malignancy.

18b. b. BI-RADS Category 2: Benign.

Axial T1 non-fat-saturation and T1 post-contrast fat saturation images demonstrate multiple oval fat-containing lesions with homogenous thin wall enhancement, consistent with benign fat necrosis. Fat necrosis involves the saponification of fat, calcification, and fibrosis. Fat necrosis is usually an asymptomatic entity but can cause skin thickening, erythema, ecchymosis, and a palpable mass. Fat necrosis has a wide spectrum of findings on MR, and it is dependent on the amount of inflammatory reaction, liquefied fat, and degree of fibrosis. Because of its varied appearance, fat necrosis can be difficult to distinguish from malignancy, especially in the setting of new calcifications in the surgical bed following resection.

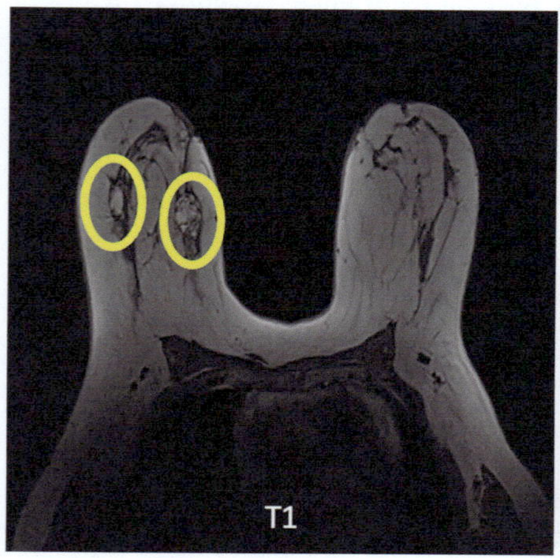

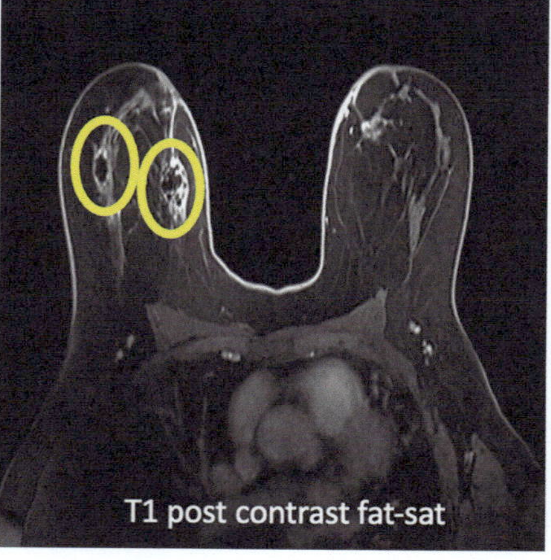

18c. d. Return to screening.

Fat necrosis is a benign finding.

19. a. Fat necrosis can be differentiated from malignancy with PET-FDG.

Fat necrosis can exhibit ^{18}F-FDG avidity [20].

20. d. Scleroderma.

In a patient with recent breast surgery, the recent surgery is the most common etiology of fat necrosis. In patients with no history of recent breast surgery, trauma is more likely the cause of fat necrosis. Patient with flaps are more likely to have fat necrosis when irradiated. Scleroderma is associated with coarse subcutaneous calcifications but is not a cause of fat necrosis.

21. a. Smooth-bordered radiolucent mass.

Fat necrosis is a benign inflammatory entity of adipose tissue, usually secondary to trauma, surgical intervention, or radiation therapy. Appearance of fat necrosis can be highly variable. On mammography, fat necrosis typically appears as a smooth-bordered lucent mass, oil cyst, or coarse calcifications. On ultrasound, the most specific sign on ultrasound is a hyperechoic oval lesion with a mobile fluid-fluid level. On MR, fat necrosis typically demonstrates a round or oval mass with hypointense T1 signal on fat-saturated images and an enhancing rim, which represents inflammatory changes. Calcifications may present as signal voids. Enhancement kinetics is variable and not specific. Fat necrosis may also present non-classically with internal septations, thick and irregular rim, associated spiculations and architectural distortion, or irregular masses [20]. Lesions with indeterminate imaging characteristics can be indistinguishable from malignancy and may require tissue diagnosis to confirm benignity.

22. d. Fat necrosis.

Axial T1-weighted nonfat saturated images demonstrate bilateral mastectomies with autologous tissue flap reconstruction. On MR, mastectomy with reconstruction is evidenced by linear T1 hypointensities running parallel to the skin (red arrow) which represent acellular dermal matrix of the allograft as well as replacement of normal fibroglandular tissue with fat (shaded area) and possible muscle. This surgery has a 5–35% incidence of fat necrosis due to inadequate bloody supply to the flap [8]. The other complications are associated with reconstruction with capsule implant.

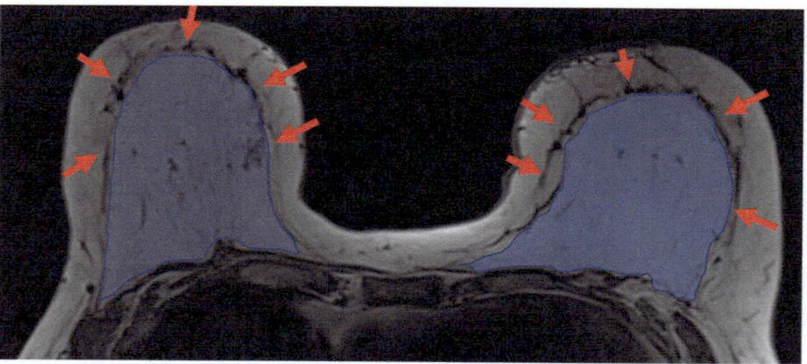

23. c. 1 year.

Post-reconstruction seromas are typically replaced by scarring and fibrosis within 1 to 1 ½ years after surgery [8].

24. b. TRAM (transverse rectus abdominis myocutaneous) flap. The image demonstrates absent right abdominus rectus muscles (arrow), which have been surgically moved to create a flap following left mastectomy. TRAM flaps may be pedicled, free, or free muscle-sparing. Latissimus dorsi flaps do not use the rectus muscles and are easier to create though less pleasing aesthetically. DIEP and SIEA flaps use only the skin and fat from the anterior abdominal wall and not the underlying muscle; they pose higher risk of ischemic complications compared to myocutaneous flaps.

Autologous tissue flaps, along with prosthetic implants and more recently autologous fat grafting, are commonly employed for breast reconstruction following mastectomies. Tissue flap techniques are varied but most commonly utilize the muscle and fat from the anterior abdominal wall. Postsurgical imaging demonstrates predominantly fatty breasts devoid of normal fibroglandular tissue. Breast cancer recurrence may occur following reconstruction since breast tissue in the chest wall and axilla are not completely surgically removed. Most recurrences present in subcutaneous tissue of the flap, superficial to the muscular component.

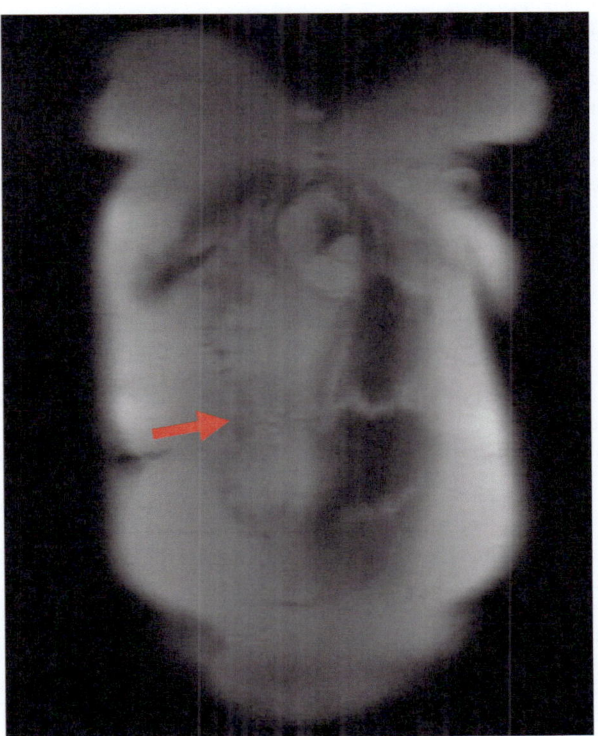

References

1. Margolis NE, Morley C, Lotfi P, et al. Update on imaging of the postsurgical breast. Radiographics. 2014;34(3):642–60.
2. Harvey J, March DE. Making the diagnosis: a practical guide to breast imaging: expert consult—online and print. W B Saunders; 2013.
3. Ibrahim NB, Anandan S, Hartman AL, et al. Radiographic findings after treatment with balloon brachytherapy accelerated partial breast irradiation. Radiographics. 2015;35(1):6–13.
4. Ojeda-Fournier H, Olson LK, Rochelle M. Hodgens BD, Tong E, Yashar CM. Accelerated partial breast irradiation and posttreatment imaging evaluation. Radiographics. 2011;31(6):1701–16.
5. Drukteinis JS, Gombos EC, Raza S, Chikarmane SA, Swami A, Birdwell RL. MR imaging assessment of the breast after breast conservation therapy: distinguishing benign from malignant lesions. Radiographics. 2012;32(1):219–34.
6. Li J, Dershaw DD, Lee CH, Joo S, Morris EA. Breast MRI after conservation therapy: usual findings in routine follow-up examinations. AJR Am J Roentgenol. 2010;195(3):799–807.

7. Galimberti V, et al. Nipple-sparing and skin-sparing mastectomy: review of aims, oncological safety and contraindications. Breast. 2017;34:S82–4. https://doi.org/10.1016/j.breast.2017.06.034.

8. Pinel-Giroux FM, El Khoury MM, Trop I, Bernier C, David J, Lalonde L. Breast reconstruction: review of surgical methods and spectrum of imaging findings. Radiographics. 2013;33(2):435–53.

9. Peng C, Chang CB, Tso HH, Flowers CI, Hylton NM, Joe BN. MRI appearance of tumor recurrence in myocutaneous flap reconstruction after mastectomy. AJR Am J Roentgenol. 2011;196(4):W471–5.

10. Yoo H, Kim BH, Kim HH, Cha JH, Shin HJ, Lee TJ. Local recurrence of breast cancer in reconstructed breasts using TRAM flap after skin-sparing mastectomy: clinical and imaging features. Eur Radiol. 2014;24(9):2220–6.

11. Lai KC, Slanetz PJ, Eisenberg RL. Linear breast calcifications. AJR Am J Roentgenol. 2012;199(2):W151–7.

12. Demetri-Lewis A, Slanetz PJ, Eisenberg RL. Breast calcifications: the focal group. Am J Roentgenol. 2012;198(4):W325–43.

13. Upadhyaya V, Uppoor R, Shetty L. Mammographic and sonographic features of fat necrosis of the breast. Indian J Radiol Imaging. 2013;23(4):366.

14. Taboada JL, Stephens TW, Krishnamurthy S, Brandt KR, Whitman GJ. The many faces of fat necrosis in the breast. AJR. 2009;192:815–25.

15. Morakkabati N, Leutner CC, Schmiedel A, Schild HH, Kuhl CK. Breast MR imaging during or soon after radiation therapy. Radiology. 2003;229:893-90114593189.

16. Mahoney MC, Sharda RG. Postoperative enhancement on breast MRI: time course and pattern of changes. Breast J. 2018; https://doi.org/10.1111/tbj.13039.

17. Heller SL, Lourenco AP, Niell BL, Ajkay N, Brown A, Dibble EH, Didwania AD, Jochelson MS, Klein KA, Mehta TS, Pass HA, Stuckey AR, Swain ME, Tuscano DS, Moy L. Imaging after mastectomy and breast reconstruction. https://acsearch.acr.org/docs/3155410/Narrative/. American College of Radiology. Accessed 2/3/2021.

18. Dashevsky BZ, Hayward JH, Woodard GA, Joe BN, Lee AY. Utility and outcomes of imaging evaluation for palpable lumps in the postmastectomy patient. AJR Am J Roentgenol. 2019;213:464–72.

19. Günhan-Bilgen I, Oktay A. Management of microcalcifications developing at the lumpectomy bed after conservative surgery and radiation therapy. Am J Roentgenol. 2007;188(2):393–8.

20. Daly CP, Jaeger B, Sill DS. Variable appearances of fat necrosis on breast MRI. Am J Roentgenol. 2008;191(5):1374–80.

Physics

12

Kayla Blunt, Yongkai Liu, and Kyung Sung

K. Blunt (✉)
Department of Radiology, Morsani College of Medicine, University of South Florida Health,
Tampa, FL, USA
e-mail: bluntk@usf.edu

Y. Liu
Departments of Radiology, and Physics & Biology in Medicine, Magnetic Resonance
Research Labs, David Geffen School of Medicine, University of California, Los Angeles,
Los Angeles, CA, USA
e-mail: YongkaiLiu@mednet.ucla.edu

K. Sung
Radiology, Bioengineering, and Physics & Biology in Medicine, Magnetic Resonance
Research Labs, David Geffen School of Medicine, University of California, Los Angeles,
Los Angeles, CA, USA
e-mail: ksung@mednet.ucla.edu

X-Ray Mammography

1. When a molybdenum (Mo) target is used, why would the Rhodium (Rh) filter be selected instead of a Molybdenum (Mo) filter to image thicker and/or denser breasts?
   (a) The K-shell binding energy of Rh is higher than that of Mo.
   (b) Rh produces less Bremsstrahlung radiation than Mo.
   (c) Rh produces characteristic X-rays with energies that are useful for clinical imaging, whereas Mo does not.
   (d) Rh allows the transmission of more low energy X-rays.

2. What is the primary advantage of digital breast tomosynthesis (DBT) compared to 2D mammography?
   (a) Improved in-plane spatial resolution.
   (b) Reduced patient dose.
   (c) Magnification of suspicious breast lesions.
   (d) Reduced anatomical noise.

3. What are typical technique factors for a 2D contact mammogram of an average-sized breast (6 cm compressed breast thickness, 15% glandularity)?
   (a) 28 kV, 100 mAs, grid, 0.3 mm focal spot.
   (b) 28 kV, 100 mAs, no grid, 0.1 mm focal spot.
   (c) 55 kV, 50 mAs, no grid, 0.3 mm focal spot.
   (d) 55 kV, 50 mAs, grid, 0.1 mm focal spot.

4. What are typical technique factors for a magnification mammogram of an average-sized breast (6 cm compressed breast thickness, 15% glandularity)?
   (a) 28 kV, 100 mAs, grid, 0.3 mm focal spot.
   (b) 28 kV, 100 mAs, no grid, 0.1 mm focal spot.
   (c) 55 kV, 50 mAs, no grid, 0.3 mm focal spot.
   (d) 55 kV, 50 mAs, grid, 0.1 mm focal spot.

5. What is the primary reason for using lower X-ray tube voltages (kV) in mammography compared with other X-ray imaging modalities?
   (a) Reduced dose to the breast.
   (b) Reduced focal spot blur.
   (c) Improved subject contrast.
   (d) Improved spatial resolution.

6. What is the primary mechanism of interaction between X-ray photons and breast tissue during a mammography exam?
   (a) Rayleigh scattering.
   (b) Photoelectric absorption.
   (c) Compton scattering.
   (d) Pair production.

7. What is the advantage of breast compression?
    (a) Reduced scatter.
    (b) Reduced geometric blurring.
    (c) Longer exposure times are permitted.
    (d) a and b.

8. Spatial resolution is improved in mammography by all of the following, except?
    (a) Smaller focal spot size.
    (b) Reduced X-ray tube voltage (kV).
    (c) Breast compression.
    (d) Reduced detector element size.

9. Match the labeled features of the clinical X-ray spectrum with the parameter that influences its position on the spectrum.

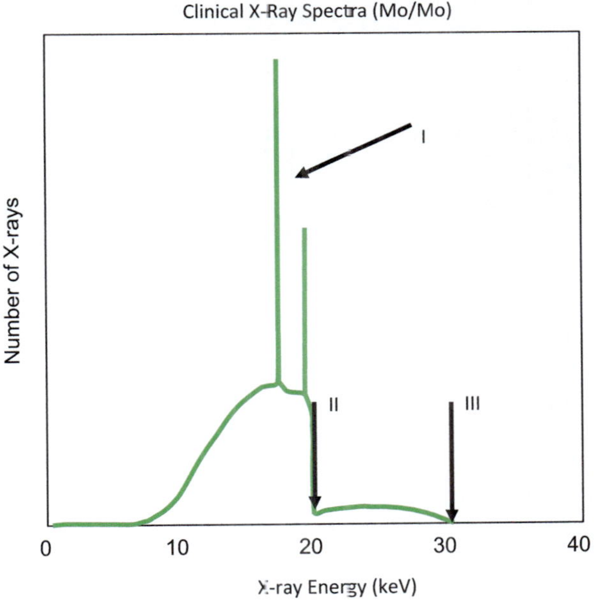

    (a) X-ray tube voltage (kV).
    (b) K-edge energy of the selected filter.
    (c) Target material.

10. Why is the chest wall aligned with the cathode side of the X-ray tube, while the nipple is aligned with the anode side of the X-ray tube?
    (a) To improve subject contrast.
    (b) To improve spatial resolution.
    (c) To achieve a more uniform exposure at the image receptor.
    (d) To increase the field of view.

11. The ACR mammography phantoms include all of the following features, except?
    (a) Fibers.
    (b) Specks.
    (c) Masses.
    (d) Line pairs.

12. Which characteristic of system performance is being evaluated in the image below?

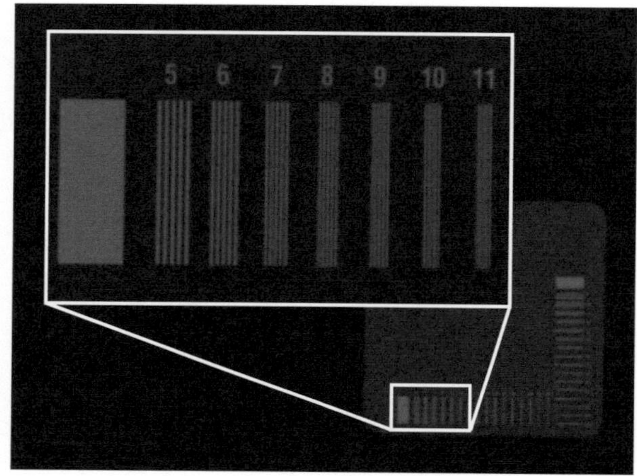

    (a) Contrast resolution.
    (b) Spatial resolution.
    (c) Noise texture.
    (d) Contrast-to-noise ratio.

13. The visibility of a 3 cm low-contrast breast lesion may be improved by which of the following?
    (a) Increasing mAs.
    (b) Reducing kV.
    (c) Reducing detector element size.
    (d) a and b.

14. What is the SI unit of average glandular dose (AGD)?
    (a) Sievert.
    (b) Gray.
    (c) Coulomb per kilogram.
    (d) Roentgen.

15. Why is a "half-field" geometry employed in mammography, as shown in the figure below?

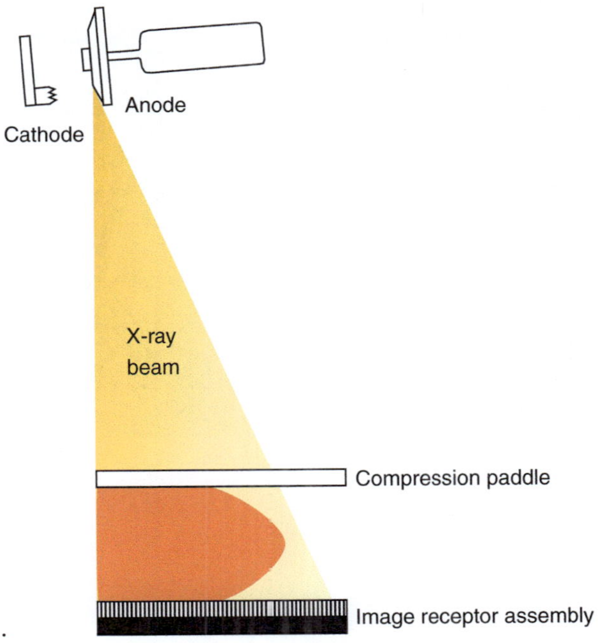

    (a) To avoid exposure of the patient's torso.
    (b) To increase X-ray field coverage at the chest wall.
    (c) To improve contrast resolution.
    (d) a and b.

16. Why does the Mammography Quality Standards Act (MQSA) require a minimum half-value layer (HVL) of clinical X-ray spectra?
    (a) To reduce patient dose.
    (b) To improve contrast.
    (c) To reduce scatter.
    (d) a and b.

17. What must be done if the average glandular dose (AGD) to a patient exceeds 3 mGy per view?
    (a) Stop clinical use of the mammography system.
    (b) Correct the issue within 30 days.
    (c) No action necessary.
    (d) a and b.

18. Identify the artifact in the image below.

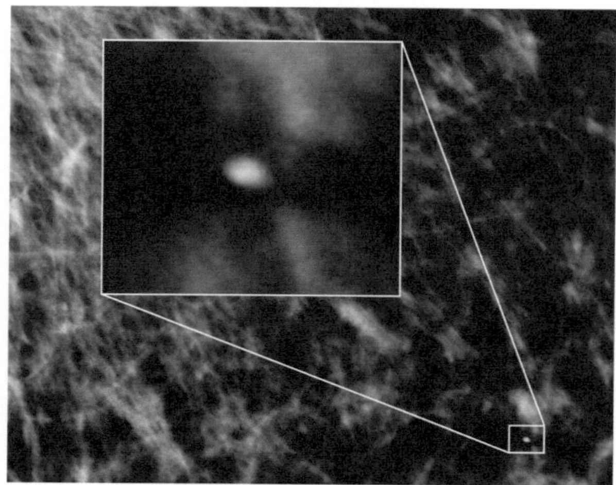

    (a) Grid lines.
    (b) Motion.
    (c) Ghosting.
    (d) Antiperspirant.

19. Identify the artifact in the image below.

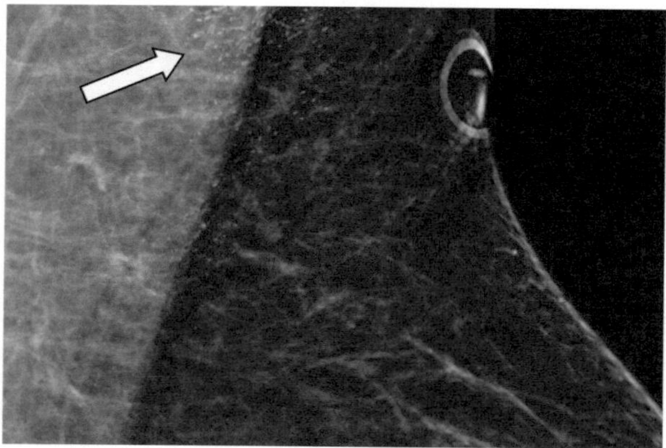

    (a) Grid lines.
    (b) Motion.
    (c) Ghosting.
    (d) Antiperspirant.

Breast Ultrasound

20. In B-mode ultrasound imaging, image brightness corresponds to which of the following?
    (a) Linear attenuation coefficient of tissues.
    (b) Electron density of tissues.
    (c) Detected ultrasound wave amplitude.
    (d) Detected ultrasound wave frequency.

21. What is the most likely ultrasound frequency emitted by a transducer used for breast imaging?
    (a) 1 MHz.
    (b) 3 MHz.
    (c) 6 MHz.
    (d) 12 MHz.

22. Ultrasound waves are strongly reflected at tissue boundaries with large differences in what?
    (a) Ultrasound attenuation.
    (b) Acoustic impedance.
    (c) Atomic number.
    (d) Electron density.

23. Identify the artifact in the image below.

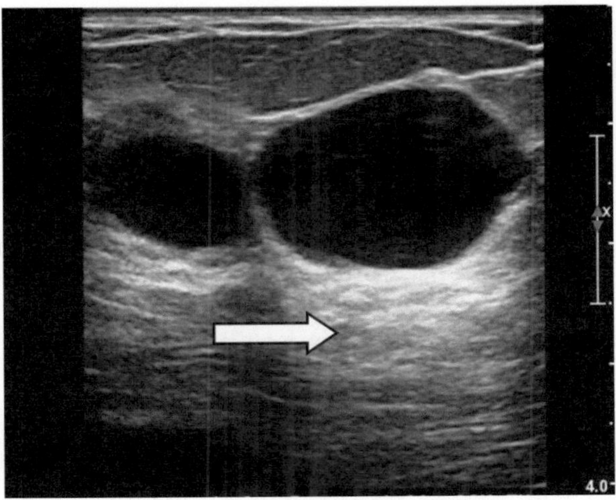

    (a) Mirror image.
    (b) Acoustic shadowing.
    (c) Acoustic enhancement.
    (d) Reverberation.

24. Identify the artifact in the image below.

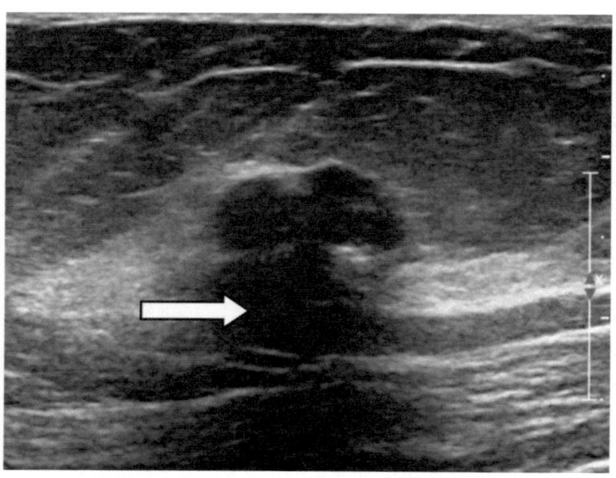

(a) Mirror image.
(b) Acoustic shadowing.
(c) Acoustic enhancement.
(d) Reverberation.

MRI

25. Which of the following statements is true?
    (a) 1 Tesla = 1000 Gauss.
    (b) Higher magnetic field strength increases polarization, which contributes to better image quality.
    (c) Exams performed at higher magnetic field strengths have lower SAR.
    (d) 1H always precesses at the same Larmor frequency.

26. Which of the following statements is false?
    (a) Spin and precession are the same.
    (b) Larmor frequency increases with larger B0.
    (c) Larmor frequency increases with higher gyromagnetic ratio.
    (d) Higher Larmor frequencies produce stronger signals.

27. A device labeled as "MRI Conditional" means:
    (a) The device should never be used in a low-field MRI environment.
    (b) The device is considered to be safe in a ≤ 1.5 T MRI environment.
    (c) The device is safe in all types of MRI environment.
    (d) Specific conditions must be met to ensure the safe use of the device.

28. What is a potential adverse health effect related to the MRI scanner?
    (a) Temporary or permanent hearing loss.
    (b) Production of small pockets of gas in body fluids.
    (c) Radiation-induced erythema.
    (d) Cancer.

29. When a spin-echo sequence is used for acquisition, what are the relative TE and TR values for proton-density weighting?
    (a) Short TE and long TR.
    (b) Short TE and intermediate TR.
    (c) Intermediate TE and intermediate TR.
    (d) Intermediate TE and long TR.

30. Which statement is false for multi-echo spin-echo imaging?
    (a) Multi-echo imaging can decrease scan times by 2x or more.
    (b) Turbo spin echo is excellent for fast T2-weighted imaging.
    (c) Short TRs are important for T2-weighted imaging because they eliminate T1-contrast.
    (d) Spin echo EPI is routine for diffusion-weighted imaging.

31. What is echo time (TE)?
    (a) The time between the middle of the first RF pulse and the peak of the spin echo.
    (b) The time between the end of the first RF pulse and the peak of the spin echo.
    (c) The time between successive pulse sequences.
    (d) Duration of first RF pulse.

32. How many RF pulses are required per TR in spin-echo imaging?
    (a) One.
    (b) Two.
    (c) Three.
    (d) Zero.

33. How many RF pulses are required per TR in gradient echo imaging?
    (a) One.
    (b) Two.
    (c) Three.
    (d) Zero.

34. The following image contains a "zipper" artifact. What is the main cause of the zipper artifact?

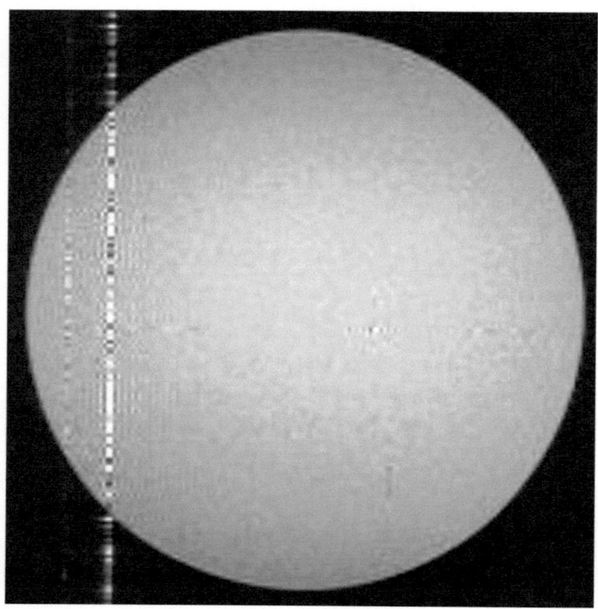

   (a) Patient motion.
   (b) Susceptibility.
   (c) Radiofrequency interference.
   (d) Low spatial resolution.

35. What is true about parallel imaging?
   (a) The is no SNR penalty in parallel imaging.
   (b) Parallel imaging can be used with single-channel coils.
   (c) Typical acceleration factors in parallel imaging are 20 to 30.
   (d) Parallel imaging can improve either spatial- or temporal resolution without increasing scan time.

Answers

1. a. The K-shell binding energy of Rh is higher than that of Mo.

   The k-shell binding energy of Mo is approximately 20 keV, while the k-shell biding energy of Rh is approximately 23 keV. The higher k-shell binding energy, and thus higher photoelectric absorption k-edge, of Rh permits higher-energy X-rays to penetrate the Rh filter and produces a "harder," more penetrating X-ray beam of a higher effective energy. This more penetrating X-ray beam reduces patient dose and keeps exposure times reasonably low when imaging thicker and/or denser breasts using automatic exposure control (AEC). Patient dose is reduced because the "harder" Rh-filtered beam results in a greater proportion of X-ray photons passing through the breast to reach the detector than a "softer" Mo-filtered beam (i.e., lower dose to achieve similar image noise) [1].

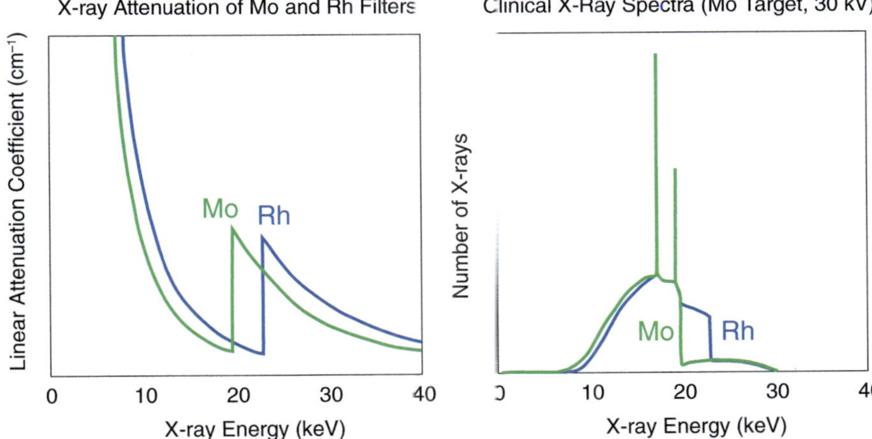

2. d. Reduced anatomical noise.

DBT involves acquiring multiple low-dose projection X-rays of the breast at various angles, then reconstructing axial slices of the breast from the acquired projection data. Each axial slice focuses on a thin (approximately 1 mm) layer of breast tissue while blurring out the under- and overlying anatomy that may otherwise obscure the structures within a given slice. This reduction in anatomical noise improves image contrast and the sensitivity of DBT. In-plane spatial resolution in DBT is often poorer than in conventional 2D mammography because signals from adjacent detector elements are binned together to improve the signal-to-noise ratio of the low-dose projection images. The radiation dose is approximately equal for DBT and conventional 2D breast exams and DBT is performed in contact mode, like 2D imaging, so there is no change in the magnification factor.

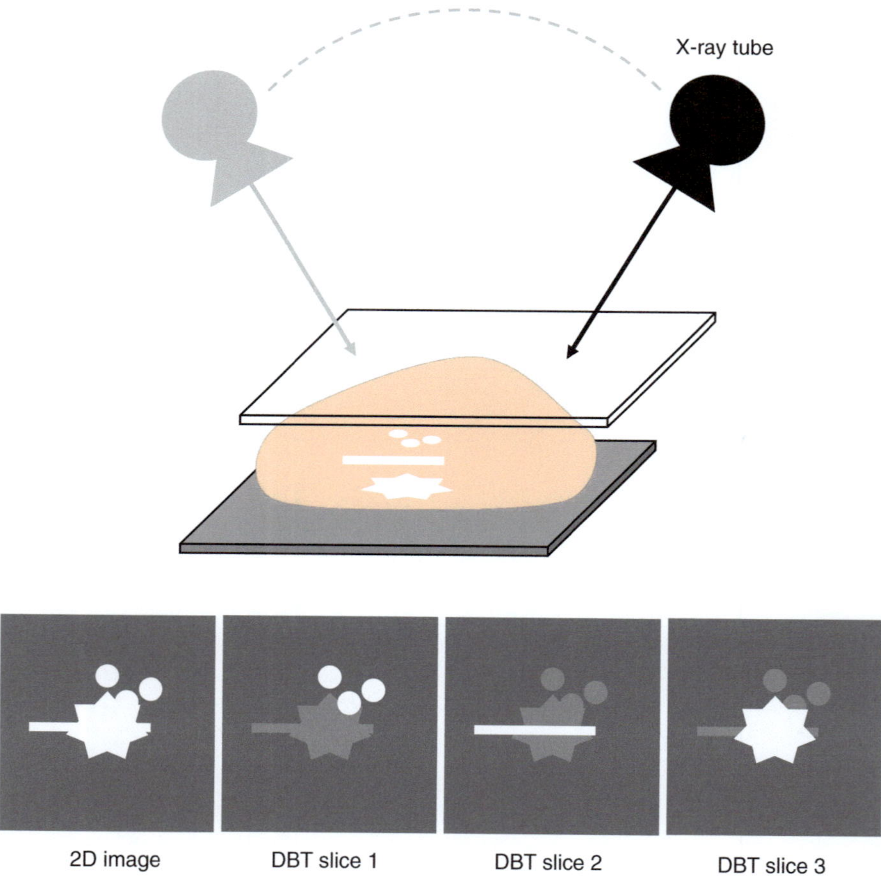

3. a. 28 kV, 100 mAs, grid, 0.3 mm focal spot.

Low X-ray tube voltages (kV) are used in mammography to maximize subject contrast between adipose-, glandular-, and cancerous breast tissues. For an average-sized breast, 28 kV and 100 mAs are typical technique factors. The grid is always utilized in 2D contact mammography to reduce the proportion of scattered radiation reaching the image receptor. The 0.3 mm focal spot size is used in contact mammography to provide excellent spatial resolution while permitting reasonably low exposure times (approximately 1 s).

4. b. 28 kV, 100 mAs, no grid, 0.1 mm focal spot.

For an average-sized breast, 28 kV and 100 mAs are typical technique factors. In magnification mammography, the breast is positioned closer to the X-ray source (focal spot) while the source-to-image distance (SID) remains constant. This geometry creates an "air gap" between the breast and the image receptor and allows space for scattered radiation travelling at oblique trajectories to miss the image receptor. The grid is removed in magnification mammography because scatter reduction is achieved via the air gap technique and use of the grid would needlessly increase radiation dose to the breast. The 0.1 mm focal spot size is utilized in magnification mammography to counteract the increased geometric blurring that is introduced as the geometric magnification factor increases. The magnification factor of a projection X-ray image is equal to the source-to-image distance (SID) divided by source-to-object distance (SOD): magnification factor = SID/SOD. Since a smaller SOD is used in magnification mammography, selection of a smaller focal spot offsets the resulting increased geometric blurring to maintain excellent spatial resolution.

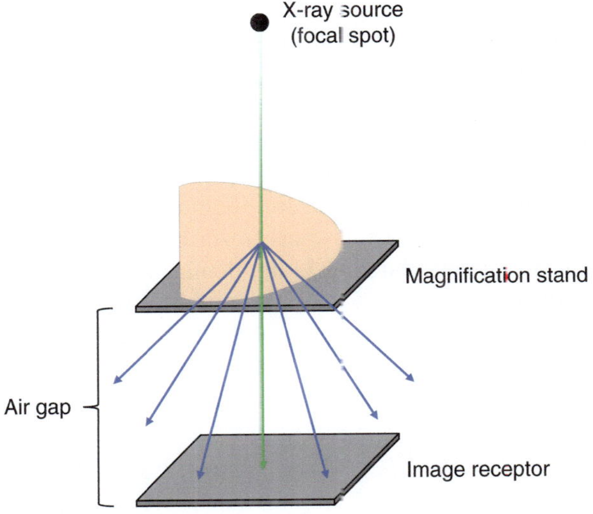

5. c. Improved subject contrast.

The kV determines the maximum energy of the polyenergetic X-ray spectrum. At lower X-ray energies, there is a greater disparity between the linear attenuation coefficients of fat, glandular tissue, and cancerous tissue, and thus improved subject contrast. Imaging at low kV is especially critical in mammography because the linear attenuation coefficients of these tissues are quite similar and difficult to distinguish at higher kV.

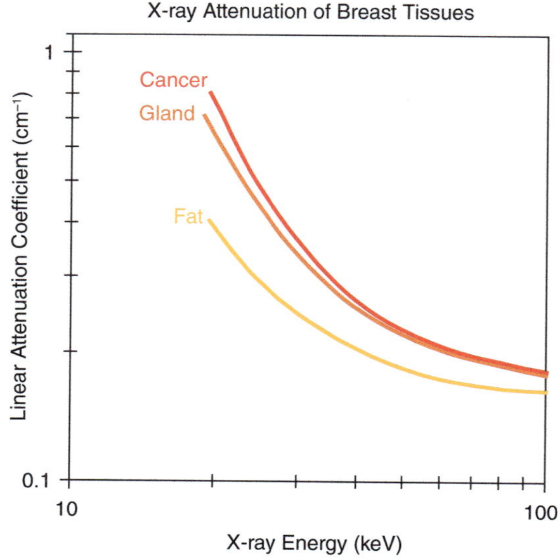

6. b. Photoelectric absorption.

Within the X-ray energy range utilized in diagnostic radiology, X-ray photons interact with matter via Rayleigh scattering, photoelectric absorption, and Compton scattering. Rayleigh scattering is only likely to occur at very low photon energies and accounts for less than approximately 10% of all X-ray interactions with tissue in mammography (and an even smaller percentage for other, higher-energy imaging modalities). A rule of thumb is that photoelectric absorption is the dominant interaction mechanism of X-rays in soft tissue below 25 keV, and Compton scattering is the dominant interaction mechanism of X-rays in soft tissue above 25 keV. For a typical mammography exam performed at 28 kV, the average energy of the polyenergetic X-ray spectrum is approximately 14 keV. Thus, the dominant mechanism of interaction between X-rays and breast tissue will be photoelectric absorption.

7. d. a and b.

There are many advantages to breast compression including reduced scatter production and reduced geometric blurring. Less scattered radiation is produced in thinner body parts, and geometric blurring is reduced as breast tissue is moved closer to the image receptor (increased SOD). Other advantages include reduced motion blurring due to immobilization of the breast, reduced patient dose, reduced anatomical noise, and reduced exposure times.

8. b. Reduced X-ray tube voltage (kV).

Spatial resolution is not significantly impacted by technique factors such as the kV and mAs. Smaller focal spot sizes reduce geometric blurring and improve spatial resolution. Breast compression improves spatial resolution by reducing both motion blurring (immobilization) and geometric blurring (reduced magnification factor: SID/SOD). Smaller detector element size allows smaller objects to be visualized.

9. I-c; II-b; III-a.

When electrons strike the target material in an X-ray tube, both characteristic X-rays and Bremsstrahlung X-rays are produced. Characteristic X-rays (I) have discrete energies which are "characteristic" of the target material in which they are produced, whereas Bremsstrahlung interactions produce a broad spectrum of X-ray energies with a shape that depends on the selected kV and mAs. The selected kV determines the maximum energy of Bremsstrahlung X-rays that can be produced in the X-ray tube (III). The k-edge of the selected filter material determines the maximum energy of X-rays that are most likely to be transmitted through the filter (II).

10. c. To achieve a more uniform exposure at the image receptor.

The heel effect describes a loss of X-ray intensity on the anode side of the X-ray field. The X-ray intensity is reduced on the anode side due to the increased pathlength and self-attenuation of X-rays within the angled anode. The thickest part of the breast (chest wall) is positioned at the more-intense side of the X-ray field and the thinnest part of the breast (nipple) is positioned at the less-intense side of the X-ray field to achieve a relatively uniform exposure of the image receptor.

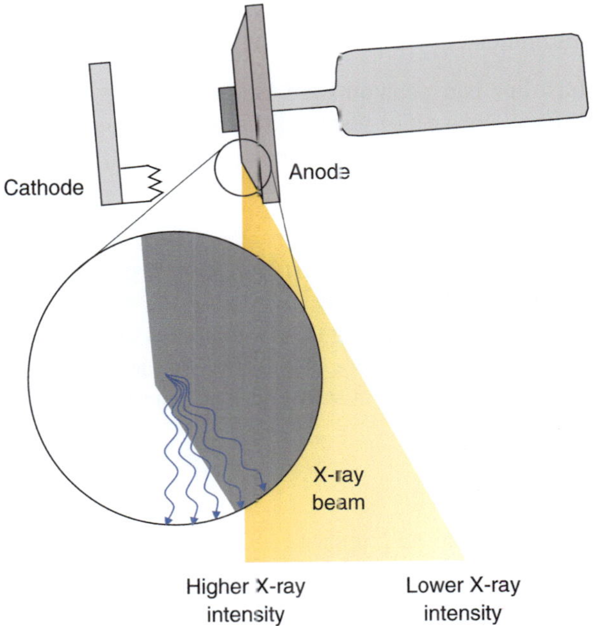

11. d. Line pairs.

The ACR mammography phantoms contain simulated fibers, specks, and masses of various sizes. There are three ACR-approved accreditation phantoms: the mini Digital Stereotactic Phantom, small ACR Mammography Phantom (pictured below), and large ACR Digital Mammography Phantom. Technologists and medical physicists acquire images of an ACR phantom and document the number of fibers, specks, and masses that can be visualized. The ACR phantoms may also be used by medical physicists to determine the average glandular dose, signal-to-noise ratio, contrast-to-noise ratio, and geometric accuracy.

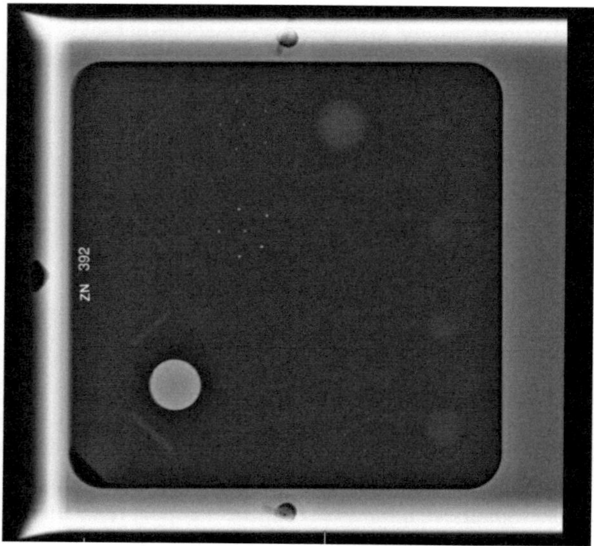

12. b. Spatial resolution.

High-contrast line pair phantoms are used to evaluate limiting system spatial resolution. Excellent spatial resolution is required in mammography so that microcalcifications as small as 100 μm may be visualized.

13. d. a and b.

Improving the contrast-to-noise ratio (CNR) of a large, low-contrast lesion will improve its radiographic visibility. Increasing the mAs reduces image noise (quantum mottle), while reducing the kV improves subject contrast. Therefore, both options A and B improve the CNR. Reduced detector element size improves spatial resolution but will not significantly impact the visibility of large, low-contrast lesions.

14. b. Gray.

The gray (Gy) is equal to 1 joule per kilogram (J/kg) and is the SI unit of absorbed dose. The sievert (Sv) is also equal to 1 J/kg, but it is reserved for the equivalent dose and effective dose (as well as older quantities that these quantities have since replaced). In other words, the Sv is used to distinguish instances where weighting factors have been applied to the absorbed dose to provide additional information about the associated risk of biological damage. The SI unit of exposure is the coulomb per kilogram (C/kg), whereas the conventional unit of exposure is the Roentgen (R).

15. d. a and b.

In mammography, the X-ray field is bisected so that central axis of the X-ray beam is perpendicular to the image receptor and aligned with the chest wall edge, as shown in the figure above. This "half-field" geometry is unique to mammography and is utilized to avoid unnecessary exposure of the patient's torso and increase X-ray field coverage of the chest wall.

16. a. To reduce patient dose.

The HVL is the thickness of material required to reduce the X-ray beam intensity to half of its initial value. High energy, more penetrating X-ray beams have higher HVLs. A minimum HVL ensures adequate removal of the low energy components of the clinical X-ray spectrum, i.e., adequate "beam hardening." It is desirable to remove the low energy components of the X-ray spectrum because they contribute to patient dose but are unlikely to reach the image receptor and contribute to image formation.

17. c. No action necessary.

The AGD limit of 3 mGy per view only applies to the ACR mammography phantom. If a medical physicist determines that the AGD to the ACR phantom exceeds 3 mGy per view, then the system cannot be used clinically until the issue is corrected. However, the AGD to patients may exceed 3 mGy per view and still be considered acceptable, particularly for large, dense breasts.

18. b. Motion.

Because the focal spot sizes used in mammography are very small, low X-ray tube currents (mA) and relatively long exposure times (approximately 1 s) are required to avoid overheating of the target material. Breast compression immobilizes the breast and significantly reduces motion artifacts; however, motion blur is fairly common because of the relatively long exposure times in mammography.

19. d. Antiperspirant.

Antiperspirants often contain highly attenuating additives such as aluminum. Antiperspirant artifacts are commonly seen in the axilla. The artifactual hyperdensities have a distinct appearance but may be mistaken for pathology or obscure actual pathology in the axilla. Cleaning the skin of antiperspirant residue will remediate the artifact.

20. c. Detected ultrasound wave amplitude.

Ultrasound transducers transmit and receive ultrasound waves by converting electrical energy into mechanical (sound) energy and vice versa. Ultrasound waves are produced and transmitted into the patient by vibrating piezoelectric transducer elements. The ultrasound waves are ultimately reflected, refracted, scattered, and/or absorbed within the patient. In B-mode ultrasound imaging, the measured amplitudes of reflected and scattered sound waves that are received by the transducer are converted into brightness levels (grayscale) in the ultrasound image.

21. d. 12 MHz.

Clinical ultrasound transducers are typically operated between 1 and 20 MHz. Transducer frequency is inversely proportional to the maximum depth of penetration of the ultrasound wave, and transducer frequency is generally selected to match the depth of the body part being imaged. The spatial pulse length is inversely proportional to transducer frequency, thus axial spatial resolution improves with increasing transducer frequency. For breast imaging, 12 MHz transducers generally provide adequate depth of penetration and relatively high axial spatial resolution.

22. b. Acoustic impedance.

Acoustic impedance (Z) is the product of physical density (ρ) of a material and its speed of sound (c): $Z = \rho * c$. Most of the ultrasound energy is transmitted through a tissue boundary when the acoustic impedances of the tissues are similar, whereas most of the ultrasound energy is reflected at a tissue boundary when there is a large mismatch in acoustic impedance. The large difference in acoustic impedance at air-soft tissue and soft tissue-bone interfaces explains why it is impractical to acquire ultrasound images beyond these interfaces. Ultrasound gel displaces air and is formulated to have an acoustic impedance similar to that of soft tissue, allowing the ultrasound beam to be transmitted into the patient to produce useful ultrasound images.

23. c. Acoustic enhancement.

Acoustic enhancement describes an increased echo intensity that occurs distal to structures of low acoustic attenuation. Acoustic enhancement can aid in the characterization of breast lesions, for example by distinguishing fluid-filled lesions from solid masses.

24. b. Acoustic shadowing.

Acoustic shadowing describes a decreased echo intensity that occurs distal to structures of high acoustic attenuation. Like acoustic enhancement, acoustic shadowing can aid in the characterization of breast lesions, for example by distinguishing calcified objects from fluids and air.

25. b. Higher magnetic field strength increases polarization, which contributes to better image quality.

$$1 \text{ Tesla} = 10,000 \text{ Gauss}$$

Certain atomic nuclei, such as the hydrogen nucleus, ^{1}H, possess a property known as "spin," and the spinning nucleus induces a magnetic field which behaves like a bar magnet. Application of a strong, external magnetic field (B_0) aligns the nucleus either in parallel or antiparallel with the B_0 field. As the strength of the B_0 field increases, a larger proportion of protons will align in parallel with the B_0 field. This increases the magnitude of the net magnetization vector and the measurable MR signal, thus the image signal-to-noise ratio.

Although a bar magnet would orientate completely parallel or antiparallel to the B_0 field, the nucleus has an angular momentum due to its rotation, so it will rotate, or precess, around the B_0 axis. The frequency of precession around the field direction is the Larmor frequency (ω), described by the Larmor equation:

$$\omega = \gamma B_0$$

where γ is the gyromagnetic ratio and the fixed constant for a specific nucleus. For example, the gyromagnetic ratio of the hydrogen nucleus is approximately 42.58 MHz/T. Thus, the precession frequency increases with a larger B_0 field for a given nucleus.

26. a. Spin and precession are the same.

Protons intrinsically have spin and precession in the presence of a B_0 field. The proton spins about its axis and precesses around the B_0 field. The spinning and precessing proton are analogous to a spinning top, which spins about its axis and also precesses around the earth's gravitation field.

27. d. Specific conditions must be met to ensure the safe use of the device [2].

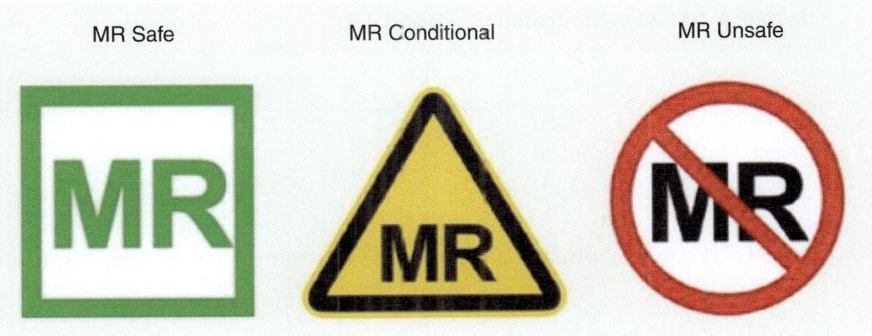

- MR Safe: Items pose no known hazards in all MR environments and are indicated by a green and white icon.
- MR Conditional: Items do not pose any known hazards in a specific MR environment with specific conditions of use. The icon consists of "MR" inside of a yellow triangle.
- MR Unsafe: Items such as any magnetic item are unsafe in all MR environments. Unsafe icon features an "MR" inside of a red circle with a bar through it.

28. a. Temporary or permanent hearing loss.

High-intensity noise produced by MRI scanners can reach peak sound pressure levels of 125.7–130.7 dB and have an average equivalent intensity of 100 to 115 dB. The intensity of noise produced by MRI scanners generally has a positive correlation with the magnetic field strength (i.e., 3 T scanners are louder than 1.5 T scanners) and is caused by motion of the gradient coils as they are rapidly switched on and off. Exposure to such high-intensity noise could result in noise-induced hearing loss if someone were to be imaged frequently or was imaged without proper ear protection [3, 4].

29. a. Short TE and long TR.

Image contrast for spin echo (S_{SE}) is proportional to the following signal equation:

$$S_{SE} \propto \rho\left(1 - e^{-TR/T_1}\right) e^{-TE/T_2},$$

where ρ is the spin density, TR is repetition time, and TE is echo time. When a long TR is used, e^{-TR/T_1} becomes close to 0, resulting in no T_1-contrast. When a short TE is used, e^{-TE/T_2} becomes close to 1, resulting in no T_2-contrast.

Please note memorization of this equation is not required material for board preparation.

In summary, different tissue contrast for spin-echo imaging can be created by selecting a certain combination of TE and TR.

	TE	TR
Spin density	Short	Long
T1-weighted	Short	T1-Short, Short
T2-weighted	T2-Long, Long	Long

30. c. Short TRs are important for T2-weighted imaging because they eliminate T1-contrast.

Long TRs should be used to eliminate T1-contrast for T2-weighted imaging.

31. a. The time between the middle of the first RF pulse and the peak of the spin echo.

The time between the center of the first RF pulse (usually 90° for spin-echo pulse sequence) and the peak of the spin echo is called the echo time (TE).

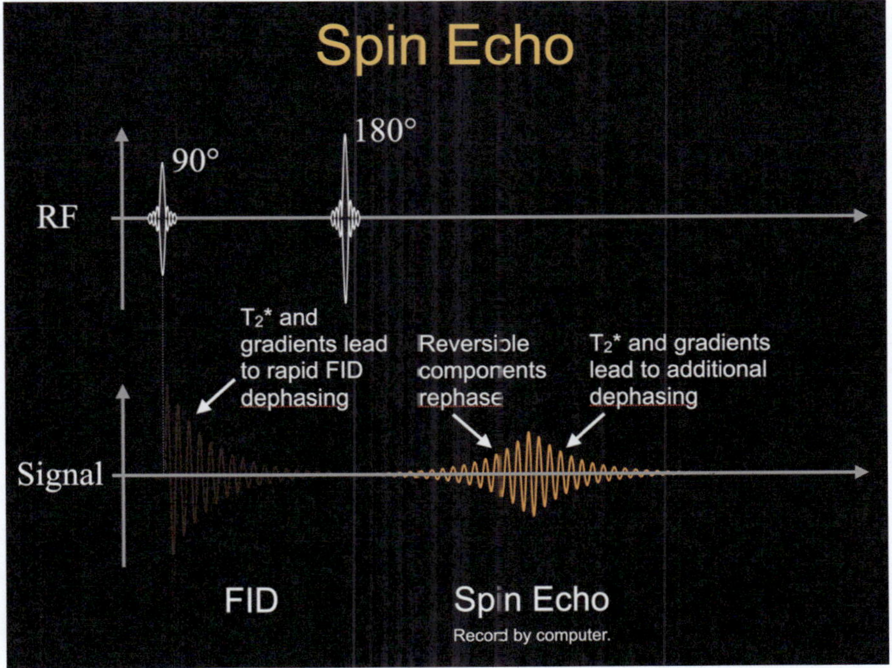

32. b. Two.

A spin echo (SE) is produced by a pair of RF pulses. The first pulse (usually 90°) rotates the net magnetization into the transverse plane. The second RF pulse is the refocusing pulse (usually 180°), which generates the spin echo.

33. a. One.

A gradient recalled echo (GRE) is produced by a single RF pulse and a gradient polarity reversal.

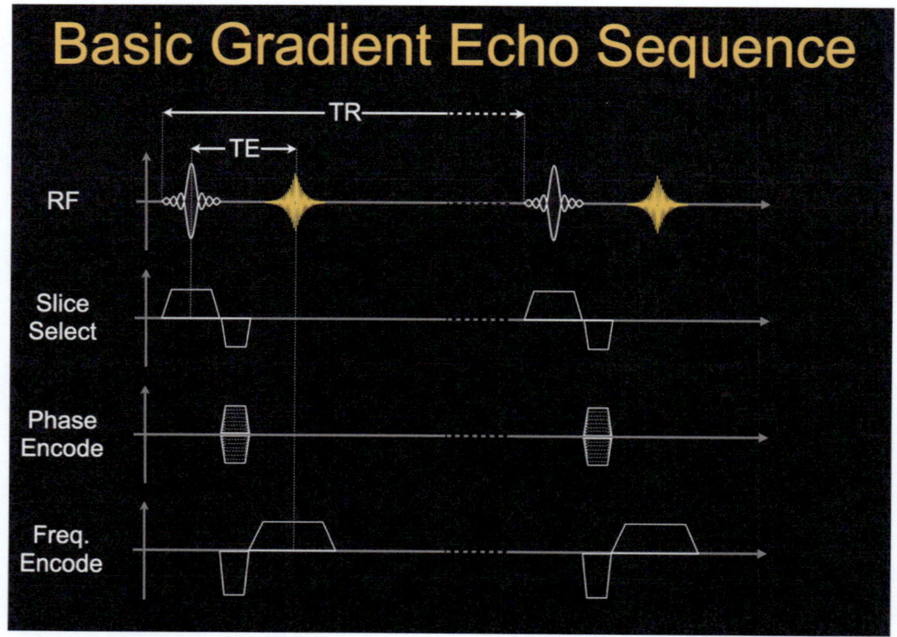

34. c. Radiofrequency interference.

Zipper artifacts are caused by radiofrequency (RF) noise contamination that enters the scanner room or from within the room itself. For example, zipper artifacts may occur when the scanner door is left open or if the room's RF shielding is compromised.

35. d. Parallel imaging can improve either spatial- or temporal resolution without increasing scan time.

Parallel imaging is a widely used technique where the placement of multiple receiver coils is used to allow a reduction in the number of phase-encoding steps during image acquisition. The typical acceleration factors in imaging time are 2–4, which come with SNR penalties [5].

References

1. Bushberg JT, et al. The essential physics of medical imaging. 3rd ed. Lippincott Williams and Wilkins; 2011.
2. Shellock FG, Woods TO, Crues JV III. MR Labeling information for implants and devices: explanation of terminology. Radiology. 2009;253(1):26–30.
3. Hattori Y, Fukatsu H, Ishigaki T. Measurement and evaluation of the acoustic noise of a 3 tesla MR scanner. Nagoya J Med Sci. 2007;69(1–2):23–8.
4. Salvi R, Sheppard A. Is noise in the MR imager a significant risk factor for hearing loss? Radiology. 2018;286(2):609–10.
5. Deshmane A, Gulani V, Griswold MA, Seiberlich N. Parallel MR imaging. J Magn Reson Imaging. 2012;36:55–72.

Index